W9-AUD-673

Tissue Engineering

Applications in Oral and Maxillofacial Surgery and Periodontics

Second Edition

Second Edition

TISSUE ENGINEERING

Applications in Oral and Maxillofacial Surgery and Periodontics

Edited by

Samuel E. Lynch, DMD, DMSc
President and CEO
BioMimetic Therapeutics
Franklin, Tennessee

Robert E. Marx, DDS
Professor of Surgery and Chief
Division of Oral and Maxillofacial Surgery
University of Miami Miller School of Medicine
Miami, Florida

Myron Nevins, DDS
Private Practice in Periodontics
Swampscott, Massachusetts

Leslie A. Wisner-Lynch, DDS, DMSc
Director, Applied Research
BioMimetic Therapeutics
Franklin, Tennessee

Quintessence Publishing Co, Inc

Chicago, Berlin, Tokyo, London, Paris, Milan, Barcelona, Istanbul,
São Paulo, Mumbai, Moscow, Prague, and Warsaw

Library of Congress Cataloging-in-Publication Data

Tissue engineering : applications in oral and maxillofacial surgery and periodontics /
[edited by] Samuel Lynch ... [et al.]. — 2nd ed.
    p. ; cm.
 Includes bibliographical references and index.
 ISBN 978-0-86715-464-1 (hardcover)
 1. Mouth—Surgery. 2. Face—Surgery. 3. Maxilla—Surgery. 4. Periodontics. 5.
Tissue engineering. 6. Dental implants. 7. Bone regeneration. I. Lynch, Samuel E.
 [DNLM: 1. Oral Surgical Procedures. 2. Tissue Transplantation—methods. 3. Bone
Regeneration. 4. Culture Techniques. 5. Dental Implantation—methods. 6. Wound
Healing. WU 640 T6159 2008]
 RK533.T55 2008
 617.5'22—dc22

                                                2007037627

quintessence books

© 2008 Quintessence Publishing Co, Inc

Quintessence Publishing Co, Inc
4350 Chandler Drive
Hanover Park, IL 60133
www.quintpub.com

Editor: Katie Funk
Design: Dawn Hartman
Production: Sue Robinson

Printed in China

Table of Contents

Preface

Great progress has been made in the clinical applications of tissue engineering since the first edition of this book was published in 1999. Two pure, recombinant (synthetic) growth factors have received FDA approval for use in orofacial indications and are now available for widespread clinical use. Recombinant human platelet-derived growth factor (rhPDGF) was the first pure recombinant growth factor to be FDA approved for use in dentistry. It is indicated for promotion of bone and periodontal regeneration and treatment of gingival recession and has been widely used by clinicians in numerous indications since its commercial introduction. More recently, recombinant human bone morphogenetic protein 2 (rhBMP-2) also received FDA approval for sinus floor augmentation and alveolar ridge augmentation associated with extraction sockets. Both rhPDGF and rhBMP-2 were tested in lengthy and rigorous large-scale randomized controlled multicenter clinical trials and were FDA approved through a premarket approval (PMA) process, the most rigorous level of approval for medical devices.

The availability of rhPDGF and rhBMP for widespread clinical use ushers in a new era in patient care in periodontics and oral and maxillofacial surgery, allowing us to move from primarily passive, often highly invasive therapies to active ones that significantly stimulate the healing and regenerative processes. Traditionally, in most bone grafting and regenerative procedures clinicians have been faced with a choice of harvesting autograft or relying on osteoconductive matrices or cell-occlusive barriers. These techniques and materials served well when used in appropriate situations, with specific surgical techniques, and in relatively uncompromised patients. However, harvesting large amounts of autograft is time consuming and leads to increased pain and potential complications for patients, and passive therapies such as osteoconductive matrices and barrier membranes may only be used successfully in the treatment of a limited number of clinical problems.

The challenge and expectation for tissue engineering incorporating pure bioactive proteins, scaffolds, and eventually a source of regenerative cells is to achieve more predictable results in more diverse and compromised patient populations more quickly and with less pain. The genesis of this second edition was a belief by the editors and authors that we have indeed made tremendous progress in realizing these clinical goals and in achieving results that were previously only possible using highly invasive and time-consuming surgical techniques—or simply not possible at all on a predictable basis.

Time will tell how significant an impact these new therapies will have on clinical practice. As with all medical advances, it is likely that these early applications will result in some failures, as well as some successes, in indications that have yet to be contemplated. This process will lead to further refinements in combining matrices, pure bioactive protein therapeutics, and cells. It is the hope of the authors and editors of this book that the information presented here will be expanded as readers continue to learn and apply their knowledge to achieve the best outcomes for family, friends, neighbors, and all in need of our care.

Samuel E. Lynch, DMD, DMSc

Contributors

Philip J. Boyne, DMD, MS, DSc
Professor Emeritus
Department of Oral and Maxillofacial Surgery
Loma Linda University
Loma Linda, California

Emil G. Cappetta, DMD
Clinical Professor of Periodontology
New Jersey Dental School
University of Medicine and Dentistry of New Jersey
Newark, New Jersey

Private Practice
Summit, New Jersey

Michael H. Carstens, MD
Associate Professor
Division of Plastic and Reconstructive Surgery
St Louis University
St Louis, Missouri

Tim R. Daniels, MD
Associate Professor
Foot and Ankle Surgery, Trauma
St Michael's Hospital
University of Toronto
Toronto, Ontario
Canada

Joshua Dines, MD
Attending Orthopedic Surgeon
Sports Medicine
Hospital for Special Surgery
New York, New York

Bruce Doll, DDS, PhD
Assistant Professor
Department of Periodontics
School of Dentistry
University of Pittsburgh
Pittsburgh, Pennsylvania

Ember L. Ewings, MD
Resident
Division of Plastic and Reconstructive Surgery
St Louis University
St Louis, Missouri

Joseph P. Fiorellini, DMD, DMSc
Professor and Chair
Department of Periodontics
School of Dental Medicine
University of Pennsylvania
Philadelphia, Pennsylvania

William V. Giannobile, DDS, DMSc
Najjar Endowed Professor of Dentistry
Department of Periodontics and Oral Medicine
School of Dentistry
Professor
Department of Biomedical Engineering
College of Engineering
Director
Michigan Center for Oral Health Research
University of Michigan
Ann Arbor, Michigan

Reinhard Gruber, PhD
Associate Professor
Department of Oral Surgery
Medical University of Vienna
Vienna, Austria

Leslie Robin Halpern, DDS, MD, PhD, MPH
Assistant Professor
Department of Oral and Maxillofacial Surgery
Massachusetts General Hospital
Harvard School of Dental Medicine
Boston, Massachusetts

Charles Hart, PhD
Chief Scientific Officer
BioMimetic Therapeutics
Franklin, Tennessee

Alan S. Herford, DDS, MD
Chairman and Program Director
Department of Oral and Maxillofacial Surgery
Loma Linda University
Loma Linda, California

Hideharu Hibi, DDS, PhD
Center for Genetic and Regenerative Medicine
Graduate School of Medicine
Nagoya University
Nagoya, Japan

Jeffrey O. Hollinger, DDS, PhD
Professor
Departments of Biological Sciences and Biomedical
 Engineering
Director
Bone Tissue Engineering Center
Carnegie Mellon University
Pittsburgh, Pennsylvania

Ole T. Jensen, DDS, MS
Private Practice in Oral and Maxillofacial Surgery
Denver, Colorado

Zvi Laster, DMD
Chairman
Department of Oral and Maxillofacial Surgery
Poriya Hospital
Tiberias, Israel

Samuel E. Lynch, DMD, DMSc
President and CEO
BioMimetic Therapeutics
Franklin, Tennessee

Robert E. Marx, DDS
Professor of Surgery and Chief
Division of Oral and Maxillofacial Surgery
University of Miami Miller School of Medicine
Miami, Florida

Michael K. McGuire, DDS
Private Practice
Houston, Texas

James T. Mellonig, DDS, MS
Professor and Director of Advanced Education Program
Department of Periodontics
School of Dentistry
University of Texas Health Science Center at
 San Antonio
San Antonio, Texas

Marc L. Nevins, DMD, MMSc
Private Practice in Periodontics and Implant Dentistry
Boston, Massachusetts

Myron Nevins, DDS
Private Practice in Periodontics
Swampscott, Massachusetts

Joshua C. Nickols, PhD
Business Manager, Sports Medicine
BioMimetic Therapeutics
Franklin, Tennessee

Isabella Rocchietta, DDS
Research Fellow
Department of Periodontology
School of Dentistry
University of Milan
Milan, Italy

Mary Beth Schmidt, PhD
Biomedical Consultant
Schmidt Technical Consulting
Pomfret, Connecticut

Julio Sekler, DMD, MMSc
Private Practice
Fort Lauderdale, Florida

Massimo Simion, MD, DDS
Professor and Chairman
Department of Periodontology
School of Dentistry
University of Milan
Milan, Italy

Myron Spector, PhD
Professor of Orthopedic Surgery (Biomaterials)
Harvard Medical School
Director, Tissue Engineering
Veterans Administration Boston Healthcare System
Director, Orthopaedic Research Laboratory
Brigham and Women's Hospital
Boston, Massachusetts

R. Gilbert Triplett, DDS, PhD
Regents Professor and Chairman
Department of Oral and Maxillofacial Surgery and
    Pharmacology
Baylor College of Dentistry
Texas A&M University System Health Science Center
Dallas, Texas

Minoru Ueda, DDS, PhD
Professor and Chairman
Department of Oral and Maxillofacial Surgery
Graduate School of Medicine
Nagoya University
Nagoya, Japan

N. Guzin Uzel, DMD, DMSc
Director of Predoctoral Periodontics
Robert Schattner Center
School of Dental Medicine
University of Pennsylvania
Philadelphia, Pennsylvania

Ulf M. E. Wikesjö, DDS, PhD, DMD
Professor of Periodontics, Oral Biology, and Graduate
    Studies
Director, Laboratory for Applied Periodontal and
    Craniofacial Regeneration
School of Dentistry
Medical College of Georgia
Augusta, Georgia

Leslie A. Wisner-Lynch, DDS, DMSc
Director, Applied Research
BioMimetic Therapeutics
Franklin, Tennessee

John M. Wozney, PhD
Assistant Vice President
Women's Health and Musculoskeletal Biology
Wyeth Research
Cambridge, Massachusetts

Yoichi Yamada, DDS, PhD
Center for Genetic and Regenerative Medicine
Graduate School of Medicine
Nagoya University
Nagoya, Japan

Introduction

Samuel E. Lynch, DMD, DMSc

The goal of tissue engineering and regenerative medicine is to promote healing and, ideally, true regeneration of a tissue's structure and function more predictably, more quickly, and less invasively than allowed by previous techniques. The desire for such improved patient outcomes is shared across medical disciplines and geographic divides. Many approaches and materials have been proposed over the past 20 years, as researchers have sought to better understand the cellular and molecular mechanisms involved in healing and regeneration in order to optimize treatments. However, the ability to regenerate tissues lost to disease, trauma, or congenital deformity with predictability and precision has been elusive, and today many clinicians skeptically approach new regenerative therapeutics as promise without predictability.

The first edition of this book[1] introduced the guiding biologic principles and potential clinical applications of tissue engineering to oral and maxillofacial surgery and periodontics. It sought to provide researchers with a clinical perspective of the challenges of patient care and clinicians with information and techniques that could be used in their practice, as well as a window into the possible future of tissue repair and regeneration. In this edition, we are indeed fortunate to describe many advances in our understanding of biologic paradigms and exciting new therapies that are fulfilling the promise of achieving better patient outcomes more quickly, less invasively, and with improved predictability. No doubt future researchers will continue to build upon the principles discussed here, and clinicians will find new applications for the recently introduced recombinant protein therapeutics beyond those for which they were initially developed—and this is

as it should be. But as we compiled the chapters of this book it became clear that our ability to speed healing and enhance bone regeneration is greater today than it was when the first edition of this book was published in 1999. Our patients are the benefactors.

A Brief Historical Perspective

Regenerative treatment modalities throughout medicine have historically included the use of three-dimensional biomaterial scaffolds, or matrices, to support the regeneration of tissues lost to disease, trauma, or congenital deformity. Autogenous bone grafts used in oral, craniomaxillofacial, and general orthopedic grafting procedures are considered the gold standard because they provide an osteoconductive matrix in addition to cells and growth-stimulating molecules. However, the quality of autogenous bone is variable depending on the health status of the patient, often resulting in the unfortunate situation in which the very patients who are in greatest need of the best material to promote bone regeneration (eg, those with osteopenia/osteoporosis, diabetes, or a history of smoking) are the ones who receive poorer quality autogenous bone grafts. Even in healthy patients, the disadvantages of a limited supply, increased procedure time and postoperative pain, and risk of surgical complications at the harvest site may in some cases outweigh the advantages provided by autogenous grafts.

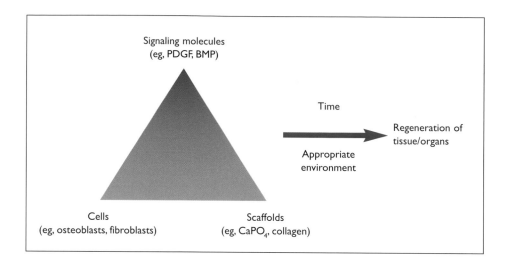

Fig 1 The active (tissue engineering) approach to regenerating tissues generally combines three key elements: scaffolds (tissue-specific matrices), signaling molecules (growth factors/morphogens), and cells. By combining these key elements, tissue regeneration often can be accomplished.

Because of the inherent limitations of autograft, substantial effort has been made to develop an off-the-shelf autograft substitute that works as well but with fewer side effects. Numerous matrices, including allogeneic, xenogeneic, and synthetic graft materials are available for use in oral surgical and orthopedic procedures; these function primarily by passively guiding, or conducting, cell migration through the matrix, eventually leading to repair of the defect. One or more of these matrices may be used in oral surgical procedures, including grafting of defects associated with periodontal disease, tooth extraction, periapical infection, implant placement, or insufficient bone height and/or width. These may be used alone; in combination with autogenous graft; or in combination with titanium cages, barrier membranes (guided tissue/bone regeneration), or other passive materials designed to act as a physical guide or barrier for cells involved in the repair and regeneration process. While these options are useful for maintaining space and a framework for tissue deposition, results obtained with passive therapeutic matrices may be variable, depending upon their inherent physical and chemical properties as well as the patient's individual healing response.

From Passive to Active—The Tissue Engineering Approach

The lack of a predictable outcome when using passive therapies, such as osteoconductive matrices and guided tissue regeneration, led to the development of treatments designed to stimulate the cells responsible for regeneration. This tissue engineering approach to bone and periodontal regeneration combines three key elements to enhance regeneration: (1) conductive scaffolds, (2) signaling molecules, and (3) cells[1] (Fig 1).

As described in the first edition of this book, a variety of naturally occurring potent bioactive proteins (signaling molecules) are known to be present in bone, platelets, and a number of other cells and tissues. As these factors have been extensively studied in the periodontal, craniomaxillofacial, and orthopedic fields, the two types of molecules that have received the greatest attention are *growth factors* that are primarily mitogenic (cell proliferative) and chemotactic (cell recruiting) agents and *morphogens* that act by altering cellular phenotype, ie, by causing the differentiation of stem cells into bone-forming cells—a process commonly known as *osteoinduction*.

Platelet-rich plasma

One of the best sources of growth factors in the body is blood platelets. Growth factors, such as platelet-derived growth factor (PDGF) and transforming growth factor-β (TGF-β), contained in the α-granules of platelets and released at sites of injury, have been shown to be important in the normal healing of bone, gingiva, and skin.[2] However, the ability to make use of concentrated forms of these proteins for routine oral surgical treatment was not possible until 1998, when Marx et al[3] introduced the technique of platelet concentration to create platelet-rich plasma (PRP) for use in dental surgery. This early example of tissue engineering in vivo, presented in the first edition of this book and updated in the current book, is accomplished by first concentrating the platelets and subsequently activating them to release their growth factor contents, including PDGF, TGF-β, platelet-derived endothelial cell growth factor (PD-ECGF), insulin-like growth factor-1 (IGF-1), and platelet factor-4. These factors, when applied to the treatment site, provide the signal to local mesenchymal and epithelial cells to migrate, divide, and increase collagen and matrix synthesis. The thrombin-calcium preparations also initiate clotting, including the conversion of fibrinogen to fibrin, resulting in clinically useful PRP gel that provides excellent handling characteristics and may enhance the efficacy of particulate autografts and bone substitutes. Today, there are a variety of platelet concentration procedures available that claim to increase platelet numbers by as much as five- to sixfold the normal circulating levels. However, studies evaluating the effect of platelet gel concentrate—alone or in combination with osetoconductive matrices—on graft maturity, bone density, and new bone formation in a number of different clinical applications have demonstrated somewhat variable outcomes, which are thought to be a result of variability in platelet concentration as well as individual patient responses.[4–7] Therefore, while clearly an advance, the use of PRP has been limited by somewhat variable outcomes and cumbersome procurement techniques. Applications for and results achieved with PRP are discussed more fully in chapter 9.

Recombinant protein therapeutics

Providing growth-modulating molecules (growth factors and morphogens) in a highly concentrated, pure, and consistent form is important in order to increase the predictability of regenerative procedures.[8] With advances in recombinant technology, proteins may now be synthesized, concentrated, purified, and packaged in large, sterile quantities under tightly controlled and regulated conditions using good manufacturing practices (GMPs), with each lot meeting strict release criteria. This rigorous manufacturing process allows for the development and commercialization of pure recombinant human growth factor–matrix combination products throughout medicine.

Table 1 US FDA-approved recombinant protein therapeutics

Recombinant protein therapeutic	Approved indications
rhPDGF-BB (gel)	Treatment of diabetic neuropathic ulcers in the lower extremities that extend into the subcutaneous tissue or beyond and have adequate blood supply
rhPDGF-BB (with β-tricalcium phosphate)	Treatment of intrabony and furcation periodontal defects and gingival recession associated with periodontal defects
rhBMP-2 (with type I collagen sponge)	Spinal fusion procedures in skeletally mature patients with degenerative disc disease at level L4-S1
	Treatment of acute, open tibial shaft fractures stabilized with intramedullary nailing in skeletally mature patients
	As an alternative to autogenous bone graft for sinus augmentations and for localized alveolar ridge augmentations for defects associated with extraction sockets

Combination products, which represent the next generation of tissue engineering therapeutics, have gained increasing attention from clinicians and researchers as a strategy to optimize tissue regeneration. These products combine tissue-specific matrices with highly concentrated bioactive proteins that actively recruit healing cells to the treatment site and expand their cell numbers. The ability to combine highly concentrated forms of individual signaling proteins with conductive matrices represents one of the most significant advances within tissue engineering and allows clinical researchers to develop improved regenerative products combining the physical and chemical characteristics required for specific cell attachment, growth, and differentiation, with the optimal binding and release profile for these bioactive proteins, in order to achieve the greatest regeneration. To date, only three recombinant growth factor products have been widely commercialized for use in tissue regeneration (Table 1).

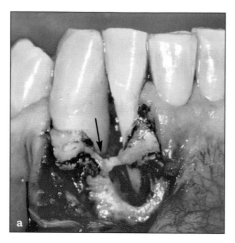 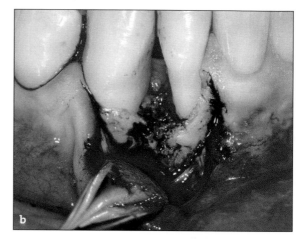

Fig 2 *(a)* Mandibular lateral incisor that has been deemed hopeless and referred for extraction and implant site development. A wide interdental crater *(arrow)* is present on the mesial surface of the canine. *(b)* Clinical appearance of the defect 11 months after treatment with mineralized allograft hydrated and mixed with rhPDGF and covered by a collagen membrane. More than 10 mm of bone fill is observed. (Figs 2a and 2b from Nevins et al.[11] Reprinted with permission.)

Recombinant human PDGF-BB

In 1997, the first recombinant (ie, synthetic) protein therapeutic was approved by the US Food and Drug Administration (FDA). The product provides recombinant human PDGF-BB (rhPDGF-BB) in a gel formulation for the treatment of recalcitrant neuropathic dermal ulcers in diabetic patients.

In 2005, an rhPDGF-BB + β-tricalcium phosphate (β-TCP) product was approved for bone and periodontal regeneration and treatment of gingival recession. This product contains approximately 1,000 times higher concentration of PDGF than the level commonly obtained through platelet concentration.[9–12] Development of rhPDGF-BB within the oral surgical field gained significant momentum when pilot human histologic studies evaluating rhPDGF-BB in combination with bone allograft for the treatment of severe periodontal intrabony and class II furcation defects provided the highest level of proof for true periodontal regeneration—human histologic evidence. These studies demonstrated that the use of highly purified rhPDGF-BB mixed with bone allograft results in robust periodontal regeneration in both class II furcations and interproximal intrabony defects.[13,14] This was the first report of periodontal regeneration demonstrated histo-

logically in human class II furcation defects. Additional clinical cases have recently been published, demonstrating complete bone fill in highly challenging periodontal bone defects following the use of rhPDGF mixed with mineralized particulate bone allograft[15] (Fig 2). The most recent findings regarding the use of rhPDGF-BB in various dental applications are highlighted below.

Gingival recession

The current approach for treatment of gingival recession most often uses a subepithelial connective tissue autograft from the palate. A recent pilot clinical study[16] evaluated the potential to eliminate the need to harvest the connective tissue from the palate by using rhPDGF-BB together with a small amount of bone graft material covered with a collagen membrane. The recombinant therapeutic appeared to provide comparable results to the connective tissue graft, without the need for a second surgical (harvest) site. A larger clinical trial is now being conducted to more fully assess the predictability of using rhPDGF in this indication, thereby potentially reducing procedure time and eliminating the morbidity and risk for postoperative complications resulting from the harvest site.

Periodontal defects

A large-scale randomized, controlled blinded pivotal clinical trial of the use of rhPDGF-BB to treat periodontal defects demonstrated rhPDGF to be a potent stimulator of alveolar bone regeneration.[17] Representative cases were presented in a follow-up report of results up to 2 years following treatment.[18] These cases demonstrate maintenance of clinical outcomes and substantial increases in radiographic linear bone gain and percent bone fill compared with 6-month observations. Radiographically, the regenerated bone matured over time, increasing in density and normal trabeculation.

Alveolar ridge augmentation and peri-implant defects

More recently, rhPDGF also has been used to promote bone regeneration around endosseous implants. In a proof-of-principle study evaluating vertical ridge augmentation in a standardized model using rhPDGF-BB in combination with block form anorganic bovine bone, the authors report results demonstrating the potential to regenerate significant amounts of new bone around dental implants placed in severely atrophic mandibular ridges.[19] Additionally, the results suggest the importance of the periosteum as a source of osteoprogenitor cells in growth factor–mediated regenerative procedures. This study clearly demonstrates the advantage of bioactive recombinant therapeutics over GBR techniques that rely on passive wound healing.

Dental clinical applications of rhPDGF are discussed in chapters 1, 3, 5 to 8, and 15. In addition, new information is provided regarding the use of rhPDGF-BB in orthopedic indications such as foot and ankle fusion and distal radius fracture procedures (chapter 19) and for regenerating tendon- and ligament-related injuries (chapter 20).

Recombinant human BMP-2

Bone morphogenetic proteins (BMPs) are morphogens and differentiation factors originally isolated from bone matrix based on their ability to induce ectopic bone formation, ie, bone formation de novo where bone does not normally exist, such as in subcutaneous or intramuscular sites.[20] The BMPs function by inducing the differentiation of cells of mesenchymal origin into bone-forming cells. Demineralized freeze-dried bone allografts (DFDBAs) have been shown to contain BMPs; however, the concentration of BMP compared with the concentration of other growth factors present in allograft, such as IGF-2 and TGF-β, is very low,[21] and the amount of BMP within quantities of DFDBA typically used in periodontal and craniomaxillofacial procedures may be suboptimal.[20] Recombinant human BMP-2 (rhBMP-2) in combination with a type I bovine collagen sponge has been approved in the US by the FDA for use in spinal fusion, tibial fracture repair, and, most recently, as an alternative to autogenous grafts in sinus augmentation and extraction socket grafting procedures in skeletally mature patients. Preclinical results do not support the appropriateness of rhBMP-2 for the treatment of human periodontal defects.[22–24] Studies indicate that rhBMP-2 may realize its best application in large defects resulting from trauma or congenital deformity (see chapters 16 and 17). This book provides the reader with extensive new information related to the use of rhBMP-2 in craniomaxillofacial procedures. Specifically, chapters 1, 11 to 13, 16, and 17 discuss the current state of knowledge on the clinical use of BMPs in oral and maxillofacial surgery.

Summary

Tissue engineering using PRP or recombinant protein therapeutics with tissue-specific scaffolds is now a clinical reality in periodontal, craniomaxillofacial, and orthopedic indications. No doubt our understanding of the biologic and physical requirements to achieve predictable regeneration of specific tissues (eg, bone, cartilage, tendon, ligament, and skin) will continue to evolve as we establish more optimal binding and release characteristics for the bioactive proteins, more conductive cell scaffolds, and eventually the use of stem cells in cases where no other options are available to treat human degenerative conditions.

We are entering a new era of regenerative medicine in which patients and the health care system will see tremendous benefits from faster and more predictable healing using less invasive and less traumatic treatments. The current availability of recombinant protein therapeutics represents a major evolution in our regenerative therapies. Dental surgeons at long last have access to pure recombinant tissue growth factors, allowing us to progress from previously passive therapies to new active treatments, thereby enhancing the opportunity for regeneration of bone and other tissues, and providing more efficient and predictable outcomes for patients.

References

1. Lynch SE. Introduction. Lynch SE, Genco RJ, Marx RE (eds). Tissue Engineering: Applications in Maxillofacial Surgery and Periodontics. Chicago: Quintessence, 1999:xi–xviii.

2. Lynch SE. Bone regeneration techniques in the orofacial region. In: Lieberman JR, Friedlaender GE (eds). Bone Regeneration and Repair Biology and Clinical Applications. Totowa, NJ: Humana, 2005:359–390.

3. Marx RE, Carlson ER, Eichstaedt RM, Schimmele SR, Strauss JE, Georgeff KR. Platelet-rich plasma growth factor enhancement for bone grafts. Oral Surg Oral Med Oral Pathol Oral Radiol Endod 1998;85:638–646.

4. Boyapati L, Wang HL. The role of platelet-rich plasma in sinus augmentation: A critical review. Implant Dent 2006;15:160–170.

5. Esposito M, Grusovin MG, Coulthard P, Worthington HV. The efficacy of various bone augmentation procedures for dental implants: A Cochran systematic review of randomized controlled clinical trials. Int J Oral Maxillofac Implants 2006;21:696–710.

6. Schlegel KA, Zimmermann R, Thorwarth M, et al. Sinus floor elevation using autogenous bone or bone substitute combined with platelet-rich plasma. Oral Surg Oral Med Oral Pathol Oral Radiol Endod 2007;104(3):e15–e25 [Epub 2007 Jul 6].

7. Weiner BK, Walker M. Efficacy of autologous growth factors in lumbar intertransverse fusions. Spine 2003;28:1968–1971.

8. Sutherland D, Bostrom M. Grafts and bone graft substitutes. In: Lieberman JR, Friedlaender GE (eds). Bone Regeneration and Repair Biology and Clinical Applications. Totowa, NJ: Humana, 2005:133–156.

9. Bowen-Pope DF, Malpass TW, Foster DM, Ross R. Platelet-derived growth factor in vivo: Levels, activity, and rate of clearance. Blood 1984;64:458–469.

10. Huang JS, Huang SS, Deuel TF. Human platelet-derived growth factor: Radioimmunoassay and discovery of a specific plasma-binding protein. J Cell Biol 1983; 97:383–388.

11. Singh JP, Chaikin MA, Stiles CD. Phylogenetic analysis of platelet-derived growth factor by radio-receptor assay. J Cell Biol 1982;95:667–671.

12. Harvest Technologies Corporation. SmartPrep 2. Available at: http://www.harvesttech.com/education/prp-brochures.html. Accessed 17 Oct 2007.

13. Nevins M, Camelo M, Nevins ML, Schenk RK, Lynch SE. Periodontal regeneration in humans using recombinant human platelet-derived growth factor BB (rhPDGF-BB) and allogenic bone. J Periodontol 2003;74:1282–1292.

14. Camelo M, Nevins ML, Schenk RK, Lynch SE, Nevins M. Periodontal regeneration in human class II furcations using purified recombinant human platelet-derived growth factor-BB (rhPDGF-BB) with bone allograft. Int J Periodontics Restorative Dent 2003;23:213–225.

15. Nevins M, Hanratty J, Lynch SE. Clinical results using recombinant human platelet-derived growth factor and mineralized freeze-dried bone allograft in periodontal defects. Int J Periodontics Restorative Dent 2007;27:421–427.

16. McGuire MK, Scheyer ET. Comparison of recombinant human platelet-derived growth factor-BB plus beta tricalcium phosphate and a collagen membrane to subepithelial connective tissue grafting for the treatment of recession defects: A case series. Int J Periodontics Restorative Dent 2006;26:127–133.

17. Nevins M, Giannobile WV, McGuire MK, et al. Platelet-derived growth factor stimulates bone fill and rate of attachment level gain: Results of a large multicenter randomized controlled trial. J Periodontol 2005;76:2205–2215.

18. McGuire MK, Kao RT, Nevins M, Lynch SE. rhPDGF-BB promotes healing of periodontal defects: 24-month clinical and radiographic observations. Int J Periodontics Restorative Dent 2006;26:223–231.

19. Simion M, Rocchietta I, Kim D, Nevins M, Fiorellini J. Vertical ridge augmentation by means of deproteinized bovine bone block and recombinant human platelet-derived growth factor-BB: A histologic study in a dog model. Int J Periodontics Restorative Dent 2006;26:415–423.

20. Wozney J, Rosen V, Celeste AJ. Novel regulators of bone formation: Molecular clones and activities. Science 1988;242:1528–1534.

21. Mohan S, Baylink D. Therapeutic potential of TGF-β, BMP and FGF in the treatment of bone loss. In: Bilezikian J, Raisz L, Rodan G (eds). Principles of Bone Biology. New York: Academic Press, 1996:1111–1123.

22. Selvig KA, Sorensen RG, Wozney JM, Wikesjö UM. Bone repair following recombinant human bone morphogenetic protein-2 stimulated periodontal regeneration. J Periodontol 2002;73:1020–1029.

23. Wikesjö UM, Lim WH, Thomson RC, Cook AD, Wozney JM, Hardwick WR. Periodontal repair in dogs: Evaluation of a bioabsobable space-providing macroporous membrane with recombinant human bone morphogenetic protein-2. J Periodontol 2003;74:635–647.

24. Sorensen RG, Wikesjö UM, Kinoshita A, Wozney JM. Periodontal repair in dogs: Evaluation of a bioresorbable calcium phosphate cement (Ceredex) as a carrier for rhBMP-2. J Clin Periodontol 2004;31:796–804.

Principles of Tissue Engineering

Protein Therapeutics and Bone Healing

Jeffrey O. Hollinger, DDS, PhD

Charles Hart, PhD

Reinhard Gruber, PhD

Bruce Doll, DDS, PhD

Over the past two decades, a significant amount of effort and money have been invested in testing the potential use of growth factors and morphogens in tissue engineering and regenerative medicine. While several other proteins show promise, only two recombinant human proteins are available for widespread use: platelet-derived growth factor BB (rhPDGF-BB) and bone morphogenetic protein 2 (rhBMP-2). rhBMP-7 is also available in special circumstances.

This chapter focuses on the roles of rhPDGF and rhBMP in periodontal and orthopedic bone healing. rhPDGF-BB, rhBMP-2, and rhBMP-7 (also known as *osteogenic protein 1 [OP-1]*) are emphasized primarily for two reasons:

1. There is a significant peer-reviewed database on the efficacy and safety of these molecules for bone regeneration.
2. The US Food and Drug Administration (FDA) has cleared the clinical use of rhPDGF-BB for chronic skin wounds in diabetic patients (Regranex, Ethicon) and for periodontically related osseous defects (GEM 21S, Bio-Mimetic Therapeutics) and rhBMP-2 (InFuse, Medtronic

Sofamor Danek) for anterior interbody spine fusion, open tibial fractures, sinus elevations, and defects associated with tooth extraction.

Regional Anatomic Domains

The concept of *regional anatomic domains* (RADs) integrates anatomic, embryologic, biomechanical, and physiologic properties in the anatomic areas of the craniofacial, axial, and appendicular skeletons. RADs have distinctive regional mechanical cues coupled with molecular and cellular information to provide guidance for osseous wound healing and, therefore, therapy design.

The RAD concept evokes compelling, clinically relevant questions:

- Will therapeutic intervention with a recombinant growth factor (eg, rhBMP or rhPDGF) have a unique and specific regional effect (ie, site effect) or a general pan-skeletal effect?

- If the growth factor works in the tibia (appendicular skeleton), will that same growth factor work in the mandibular-dental region (craniofacial skeleton) and vice versa?

Clinical experience and the literature have answered these questions. There does not appear to be a different healing outcome between the appendicular (eg, tibia) and the craniofacial (eg, mandibular-dental) site. However, the biologic healing process in appendicular endochondral bone involves a chondrogenic element. The biologic healing process in the dental and maxillofacial intramembranous bones does not involve chondrogenesis. However, a chondrogenic phase will occur if the fracture fixation in intramembranous bone is unstable.

The classic example underscoring the similarity across RADs in response to therapeutics is the autogenous bone graft. Autogenous bone grafts are effective panskeletally. The healing of a bone gap or fracture occurs by similar biologic processes regardless of the RAD (appendicular, axial, or craniofacial skeleton) or the embryologic origin (either intramembranous, such as the curved bones of the skull as well as the mandible and maxilla, or endochondral, such as the tubular long bones [tibia, radius, and femur]). Distinguishing endochondral and intramembranous bone biology is an absence of chondrogenesis during intramembranous embryogenesis and healing.

RAD sites have distinctive mechanoanatomic units (MAUs) as a consequence of regionally specific mechanical input. For example, mechanical cues of the alveolar bone of the periodontium will be different from those of the distal tibia because of differences in force vectors, movement envelopes, and tissue attachments.

Despite having different MAUs, RADs have common features that include cellular phenotypes (eg, osteoblasts, osteoclasts, and osteocytes) and molecular signals (eg, BMPs and PDGFs).

Therefore, it is reasonable to expect that RADs will respond similarly and predictably to the same therapeutic growth factor (eg, rhBMP-2, rhBMP-7, or rhPDGF-BB). However, it is not unreasonable, in light of the physiologic complexity of RADs, to assume and expect that fundamental biologic differences exist during the process of bone regeneration.

The RAD and MAU concepts were inspired by developmental skeletal biology[1–6] and were recognized first by Urist[7] and Reddi.[8] Reddi, in 1975, underscored the anatomic field from which bone matrix was derived and stated: "The transforming potency [of bone matrix] varies widely in matrices of different bones."[8] Urist, in 1980, wrote: "Every bone and every part of the human skeleton responds to injury in its individual way and incorporates a bone graft at its own rate of repair. The factors intrinsic to the repair process are age, anatomical pattern of vascularity, immobolization, contact compression, and pathologic condition."[7]

At the writing of this chapter, the hypothesis that RAD sites respond differently to the same growth factor has not been tested. The next section will reveal that the fundamental biologic processes of bone healing across RAD sites are strikingly constant across different regions. Consequently, dividing the skeletal system into RADs (sites) and MAUs (functional loading zones) does not limit the opportunities for the same beneficial clinical outcome from the same growth factor therapy. However, in the future, the RAD and MAU concepts could enhance effectiveness and efficiency in therapeutic design.

Unique functional loading characteristics

The design and development of rhPDGF and rhBMP therapeutics must integrate basic elements of the size of the bone injury, the release kinetics of the growth factor from the delivery system, and the physiologic determinants of the patient; these factors will distinguish clinical outcomes across specific sites. The size of the injury is the distance between bone ends following injury. Physiologic determinants include age, clinical conditions such as diabetes, osteoporosis, steroidal medications, and use of tobacco products. Physiologic determinants and size will affect the biologic process of bone wound healing. Figure 1-1 illustrates the concepts of RAD (sites), MAU (functional units), physiology, and injury.

Physiologic determinants, growth factor release kinetics, and delivery systems merit significant independent attention exceeding the scope of this chapter. The size of the wound (ie, fracture versus gap) has been addressed in other publications.[9–11]

In this chapter, the biologic process of bone healing in the appendicular and craniofacial skeletons is highlighted. The periodontal location (ie, the alveolar bone in the mandible and maxilla) will be the focus in the craniofacial skeleton.

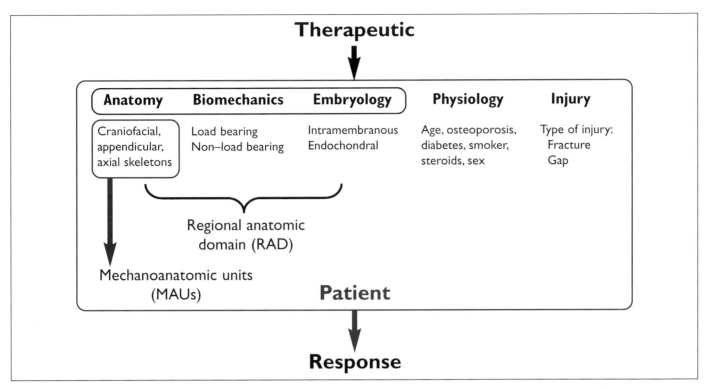

Fig 1-1 A patient's response to a therapeutic will depend on the integration of anatomic location, biomechanics, embryology, physiology, and the nature of the clinical injury. The concepts of the RAD and MAU will provide important guidelines to the design and development of effective therapeutics.

Bone Healing

Several compelling reviews on bone healing have explained fracture healing in the appendicular skeleton.[12–16] These reviews are the basis for the following discussion.

There are numerous similarities in the process of osseous wound-healing biology among different sites. However, there may be subtle differences. It is not known if these differences will influence therapeutic outcome. Furthermore, a number of other questions must be considered:

- Are there fundamental healing differences between fractures and bone gaps? Fundamental biologic differences exist in bone healing as the size of a bone wound increases from a fracture, which will heal spontaneously following reduction and fixation, to a gap that becomes a critical sized defect (CSD).[9] The CSD will not regenerate with bone spontaneously because of qualitative and quantitative biologic deficiencies.[17] Consequently, a CSD heals by fibrosis.

- Does the tibia heal differently from the periodontal alveolar bone? The basic biologic events at a healing tibial and alveolar bone wound are strikingly similar. However, the chondrogenic phase of healing for endochondral-derived appendicular bone distinguishes it from the direct bone formation that will occur during the healing process of intramembranous-derived craniofacial bone.

- Will a bone wound in the tibia respond to a growth factor differently from one in the periodontal alveolar bone? There is neither clinical nor mechanistic research evidence that growth factors promote a unique outcome at different sites or that a growth factor will be effective only at one site but not at another.

Growth factor biology influences bone-healing outcomes. The response at the recipient site (ie, spine fusion bed or alveolar bone) to the growth factor is modified by physiologic determinants of the patient and the type (eg, size) of bone injury. Moreover, the release kinetics of the delivery system determine the dose and timing of growth factor delivery at any particular site. Dosing and timing must be calibrated to the wound-healing process at the specific site.

With these fundamentals stated, the following sections review the process of bone healing. A general discussion of bone wound healing at orthopedic and periodontal sites provides the basic foundational guidance for clinical applications of rhPDGF-BB, rhBMP-2, and rhBMP-7 in orthopedics, maxillofacial surgery, and periodontics. Moreover, it is shown that in light of the nearly universal process of bone healing, rhPDGF and rhBMPs should support bone regeneration across orthopedic, maxillofacial, and periodontal sites.

Orthopedic fracture healing

Repair

A predictable sequence of biologic events follows bone fracture and gap injuries (Fig 1-2). Fracture models have identified cells and soluble factors and their temporal and spatial relationships.[12–16]

Bone injury (eg, fracture) incites an inflammatory response; complement activation ensues, and damage to blood vessels (ie, laceration) at the injury locus causes extravasation. Proteolytic degradation of extracellular matrix produces chemotactic remnants, attracting monocytes and macrophages to the wound bed. Activated macrophages release basic fibroblast growth factor (bFGF) and vascular endothelial growth factor (VEGF), stimulating endothelial cells to express plasminogen activator and procollagenase. Growth factors released from the alpha granules of degranulating platelets include the three isomeres of PDGF—transforming growth factor β1 (TGF-β1), TGF-β2, and VEGF—which start the wound-healing module.

The extravasated, localized collection of blood will clot, form a hematoma, establish a hemostatic plug, and prevent blood volume depletion. Orchestrating the clotting cascade are platelets, which have the dual function of hemostasis control and mediator signaling, specifically signaling of PDGF, TGF-β, and FGF.

The initial osseous wound environment is characterized by a decrease in oxygen tension and pH (to approximately pH 4 to 5), conditions needed for the operational activities of polymorphonuclear neutrophil leukocytes and macrophages. Polymorphonuclear neutrophil leukocytes remove microbial infestations and microdebris, whereas the macrophages purge the injury site of larger, insidious debris and may develop into polykaryon (multinucleated giant cells) to manage a sustained barrage of invaders and necrotic bone shards. Macrophages provide a formidable synthesis capability to the wound site, manufacturing and secreting growth factors to fortify cellular activity, recruit cells, and provoke mitogenesis and chemotaxis throughout the injury repair cascade until abatement.

By days 3 to 5 following bone fracture and injury, an organized repair system develops, consisting of new blood vessels, collagen isotypes, and cells (eg, fibroblasts and macrophages). It is likely that selective binding of growth factors to collagens may localize, protect, and temporally position growth factors to optimize cellular interaction. Therefore, the collagenous component of the repairing wound is a key instructional substratum to present modulating factors, such as TGF-β, FGF, PDGF, and the BMPs to receptive cells. Furthermore, the collagenous substratum functions as a provisional solid-state matrix for differential cellular attachment. For example, undifferentiated cells traversing new blood vessels and osteoprogenitor cells localized to periosteum and endosteum—beckoned to the fracture site by chemotactic signals (eg, TGF-βs and PDGF)—anchor to the granulation tissue collagen and differentiate into chondrocytes and osteoblasts under the influence of differentiating molecules, such as TGF-βs and BMPs (Fig 1-3). The combined activities of cellular anchorage, transduction, and cell-factor interaction promote cellular differentiation to specific phenotypes, leading to bone repair.

The gradual differentiation of cells, accumulation of cell expression products, and maturation of the extracellular matrix over the course of several weeks result in callus formation. Components of the callus are vascular elements, stromal products, cartilage, and cells. Cartilage is replaced by woven bone: cellular, randomly oriented spicules of immature bone. Woven bone matures to lamellar bone, which is less cellular than woven bone, consisting of bony sheets directed to buttress fracture fragments. The functional role of a callus is to stabilize the bone fragments.

Teams of cells and a consortium of molecular signaling factors (parathyroid hormone, TGF-β, FGFs, VEGF, the BMPs, PDGF, cytokines, and metalloproteases) constitute the repertoire of ingredients to ensure that fracture healing in the adult is completed about 6 to 8 weeks postinjury. However, if sufficient quantities of cells are not resident at the injury locus, they must be recruited, expanded in number, and acted upon by the proper combination of growth factors. At the injury locus, the lure for

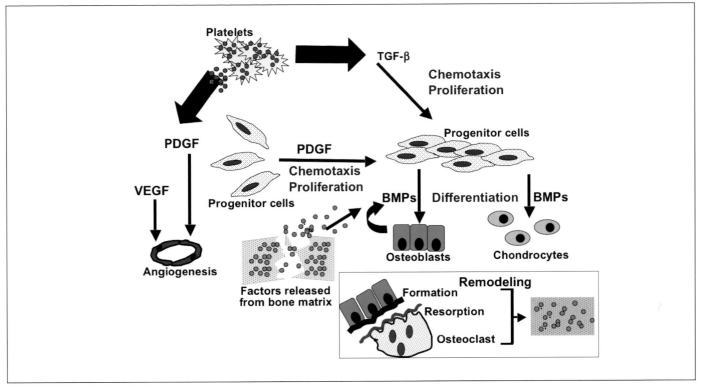

Fig 1-2 Many signaling molecules and cells are involved in bone healing. The emphasis on PDGF and BMP are underscored during the osseous wound-healing process from initiation through remodeling. The platelets jettison alpha granules containing PDGF for angiogenesis, chemotaxis, and mitogenesis. BMPs become locally available at the bone wound as they are released from the damaged bone matrix and promote osteoblast differentiation. BMPs and PDGF contribute powerful coregulatory control over the remodeling process to restore form and function. (VEGF) Vascular endothelial growth factor; (TGF-β) transforming growth factor β.

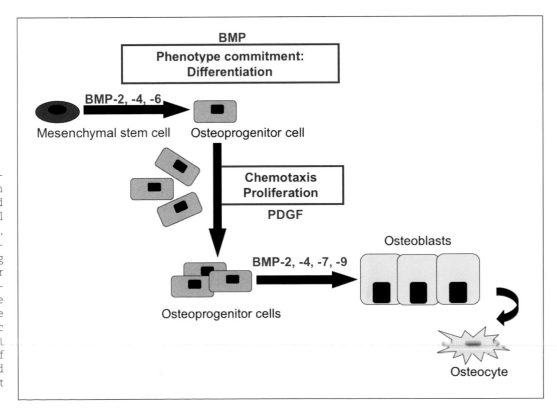

Fig 1-3 Recruitment (chemoattraction) and proliferation of cells at the bone wound are directed by PDGF. Several BMPs (BMP-2, BMP-4, BMP-6, BMP-7, and BMP-9) are responsible for differentiating stem cell and osteoprogenitor cells to osteoblasts. The impact of the BMPs would be significantly nullified if the chemotactic and mitogenic properties of PDGF did not encourage recruitment of sufficient cells to the wound site as well as subsequent amplification.

monocytes that will convert into osteoclasts appears to be fragments of the ubiquitous attachment factor fibronectin and degradation products from the extracellular matrix. Moreover, macrophages at the wound site express FGF and VEGF and, in combination with PDGF, instigate neoangiogenesis for vascular renewal. Formation of new blood vessels and blood flow provide transit for cells to replenish those lost to injury, for instance, osteoblasts, whose origins may be traced to bone marrow stromal cells; vascular pericytes; and undifferentiated precursor cells from endosteum and periosteum.

The clinical relevance of cells in wound repair is that they represent the final common pathway of the elements that contribute to tissue regeneration. That is, the combination of growth factors, cellular attachment molecules, and matrix substratum must interact to drive the cellular machinery responsible for synthesizing new bone. When cellular machinery is either limited in quantity or defective, indicative of the aging process,[18–20] corruption in bone regeneration dynamics is predictable. Consequently, therapeutic growth factor intervention has great promise, and unique opportunities may be predicted for the use of growth factor therapy.

Remodeling

Remodeling is the final phase of bone healing that "sculpts" a fracture callus and restores form and function, producing a structure that is biologically and mechanically indistinguishable from the preinjury state. The remodeling process involves an array of cellular and molecular elements intertwined over space and time in discrete, predictable steps[21] (Fig 1-4).

Through a precise sequence of cellular-molecular interactions bundled in time, osteoblasts and osteoclasts add and subtract bone. An activating signal must be evoked to jump-start the remodeling process. The signal can be either humoral (eg, parathyroid hormone) or biomechanical (eg, strain) or both.

The effector for the signal is a cell. The signal will activate the cell, the osteoblast, which vacates the bone surface, leaving behind a lure for osteoclasts.[22] The osteoclast arrives to the osteoblast-free surface, docks via integrin-like binding, resorbs a volume of bone (up to 5 μm per day[23]), and, for reasons yet to be determined, ceases activity, succumbs to programmed cell death, and detaches. Attracted to the osteoclast-free site are osteoblasts. Osteoblasts attach to a remaining osteopontin-rich cement line and in a sheetlike fashion secrete an osteoid

matrix that calcifies. Osteoid is produced at a rate of about 1 to 2 μm per day and, achieving a thickness of approximately 20 μm (after a maturation period of about 10 days), mineralizes at a rate of 1 to 2 μm per day.[24]

Remodeling is partitioned into an activation-resorption-formation pathway.[25] Osteoblasts are activated, vacate, and are replaced by osteoclasts. These osteoclasts in turn resorb bone, vacate, and are replaced by osteoblasts that deposit bone. While some of the cues that turn on and off the functional activity of these cells have been elucidated, many more must be discovered.[26]

Cells responsible for remodeling constitute the basic multicellular unit (BMU), and the temporal duration (lifespan) of a BMU is called *sigma*.[3,23]

Craniofacial and periodontal bone healing

At the time of preparation of this chapter, no study directly comparing the biology of long-bone fracture healing to that of craniofacial or periodontal bone healing was available. It is highly likely that the biologic process of healing across appendicular and craniofacial sites is very similar, based on the favorable clinical outcome from bone grafts. Moreover, independent reviews of bone healing underscore the similarity in the biologic process of healing between appendicular and craniofacial bone.[12,21,27,28]

The periodontal ligament, teeth, and gingiva are a distinguishing set of structures in the periodontal site of the craniofacial skeleton. In a comprehensive review by Wong,[27] the phases of periodontal alveolar bone healing are thoroughly described in terms of the hemorrhagic and inflammatory responses and subsequent coagulative, destructive, proliferative, osteogenic, and remodeling phases. Temporal and spatial aspects of osseous wound healing between the alveolar bone and appendicular bone appear to be strikingly similar.[28]

However, there are features that distinguish the periodontal site from orthopedic sites. Noteworthy is the periodontium, which includes epithelial-mesenchymal interactions, the periodontal ligament, cementum, dentin, enamel, and junctional complexes between teeth and connective tissues.[29] The outcome of periodontal bone healing can result in regeneration of all those structures, with the exception of dentin and enamel.

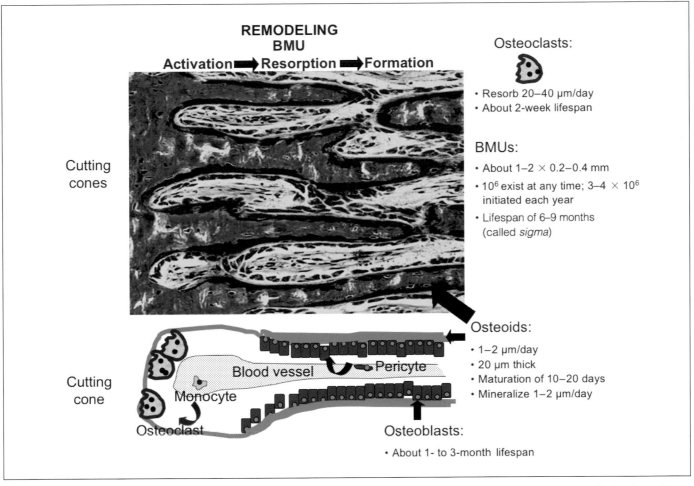

Fig 1-4 Remodeling involves a tightly controlled sequence of cellular and molecular activity collectively known as the basic multicellular unit (BMU). BMUs operate through an activation-resorption-formation pathway. BMUs are sustained during metabolic bone homeostasis for 6 to 9 months. This operational lifespan is called *sigma*. However, there is an acceleration of the sequence (known as *regional acceleratory phenomenon*) as a consequence of bone trauma. Remodeling to sculpt bone can occur by cutting cones, which include a vanguard of osteoclasts followed by osteoblasts. Replenishment of osteoclasts is accomplished by blood-borne monocyte precursors. Osteoblasts can be derived from blood vessel pericytes.

There are common cellular and biologic healing pathways between periodontal and orthopedic anatomies. Therefore, it is highly likely that common therapeutic strategies can be exploited.

The skeleton has the intrinsic capacity to regenerate functional integrity after injury, which contrasts with soft tissue wound healing, in which the final product is scar tissue.[30] There are biologic cues common and unique to soft tissue and bone that result in this distinguishing outcome. It is not the purpose of this chapter to review all of the biologic cues, but rather to emphasize rhPDGF-BB, rhBMP-2, and rhBMP-7, which have proven therapeutic value.

Platelet-Derived Growth Factor

Expression and function in wound healing

The PDGF family includes PDGF-AB, PDGF-AA, PDGF-BB, PDGF-CC, and PDGF-DD.[1,13] These molecules can stimulate formation of granulation tissue, which is a prerequisite for wound healing and bone regeneration. Bone regeneration is initiated by activation of the coagulation cascade and culminates in blood clot formation that fills the defect site. Platelets aggregate and release their granules into the developing blood clot, including varying amounts of PDGF-AB, PDGF-AA, PDGF-BB, and PDGF-CC.[30–33]

PDGFs attract and activate neutrophils and macrophages[34–37] with PDGF receptors expressed by human monocyte-derived macrophages, enabling them to respond chemotactically to their ligands.[38] Macrophages provide a continuous source of PDGFs and other growth factors that orchestrate granulation tissue formation.[30]

Granulation tissue replaces the fibrin-rich blood clot with fibroblasts, osteogenic cells, and new capillaries.[30,39,40] Chemotaxis and mitogenesis of osteogenic cells inspired by localized release of PDGF into the wound-healing milieu are antecedent to osteoblastic differentiation.

Significantly, treatment of diabetic ulcers[41] with rhPDGF-BB has been effective, likely as a consequence of the role of PDGF in granulation tissue formation. Therefore, benefits from rhPDGF are expected for bone healing,[15] at tooth extraction sites,[40] at peri-implant bone areas,[39] and in situations of compromised bone healing in elderly, osteoporotic, and diabetic individuals.

It is noteworthy to consider the therapeutic role for rhPDGF for compromised bone wound healing in the patient with diabetes. It has been shown there is a decrease in cellular proliferation in the fracture callus and a decrease in levels of PDGF transcripts in diabetic rats, suggesting a correlation between PDGF levels and fracture-healing response.[42] Moreover, platelets from diabetic patients have less PDGF than do those from nondiabetic patients.[43] Consequently, rhPDGF therapy could profoundly aid bone healing in patients with diabetes.

Isoforms and signaling

The PDGF polypeptide growth factor family currently represents four genes located on different chromosomes. The genes encode PDGF-A, PDGF-B, PDGF-C, and PDGF-D isoforms. PDGF-A and PDGF-B can be homodimers or heterodimers, whereas PDGF-C and PDGF-D exist as homodimers.[44]

PDGFs have a common structure of eight conserved cysteine residues that are involved in the spatial conformation of the monomers and their dimerization. Before processing into functional active molecules, the precursor molecules of PDGF-A and PDGF-B undergo N-terminal proteolytic cleavage within the cytoplasm, whereas extra-

cellular proteases are required for cleavage-induced activation of the CUB domain of PDGF-C and PDGF-D. PDGF-B and one of the two spliced versions of PDGF-A have a retention motif at the C terminus, allowing binding to collagen, thrombospondin, osteopontin, and heparin sulfate. This enables local concentration gradients that are especially noteworthy for wound healing. Biologic concentration gradients are a significant and powerful element of the wound-healing process. For example, if endothelial cells expressing PDGF-BB lack the retention motif, insufficient numbers of pericytes and smooth muscle cells will migrate to the wound site, and blood vessel formation will be impaired.[45,46]

The five possible combinations of PDGFs can interact with three possible combinations of receptors (PDGFRs), which also form homodimers and heterodimers. PDGFR-α/α has the highest affinity for PDGF-AA, PDGF-AB, PDGF-BB, and PDGF-CC, whereas PDGFR-β/β binding is restricted to the PDGF-BB and PDGF-DD isoforms.[33,44] All other ligands, except PDGF-AA, can signal via the heterodimeric receptor configuration. Only PDGF-BB can activate all three configurations of PDGF receptors. Ligand binding causes dimerization and autophosphorylation of tyrosine residues in the cytoplasmic domain, which provides docking sites for signaling molecules and adapter proteins that contain Src homology 2 (SH2) and SH3. Among the signaling molecules are Src-family tyrosine kinases, phosphatidylinositol-3 kinases (PI3K), phospholipase Cγ (PLC-γ), and the adapter protein growth factor receptor-bound protein 2 (Grb2) for extracellular signal-regulated protein kinase (ERK) that activates downstream signaling.[46–48]

Cellular targets

Osteogenic cells respond to PDGF ligand binding by activation of Src tyrosine kinases.[49–51] PDGF also activates AKT kinase (also known as *protein kinase B*) and Grb2-mediated ERK signaling in osteogenic cells.[51] Activation of c-Jun N-terminal kinase (JNK) and p38 mitogen-activated protein kinase (MAPK) signaling has been reported for vascular smooth muscle cells but not for osteoblasts,[44] and both pathways are involved in osteoblastic differentiation.[52–54]

PDGFs exert mitogenic and chemotactic activity on osteogenic cells derived from calvaria,[55–57] periosteum of long bones,[58] trabecular bone,[59,60] and bone marrow stromal cells.[61–63] This observation underscores the concept of functional loading discussed earlier in the chapter, whereby MAUs among the three sites may invoke different regulatory gates that control the interactions of cell-signaling molecules.

Continuous incubation of osteoblast-like cells with PDGFs can suppress osteogenic differentiation.[51,55–57,64] Nevertheless, the cells will differentiate into osteoblasts.[65,66] Further, sequential incubation of osteogenic cells with PDGF increases in vitro mineralization.[66] These findings suggest a significant therapeutic consideration: The delivery of PDGF in either a continuous or pulsatile manner will affect lineage progression and function of the cell.

At the osseous wound-healing site, PDGF increases the pool of osteogenic cells (ie, acts as a chemotactic agent and mitogen), whereas their subsequent differentiation into osteoblasts or chondrocytes is directed by the BMP family,[67,68] hedgehog proteins,[1,69] and activation of the Wnt-signaling pathway.[70]

PDGFs exert indirect effects on bone regeneration by increasing the expression of angiogenic molecules such as VEGF[71] and hepatocyte growth factor/scatter factor,[72] as well as the proinflammatory cytokine interleukin 6.[73] VEGF is a key molecule in bone regeneration.[74]

PDGFs can modulate the responsiveness of osteogenic cells to BMPs by increasing the expression of gremlin (but not noggin[75,76]) and IGF signaling.[77] The responsiveness of osteogenic cells to PDGFs can be regulated by the inflammatory cytokine interleukin 1, which inhibits PDGFR-α expression in MG-63 cells[78–80] and human osteoblastic cells.[81] In rat calvaria-derived cells and MC3T3-E1 cells, interleukin 1 cytokine has opposite effects.[55,56,82]

Angiogenesis and vasculogenesis

Angiogenesis and vasculogenesis are cellular and matrix-related processes that result in the formation of new capillaries from existing blood vessels. Development of new blood vessels and blood flow comprise a multistep process initiated by destabilization of existing blood vessel walls and degradation of the basal membrane.[83] Capillaries grow into the extracellular granulation matrix during wound healing and are essential for bone regeneration.[20,39,19]

PDGF-BB secreted from endothelial cells is a strong chemoattractant and a potent mitogen for mural cells (ie, pericytes and smooth muscle cells).[84] Genetic models demonstrate that endothelial cell–derived PDGF-BB is required to recruit PDGFR-β–positive cells and stimulate blood vessel maturation.[85,86]

Furthermore, locally applied PDGF-BB destabilizes blood vessels, purportedly because mural cells will follow the PDGF chemotactic gradient.[87] The outcome is that blood vessels adjacent to the healing wound are enabled to "sprout," and a filamentous web of neovasculature grows into the granulation tissue. Granulation tissue is a mandatory antecedent to bone healing.

When PDGF-BB is coadministered with VEGF and bFGF, corneal and ischemic limb revascularization is observed.[88,89] The mechanism involves the upregulation of PDGF receptors α and β by bFGF, leading to improved survival of endothelial cells and increased proliferation of smooth muscle cells and subsequent stabilization of newly formed capillaries.[89] Moreover, PDGF-BB can increase VEGF expression in mural cells, which in turn target endothelial cells and induce a potent angiogenic response.[90,91]

Application in calvarial bone defects and with demineralized bone matrix

PDGF-BB, delivered with a chitosan–tricalcium phosphate sponge and collagen, stimulated osseous healing in rat calvarial defects[92,93] and enhanced bone formation when applied in a methylcellulose gel.[94]

However, partially purified PDGF did not appear to affect bone formation in a rat cranial defect model and may have decreased the activity of partially purified osteogenin.[95,96] Similarly, rhPDGF-BB at 10 µg/10 mg, mixed with human demineralized bone matrix (DBM) and implanted subcutaneously in athymic mice, suppressed cartilage and consequently bone formation in a nude mouse model.[97] These study outcomes at orthotopic and heterotopic sites do not undermine the utility of PDGF as a therapeutic agent; rather they underscore normal biologic control. Exogenous PDGF administered to normal adult rodents may cause a downregulation of cellular activity and may decrease the healing response. Mechanistically, this outcome is normal biology.

In contrast with the studies cited above, Howes et al[98] determined an enhanced bone response in elderly rats when rhPDGF-BB was implanted subcutaneously with DBM. The rhPDGF-BB–supplemented DBM enhanced bone formation and upregulated biochemical bone markers, and the combination increased bone formation and associated bone markers in older animals twofold compared with DBM alone. In younger rats, the effect of rhPDGF-BB–amended DBM was not significant compared to DBM alone. These results suggest that compromised bone healing may be improved by rhPDGF-BB in aged individuals. This logic is underscored by reports of a significant decrement in osteoblast function[99] and fracture healing with age[19] as well as gene expression from bone marrow stromal cells.[20]

Periodontal applications

Periodontium is composed of gingival epithelium, connective tissue, and cementum, which is connected to alveolar bone by the periodontal ligament, a narrow band of dense, fibrous connective tissue. Chronic inflammation is the main cause of catabolic processes in the periodontium, leading to periodontal disease. If chronic inflammation is untreated, loss of periodontal structures will result. This outcome, periodontal disease, occurs in 87% of adults older than 70 years.[100] Approximately 2.1 million periodontal surgeries for the treatment of periodontal disease are performed annually in the United States.[101]

Periodontal disease treatment has included guided bone regeneration (GBR), in which a membrane is surgically placed into the area to be regenerated to prevent epithelial ingrowth.[102] However, even with a GBR technique, cementum and periodontal ligament usually do not reach their original height, and fibrosis with inappropriate mechanical function results. Further, the membrane does not satisfactorily prevent epithelium, rather than a periodontal apparatus, from developing.

Additional options to regenerate the periodontium have included rhBMP-2.[103] To date, rhBMP-2 periodontal therapy has not produced sufficiently compelling results, nor has rhBMP-2 been cleared by the FDA for periodontal application.

rhPDGF-BB has been successful in regenerating periodontal tissues and has received FDA clearance for use (GEM21S). Success with rhPDGF-BB in periodontics is underscored by the fundamental principles of bone wound biology reviewed in this chapter. Specifically, PDGF is chemotactic and mitogenic for cells that will differentiate into osteoblasts, cementoblasts, and periodontal-ligament cells. Moreover, the exogenous PDGF (in GEM21S) and endogenous VEGF promote angiogenesis and vascularogenesis, which will provide a normoxic and metabolically suitable environment for periodontal regeneration.

Homodimers PDGF-AA and PDGF-BB have been detected in epithelium and the fibrin clot during wound healing of periodontal lesions.[104] Data indicate that gingival epithelium may be a source of PDGF-AA and PDGF-BB, and expression of PDGF-receptors is a consequence of tissue injury.[104]

The PDGF-AB heterodimer concentration in the total protein extract from gingival biopsies was approximately three times higher in inflamed sites.[105] In a rat model of periodontitis, PDGF-BB levels were increased, but not in diabetic rats, thus suggesting that the PDGF-BB–driven repair process is suppressed under diabetic conditions.[106]

The mitogenic responsiveness of periodontal cells to local application of PDGF-BB was confirmed in a dog model.[107] In fenestration defects in alveolar bone, recombinant PDGF-BB applied to root surfaces increased proliferation of periodontal ligament, cementoblasts, osteoblasts, perivascular cells, and endothelial cells.[107]

The proper delivery system for PDGF therapy has been a key accomplishment and recognized as a crucial step to clinical effectiveness.[108] The delivery system material for GEM21S is tricalcium phosphate. Tricalcium phosphate fulfills PDGF pharmacokinetics, is calibrated to wound-healing biology, and provides localization of PDGF at the wound site for the appropriate period of time, and at an optimal and biologically active dose.

PDGF has a half-life of approximately 4 hours[109,110]; therefore, the delivery system has a key clinical consequence. Moreover, another report states that PDGF is undetectable in plasma and is cleared from baboon blood with a half-life of less than 2 minutes.[111]

The clinical effectiveness of PDGF requires that the delivery system scaffold release a therapeutic dose of PDGF at the right time for a regenerative outcome. A scaffold designed for PDGF and periodontal regeneration should be based on the wound healing biology of the clinical target. During the first few hours following injury, the biologic environment is in the destructive phase of wound healing. The environment is hypoxic and acidotic; lytic enzymes secreted by macrophages erode extracellular matrix and necrotic debris; vascularity is insufficient; and the constructive cells that will react with PDGF have not yet arrived. Release of exogenous PDGF during the first few hours of wound healing must be carefully calibrated.

After the first 4 hours of its release, the therapeutic dose of PDGF may decrease by 50%. It is not until approximately 24 to 36 hours following bone injury that oxygen tension and pH as well as neovasculature enable a permissive wound-healing environment for the constructive phase of healing.[12,112] Consequently, delivery system selection for rhPDGFs and rhBMPs must be guided by wound-healing biology at the specific site of application.

Several types of delivery system have been investigated for PDGF. A gel has been used for rhPDGF-BB and insulin-like growth factor 1 (IGF-1) and has been applied to root surfaces in a dog model.[108,110] The outcome was an increase in bone and cementum.[108,100] Similar findings were observed in nonhuman primates.[80] Furthermore, an rhPDGF-BB/IGF-1 combination increased osseointegration of dental implants[109,110] and bone regeneration of peri-implant buccal dehiscence defects.[113]

PDGF-BB has promoted regeneration of periodontium in cynomolgus monkeys.[114] In horizontal class III furcation defects in teeth in beagle dogs, the combination of rhPDGF-BB and GBR therapy led to bone fill of 80% at 8 weeks and 87% at 11 weeks, compared with 14% and 60%, respectively, when GBR therapy was used alone.[115] The addition of rhPDGF-BB increased periodontal ligament from 5% to 20%, and fibrosis was undetectable at 8 weeks.[115]

In a clinical study,[116] 38 human subjects with bilateral osseous periodontal lesions were treated with rhPDGF-BB/IGF-1 in a gel delivery system. In patients treated with 150 µg/ml PDGF-BB/IGF-1, alveolar bone after 9 months increased to 2.08 mm of vertical bone height and 42.3% osseous defect fill versus 0.75 mm and 18.5%, respectively, in controls. Neither local nor systemic safety issues were reported.[117,118]

rhPDGF-BB allografts administered to intrabony defects in patients reduced probing depth by 6.4 mm, with a clinical attachment of 6.2 mm and a gain of 2.1 mm in bone height.[119,120] rhPDGF-BB treatment of furcation defects similarly improved clinical outcome, resulting in a probing depth reduction of 3.4 mm and a gain in clinical attachment of 4.0 mm.[119,120] Histologic analysis of intrabony and furcation defect sites indicated regeneration of cementum, periodontal ligament, alveolar bone, and blood vessels and the absence of root resorption, ankylosis, inflammation, and adverse tissue responses.[120]

In a dog model, β-tricalcium phosphate (β-TCP) appeared to produce a better clinical outcome than particulate allogeneic mineralized bone matrix, either alone or in the presence of rhPDGF-BB, with regard to periodontal regeneration.[101,121] About 45% of the rhPDGF-BB was released from β-TCP after 10 days, while approximately 30% of rhPDGF was released from mineralized matrix in 10 days.[101,121] Moreover, 300 µg/mL rhPDGF-BB was

superior to 1 mg/mL, suggesting that a high dose may be detrimental to the clinical outcome. This point was emphasized earlier by the two studies that appeared to indicate a decreased bone-healing response when PDGF was used to alter demineralized bone matrix or partially purified osteogenin.[95–97]

A prospective, blinded, and randomized controlled clinical trial tested the safety and efficacy of rhPDGF-BB delivered with β-TCP for advanced periodontal osseous defects.[122] Eleven clinical centers enrolled 180 subjects, each requiring surgical treatment of a 4-mm or greater intrabony periodontal defect. The β-TCP combined with rhPDGF-BB at 300 µg/mL promoted a larger gain of clinical attachment level than did β-TCP alone after 3 months (3.8 mm versus 3.3 mm), although by 6 months the difference between the two groups was not statistically significant. The rhPDGF-BB–treated sites also had greater linear bone gain (2.6 mm versus 0.9 mm) and percentage of defect fill (57% versus 18%) than did the sites receiving the β-TCP with buffer at 6 months.

It is noteworthy that the safety profile of rhPDGF-BB has been well established and the FDA has cleared Regranex, an rhPDGF-BB–containing formulation, for topical application in diabetic ulcers. No antibody formation or immunologic responses were observed in patients receiving a daily dose of Regranex over a 4-month period.[123] Moreover, neither systemic reactivity nor gene toxicity was observed when the topical drug was tested using in vivo models.

Autogenous platelet therapeutics

Autogenous platelet concentrates and platelet-rich plasma (PRP) may stimulate bone regeneration of large bone defects, sinuses, and periodontal defects. The effectiveness of PRP at these sites is attributed to the fact that, in addition to PDGFs, PRP contains chemokines and other growth factors important for wound healing.[124]

However, the overall beneficial effects of PRP are controversial.[125–127] The number of platelets that can be recovered varies among commercially available preparations as well as among patient donors.[125] Significantly, PRP is not a standardized source of growth factors.[43] PRP contains seven growth factors, including PDGF-BB, as well as all of the cell adhesion molecules as a consistent source of growth factors. Consequently, both PRP preparations and patients' responses to the PRP may be unpredictable and varied.[125,128] For a comprehensive discussion of PRP, see chapter 9.

Orthopedic applications

A study of fracture repair evaluated rhPDGF-BB delivered with tricalcium phosphate on healing of transverse tibial fractures in ovariectomized female rats aged 18 months, mimicking an osteoporotic and geriatric condition.[129] Biomechanical results suggested that, 5 weeks postsurgery, fractures treated with rhPDGF-BB and tricalcium phosphate demonstrated torque-to-failure biomechanics equivalent to that of the nonfractured contralateral limbs.

In another study, ovariectomy-induced osteoporosis was produced in rats.[130] Treatment was rhPDGF-BB, vehicle alone, or alendronate, or a combination of rhPDGF-BB and alendronate, administered by tail vein injection every other day for 6 weeks. Spine bone mineral density decreased 5% after ovariectomy in vehicle-only treated rats, and bone mineral density increased by 9% in animals treated with either rhPDGF-BB or alendronate. In contrast, the alendronate/rhPDGF-BB combination increased spine bone mineral density by 18%. Furthermore, quantitative computerized tomography (CT) of axial and appendicular bones indicated significant enhancement in bone mass. Histologically, the rhPDGF-BB recipients had a substantial increase in osteoblasts, without a change in osteoclasts, when compared with the untreated group. Biomechanically, rats treated with rhPDGF-BB had significantly enhanced vertebral body compressive strength and femoral shaft torsional stiffness. The combination of alendronate with rhPDGF-BB further increased these indices.

rhPDGF-BB delivered in a collagen gel was administered to rabbits to treat tibial osteotomies.[131] Radiographically, callus density and volume around the rhPDGF-BB–treated osteotomies were greater than those in rabbits receiving only collagen. Tibiae treated with collagen alone were significantly weaker biomechanically than were nonosteotomized tibiae. In contrast, tibiae treated with a combination of rhPDGF-BB and collagen had increased strength and were not significantly different from contralateral tibiae that had not received an osteotomy. Histologically, the rhPDGF-BB/collagen combination produced more robust and advanced osteogenesis, both endosteally and periosteally, than did colla-

gen alone. Overall the radiographic, biomechanical, and histologic data indicated that locally administered rhPDGF-BB delivered in an injectable collagen gel to tibial osteotomies enhanced functional fracture repair and significantly stimulated osteogenesis.[131]

Bone Morphogenetic Proteins

BMPs are part of the TGF-β superfamily, and their relevance in bone healing has been reviewed extensively.[15,132–144] The BMPs may be divided into subfamilies (Table 1-1).

Historical perspective

Understanding of the broad functional roles for BMPs began with the study of ectopic ossification. First Ray and Holloway[147] and then Urist[148] determined that ectopic osteogenesis (equivalent to ectopic ossification) occurred when DBM was implanted in a nonbony muscular (ie, heterotopic) site in a rodent.

In 1965, the process of ectopic osteogenesis was elucidated by Urist[148] in his landmark article, and the term *autoinduction* was coined. Urist and Strates[149] introduced the terms *bone morphogenetic protein* and *osteoinduction* to the scientific and clinical communities in 1971.

Reddi and Huggins[150,151] clearly explained the cellular and molecular biology of ectopic osteogenesis. In 1976, Reddi and Anderson[152] further refined and polished Urist's work[148,149] on induced osteogenesis. Subsequently, Muthukumaran and colleagues[153] identified factors in the soluble extract of bone and, in respect to the hallmark work of Lacroix,[154] they called one of these factors *osteogenin*, later also identified as BMP-3. BMP-3 is the most abundant BMP in DBM.[155]

This comprehensive research on DBM[150–153] enabled the cloning and expression of rhBMPs. Moreover, in 2000, Reddi[156] acknowledged the earlier incisive work of Wozney and colleagues,[157] who cloned BMP-2 and BMP-4 in 1988. This accomplishment was followed in 1990 by Özkaynak and coworkers,[158] who cloned BMP-7 and BMP-8 (also called *OP-1* and *OP-2*, respectively).

Table 1-1 Subfamilies of BMPs[145,146]

Subfamily name	BMP	Function
Procollagen C proteinase related to *Drosophila tolloid*	BMP-1	Collagenase
BMP-2A	BMP-2	Osteoinduction; chondrogenesis; osteogenesis
Osteogenin	BMP-3	Modulation of BMP-2 activity
BMP-2B	BMP-4	Osteoinduction; chondrogenesis; osteogenesis
BMP-5	BMP-5	Osteoinduction; chondrogenesis; osteogenesis
Vgr-1	BMP-6	Osteoinduction; chondrogenesis; osteogenesis
OP-1	BMP-7	Osteoinduction; chondrogenesis; osteogenesis; nephrogenesis
OP-2	BMP-8	Osteoinduction; chondrogenesis; osteogenesis; spermatogenesis; placental development
OP-3	BMP-8B	Osteoinduction; chondrogenesis; osteogenesis
GDF-2	BMP-9	Hepatogenesis; osteoinduction
BMP-10	BMP-10	Osteogenic?
GDF-11	BMP-11	Osteogenic?
GDF-7; CDMP-3	BMP-12	Chondrogenic
GDF-6; CDMP-2	BMP-13	Chondrogenic
GDF-5; CDMP-1	BMP-14	Chondrogenic
BMP-15	BMP-15	Osteogenic?

(Vgr-1) Vegetal-related 1; (GDF) growth differentiation factor; (CDMP) cartilage-derived morphogenetic protein.

Secretion

BMPs are synthesized as precursor molecules that include a signal peptide, a prodomain, and a carboxy-terminal domain comprising the mature protein. In the mature domain (approximately 30 kD) are seven conserved cysteine residues, collectively known as a *cysteine knot*. The seven cysteines are universally found among all BMPs. Moreover, the sequence is conserved through species, where human equivalents to BMP include decapentaplegic and 60A genes of the fruit fly (*Drosophila melanogaster*), Xnr1-3 in *Caenorhabditis elegans*, and growth differentiation factor 5 (GDF-5)/brachypodism/BMP-14 in the short-eared mouse.[159–164]

The mature domain of BMP is processed intracellularly, where it either homodimerizes or heterodimerizes through a cysteine bond (Fig 1-5). The secreted molecule is an active dimer, for example a BMP-2/BMP-2 homodimer or BMP-2/BMP-7 heterodimer.[134]

Signaling

BMP activity occurs through a serine–threonine kinase transmembrane dimeric receptor binding complex.[136,144,165–167] The receptors are types I and II.[168] Both receptors have a cysteine-rich extracellular domain and an intracellular serine–threonine kinase–rich domain (GS domain).[140] There are three distinctive type I receptors: activin receptor-like kinase 2 (ALK-2), BMP receptor type IA/activin receptor-like kinase 3 (BMPR-IA/ALK-3), and BMP receptor type IB/activin receptor-like kinase 6 (BMPR-IB/ALK-6). Likewise, there are three type II receptors: BMP receptor type II (BMPR-II), activin type II receptor (ActR-II), and activin type IIB receptor (ActR-IIB). Different BMPs bind with different affinity to the BMP receptor complexes.

Following receptor phosphorylation activation, intracellular signals are transduced through a receptor-regulated SMAD-dependent or SMAD-independent ERK-MAPK pathway[144] (Fig 1-6). The name *SMAD* is derived from the *D melanogaster* gene, Mothers against decapentaplegic, and is the human homolog. A SMAD-interacting protein called *SMAD anchor for receptor activation (SARA)* facilitates signaling interaction.

There is cross-talk between the BMP-SMAD signaling pathway and the ERK-MAPK pathway.[144] There is some evidence indicating that BMP signaling may occur through a MAPK pathway as well.

BMP activity can be modulated by anti-BMPs: chordin, noggin, cerebrus, follistatin, and fetuin.[169] Gremlin and sclerostin, members of the DAN family of proteins, also are anti-BMPs. These molecules either bind to the BMP complexes (the mode of action of chordin, noggin, sclerostin, and gremlin), changing the conformation, or bind to the serine–threonine kinase transmembrane receptor (the mode of action of follistatin, cerebrus, and fetuin), preventing BMP docking. Osteoblasts may secrete anti-BMPs to provide self-regulatory control (ie, an autoregulatory loop). Moreover, secretion of anti-BMPs by chondrogenic cells may influence endochondral bone formation.

Intracellularly, BMP-SMAD signaling is regulated through a negative feedback loop. A BMP and activin membrane–bound inhibitor (BAMBI) has been identified in *Xenopus*, mouse, and zebra fish.[136] Moreover, inhibitory SMADs, SMADs 6 and 7, can bind to BMP receptors (intracytoplasmically) and prevent phosphorylation of the receptor SMADs (2, 3, 4, and 5). Furthermore, SMAD 6 can bind with activated intracellular SMAD complexes and deactivate signal transduction. The inhibitory SMADs constitute a negative BMP signaling feedback loop. SMAD-ubiquitin regulatory factor I, a member of the class of E3 ubiquitin ligases homologous to E3-associated protein C terminus, interacts with SMADs I and 5 and also provides regulatory control of intracellular signaling.

In the nucleus, the molecule Ski appears to act as a transcriptional repressor for BMP-SMAD signaling. Similarly, Tob and OAZ (a zinc fingerlike protein) control the BMP signaling process within the cell nucleus.

Physiologic and cellular roles

Urist[148] first realized the pivotal role a soluble signaling protein in bone matrix had in autoinduction. Urist and Strates[149] refined the autoinduction concept as osteoinduction. They captured the essential physiologic role of BMP embodied by the term *osteoinduction*, which they defined (with slight modification) as the recruitment and differentiation of pluripotential mesenchymal-like cells at a nonbony site (eg, a heterotopic muscle site) and the subsequent differentiation into chondrocytes and osteoblasts and formation of an ossicle.

The hallmark property of BMP is a differentiation factor. BMP will differentiate an undifferentiated mesenchymal cell into an osteoblast. In contrast, PDGF is a chemotactic and mitogenic factor for osteoblast-like precursors.

BMPs, like PDGF, play a role in blood vessel formation. They upregulate angiogenic peptides such as VEGF. Moreover, BMPs may bind to endothelial cells, stimulate their migration, and promote blood vessel formation.[140]

BMPs have diverse physiologic functions. BMPs are pivotal during embryologic development in specifying positional information to the embryo for dorsal and ventral relationships of the skeletal and nonskeletal systems.[139,170] During embryogenesis, unique roles for select BMPs have been suggested through gene knockouts. For example, null mutant mice for BMP-7 have developmental abnormalities of the kidney and eye along with skeletal malformations.[139] Mutations in mice for BMP-5 have the short-ear mouse phenotype as well as impaired fracture healing. BMP-8 mutations lead to defects in spermatogenesis and placental development.[139]

In this chapter, the functional role of many of the BMPs in bone formation has been emphasized. However, despite the bone-forming utility of certain BMPs (eg, -2, -4, -6, and -7), BMP-2 and BMP-4 have a direct osteoclastic stimulatory impact that can result in bone resorption.[171]

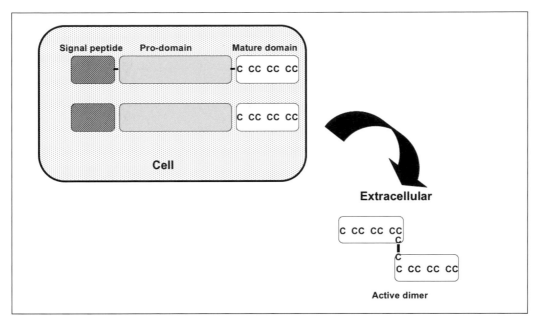

Fig 1-5 BMPs include a signal peptide involved with secretion from the cell, and the prodomain directs folding, dimerization, and biologic activity. The mature domain is secreted as an active dimer. Dimerization can result in various combinations of BMPs, for example, the BMP-2/7 heterodimer and the BMP-2/2 homodimer.

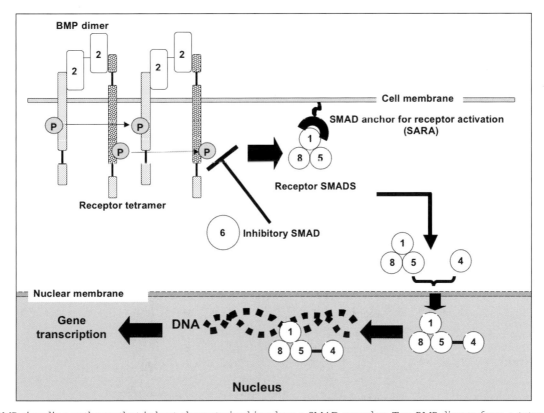

Fig 1-6 The BMP signaling pathway that is best characterized involves a SMAD complex. Two BMP dimers form a tetra complex with BMPR-IA, BMPR-IB, and BMPR-II. Following binding, the type II receptor phosphorylates the type I receptor, which in turn phosphorylates the receptor SMADs (1, 5, and 8). Inhibitory SMAD 6 may block this process. Receptor SMADs 1, 5, and 8 bind to receptor SMAD 4, translocate to the nucleus, and interact with the DNA, initiating gene transcription that can result in osteoblastic differentiation. (Based on data from several sources.[144,165–167])

Expression systems

Most rhBMPs have been manufactured in mammalian cell systems for large-scale production. rhBMP-2 has been expressed in Chinese hamster ovarian cells, and a mouse myeloma cell line was used to produce rhBMP-4. Chinese hamster ovarian cells and a primate cell line have been used for rhBMP-7. In contrast with the cell expression systems for BMPs, rhPDGF can be expressed in large-scale production volumes by yeast. This method significantly reduces manufacturing cost. To offset the high production expense of rhBMP expression, *Escherichia coli* are being tried. However, monomeric BMP must be expressed and purified, renatured, and further purified to remove unfolded monomers and *E coli* contaminants. Renaturation and refolding are not trivial, and low yields of active BMP are problematic.

Table 1-2 provides a comparison between the basic biology of PDGF and BMP.

Delivery systems

The discussion on PDGF underscored the significance of the delivery system for therapeutic effectiveness. The same theme must be emphasized for BMP delivery. Again, the delivery system must fulfill clinical and wound-healing functions:

• Provide a convenient vehicle for the surgeon to place the growth factor at the clinical target
• Be biocompatible prior to biodegradation; the biodegradation products should be biocompatible as well
• Localize, protect, and release the required dose of the growth factor at the appropriate time or times for therapeutic effect
• Enable bone growth (osteoconduction), prevent soft tissue prolapse, and biodegrade in register with new bone formation

These fundamental, but undefined, general performance targets are well known to surgeons and scientists designing and developing growth factor delivery systems.[201] Regrettably, specific details for performance targets have not been sufficiently defined. Consequently, rather than having a programmable delivery system available for PDGF and BMP, contemporary scaffolds are non-programmable and arbitrary. Details on performance design targets are lacking.

The specifics that must be defined for the delivery system for each growth factor, for each clinical target, and for each set of physiologic determinants and type of bone wound include:

• The period after injury in which the delivery system should release the growth factor, that is, pharmacokinetics.
• The temporal delivery, for example, pulsatile, bolus.
• The dose of the growth factor to be delivered.
• The rate at which the delivery system must be removed from the clinical target. How fast will bone form at a designated clinical target and, therefore, at what rate must the delivery system biodegrade?

Unfortunately, specific details, data, and quantitative information have not been satisfactorily elucidated for each of these issues. Unless the delivery system specifics are clearly defined, optimal performance targets for the delivery system and growth factor therapeutics will not be achieved. For example, in the clinic, a growth factor such as BMP may be released too soon from the delivery system after the surgeon places it at the clinical target. Therefore, a therapeutic (ie, physiologic) dose may not be realized. Consequently, to compensate for this mismatch, a supraphysiologic dose will be required. This problem occurs at present when milligram doses of rhBMP are needed for spinal fusions.

The dilemma of the mismatch between delivery system properties and clinical target requirements has been a serious issue that merits significant attention.[135,138,143,202–204] Recent, lucid reviews on delivery systems for BMPs and other growth factors[137,142,201,204–206] have discussed poly(α-hydroxy acids): polylactides and polyglycolides, demineralized bone matrix, hyaluronan, gelatin, a hyaluronan–polyethylene glycol combination, calcium phosphates (tricalcium phosphate and apatitic hydroxyapatites), and collagen. Each material has virtues and liabilities.

Collagen (Integra Life Sciences) has been selected as a delivery system scaffold for rhBMP-2 for the InFuse product. The logic for using collagen is that type I bovine collagen is cleared by the FDA, and collagen carriers typically have a biphasic release profile characterized by an initial release of rhBMP with a sustained release thereafter.[134] This profile may permit rhBMP availability for responding cells at the bone wound during the constructive phase of healing.

Table 1-2 Basic biology of PDGF and BMP

Attribute	PDGF	BMP
Mechanism of action	Intracellular signaling via Ras, mitogen-activated protein, Src, PI3K, and PLC-γ mediates cellular proliferation; PI3K and PLC-γ/PKC also mediate chemotaxis[48]	SMAD-dependent (via Runx2 in osteoblast precursors) or p38-dependent mediation of cellular differentiation[168,172,173]
Receptor signaling	PDGFR subunits α and β that dimerize to form αα, αβ, and ββ; tyrosine kinase receptor signaling[50,174]	BMPR-IA, -IB, and -II, ligand-binding leads to formation of heterotetrameric complexes; serine/threonine kinase receptor signaling[173]
Functional roles	Mitogenesis; chemotaxis; supports neovascularization[34,84,175,176]	Differentiation[139]
Expression systems	E coli; yeast; insect[177-179]	Mammalian; insect; E coli[180-183]
Regulatory controls/ antagonists	STI571/Gleevec (Novartis); triazolopyrimidine (trapidil); endothelin 1; angiotensin II; endostatin; soluble receptors[184-190]	Noggin; chordin; follistatin; gremlin; cerberus; fetuin; ectodin[191-195]
Knockout phenotypes	PDGF-BB: perinatally lethal; loss of microvascular pericytes and kidney glomerular mesangial cells PDGF-AA: embryonically lethal; severe cardiovascular abnormalities[196-199]	Embryonically lethal (BMP-2, BMP-4); skeletal malformations; impaired fracture healing; abnormalities of kidney and eye[200]

(PI3K) Phosphatidylinositol-3 kinase; (PLC-γ) phospholipase Cγ; (PKC) protein kinase C.

However, it may not be optimal to have a rapid bolus release from collagen during the destructive phase of osseous wound injury repair. In the destructive phase, the environment is acidotic, hypoxic, and lytic, and constructive cells may be inadequate to respond to rhBMP. Moreover, rhBMP may be squandered by lytic degradation. Therefore, to achieve a clinically effective rhBMP dose, potentially supraphysiologic loading (in milligrams) of rhBMP is required. This substantially escalates the cost and risk to the patient. There is a compelling clinical need to design and develop a programmable delivery system scaffold that will release rhBMP (or rhPDGF) during the constructive phase of wound healing.

Orthopedic and spinal applications

There have been hundreds of peer-reviewed publications detailing preclinical studies of rhBMPs in orthopedic and spinal applications. Therefore, rather than focusing on pre-

clinical work that has been reviewed, this discussion will highlight clinical studies.

rhBMP-7 (rhOP-1) has been tested in a randomized controlled trial of 122 patients with 124 tibial nonunions.[207] The nonunions were at least 9 months old with no progress toward healing during the 3 months prior to the study. Patients were treated with an intramedullary nail plus rhOP-1 in a type I collagen carrier or with autogenous bone graft alone. After 9 months, 81% of the patients treated with rhOP-1/collagen and 85% of the patients treated with autogenous bone graft were judged by clinical criteria to be healed. Consequently, the conclusion was that rhOP-1 in a type I collagen carrier is safe and effective to treat tibial nonunions.[207]

In another investigation using rhBMP-2, a prospective randomized controlled trial in 450 patients with open tibial fractures was conducted. The fractures were irrigated and debrided and treated with a statically locked intramedullary nail or supplementation with one or two doses of rhBMP-2. After 12 months' follow-up, the patients treated with the higher dose of rhBMP-2 showed a 44% reduction in the risk of secondary interventions and presented with fewer hardware failures and infections.[208] The combination of rhBMP-2 and type I bovine collagen (absorbable collagen sponge [ACS]) has been approved by the European Union for open tibial diaphyseal fractures and is marketed as InductOs (Wyeth).[143] InductOS has also been approved by the European Union for single-level (L4-S1) anterior lumbar spine fusions.

In the United States, the rhBMP-2/ACS composition (InFuse) has been cleared by the FDA for anterior lumbar interbody fusions. Boden et al[209] did the original clinical work and reported on the first pilot study examining the osteoinductive capacity of rhBMP-2 for a human spinal fusion application. In a randomized multicenter study involving 14 patients, threaded interbody fusion cages were filled with either an rhBMP-2/collagen sponge or autogenous iliac crest bone graft and implanted for anterior lumbar interbody fusion.

Patients administered rhBMP-2 had a shorter hospital stay than did the autograft control patients (2 days versus 3.3 days). Moreover, 10 of 11 patients receiving rhBMP-2 were judged fused by 3 months after surgery, and all 11 were fused by 6 months. One of the three control patients had a nonunion after 1 year. CT images indicated that rhBMP-2–induced fusions had new bone growth through and anterior to the cages at 6 and 12 months postsurgery.[209] Subsequently, a more comprehensive population was treated, and similar results were confirmed[210]; this led to FDA clearance of InFuse in 2002.

The efficacious dose of rhBMP-2 in InFuse is 3 to 5 mg at a cost of approximately US $5,000 at the time of writing. The natural content of BMP in bone is about 1 μg/g.[138] Moreover, nanogram doses of BMP are required in vitro to upregulate osteoblast-like gene expression, and microgram doses are needed in vivo in rodents for osteoinduction.[211] The disparity between the delivered dose of the rhBMP-2 and the clinical outcome for spine fusions underscores the significant deficiencies of ACS (type I bovine collage) as a delivery system and indicates the need for something better.

The efficacy of rhBMP-7 in human spinal fusion procedures has been demonstrated. Vaccaro et al[212] used rhOP-1 for posterolateral spine fusion in 12 patients. No adverse effects were observed, and the radiographic fusion rate was slightly more that the 50% fusion rates obtained with autograft alone. Jeppsson et al[213] evaluated rhBMP-7 (rhOP-1) in cervical spine posterior fusion in four patients with rheumatoid disease. No bone formation was reported in three of the four patients. The absence of bone formation may be a consequence of dosing, delivery system, or the effect of rheumatoid arthritis.

Craniofacial and dental applications

A rich preclinical database exists for the use of rhBMP-2 in the craniofacial complex, which includes the mandible, maxilla, and calvaria. These preclinical studies have been extensively reviewed in the literature and suggest that rhBMP-2 has substantial benefit for the treatment of osseous defects in the craniofacial complex, but that it is inappropriate to apply rhBMP-2 in the treatment of periodontal defects. This discussion will follow a strategy similar to that in the orthopedic and spinal section, highlighting clinical studies rather than rereviewing preclinical reports.

Osteogenesis has been accomplished in a series of human studies using rhBMP-2 for application in sinus floor and alveolar ridge augmentation procedures. Maxillary sinus floor and alveolar ridges have been augmented with rhBMP-2 in doses of 1.8 to 3.4 mg. At a dose of 0.43 mg/mL, there were no serious or unexpected immunologic or adverse effects. The most frequent adverse effects were facial edema, oral erythema, pain, and rhinitis. Eleven of 12 patients received dental implants, and the authors reported that histologic analysis "tend[ed]" to indicate that rhBMP-2 in ACS may provide an acceptable substitute for autogenous—or other bone—graft materials used in sinus augmentation procedures.[214]

Boyne and colleagues[215] compared rhBMP-2 at 0.75-mg/mL and 1.5-mg/mL concentrations (average total dose: 8.9 mg in the low-dose group and 20.8 mg in the high-dose group) delivered in an ACS to a mixture of autogenous and allogeneic bone graft for maxillary sinus floor augmentation in 48 patients. Patients were followed for at least 36 months after functional dental implant loading, and the total treatment time course lasted 52 months. The study assessed treatment results clinically, radiographically, with CT, and histologically. Implant survival in the absence of mobility or chronic pain was also assessed.

There were no statistical differences among the treatments for ridge height gain and histology; ridge width and bone density were superior following bone graft treatment. Implant function was similar across the three treatments after 36 months. rhBMP-2 delivered in the ACS sponge promoted sufficient bone formation to support dental implant placement and functional loading of dental implants in approximately 75% to 80% of treated patients. There was no indication of adverse events nor safety issues. Consequently, this 48-patient study indicates that 9 to 21 mg of rhBMP-2 in ACS is safe and may be equivalent to a bone graft for promoting bone formation in the maxillary sinus floor.

Cochran and colleagues[216,217] and Howell et al[117,118,218] have reported favorable results with rhBMP-2 for alveolar ridge augmentation. However, the results did not demonstrate a clear advantage to the use of rhBMP-2, suggesting inadequate rhBMP-2 dosing and/or delivery system properties.

In a multicenter clinical study, Fiorellini et al[219] used rhBMP-2/ACS with rhBMP-2 concentrations of either 0.75 mg/mL or 1.50 mg/mL in patients with buccal wall defects in the alveolar ridge following dental extractions. There were two sequential cohorts of 40 patients (total of 80 patients) divided among four treatments: one of the two doses of rhBMP-2/ACS; ACS alone (placebo); or no treatment. Outcome efficacy was determined by CT after 4 months of treatment. The CTs were evaluated for the amount of bone induction, bone competency to support an endosseous dental implant, and the need for secondary augmentation. The results suggested that patients treated with the 1.50 mg/mL dose of rhBMP-2/ACS had significantly greater bone augmentation ($P \geq .05$) than did the placebo ACS control. Moreover, the competency of the regenerated bone was approximately twice as great for the rhBMP-2/ACS doses as for either no treatment or the ACS control (see chapter 12).

It was reported in the clinical study that 68% of the patients reported oral pain and 75% exhibited oral edema. Antibodies to bovine type I collagen (the ACS) were detected in 11 of 80 patients, suggesting the need for further investigation regarding use of collagen.

Conclusion

PDGF and BMP have profound roles in osseous wound healing. In light of the conserved process of bone healing, it is anticipated that rhPDGF and rhBMP should be exploited across orthopedics and periodontics. A substantial peer-reviewed database indicates the efficacy and safety of these molecules for bone regeneration. Furthermore, the FDA has cleared the clinical use of rhPDGF-BB for wound healing in compromised patients and treatment of periodontal bone and gingival defects and rhBMP-2 for anterior interbody spine fusion, sinus lifts, and extraction wounds. Although important questions remain regarding optimizing clinical doses and delivery

systems, as will be discussed further in other chapters of this book, these protein therapeutics are making a significant impact in clinical practice.

Acknowledgments

Partial funding for this work was provided by the National Institutes of Health grant NIH RO1 DE15392 (JOH). The authors wish to thank Conan Young, PhD, for his contributions to Table 2-2.

References

1. Ferguson C, Alpern E, Miclau T, Helms JA. Does adult fracture repair recapitulate embryonic skeletal formation? Mech Dev 1999;87(1–2):57–66.
2. Schneider DJ, Hu D, Helms J. From head to toe: Conservation of molecular signals regulating limb and craniofacial morphogenesis. Cell Tissue Res 1999;296:103–109.
3. Thompson Z, Miclau T, Hu D, Helms J. A model for intramembranous ossification during fracture healing. J Orthop Res 2002;20:1091–1098.
4. Eames F, de la Fuente L, Helms J. Molecular ontogeny of the skeleton. Birth Defects Res 2003;69(C):93–101.
5. Helms J, Schneider R. Cranial skeletal biology. Nature 2003;423(15 May):326–331.
6. Franceschi RT. Biological approaches to bone regeneration by gene therapy. J Dent Res 2005;84:1093–1103.
7. Urist MR. Fundamental and Clinical Bone Physiology. Philadelphia: Lippencott, 1980.
8. Reddi AH. The matrix of rat calvarium as transformant of fibroblasts (39028). Proc Soc Exp Biol Med 1975;150:324–326.
9. Schmitz JP, Hollinger JO. The critical size defect as an experimental model for craniomandibulofacial nonunions. Clin Orthop 1986;205:299–308.
10. Hollinger JO, Schmitz JP, Mark DE, Seyfer AE. Osseous wound healing with xenogeneic bone implants with a biodegradable carrier. Surgery 1990;107:50–54.
11. An YH, Friedman RJ. Animal models of bone defect repair. In: An YH, Friedman RJ (eds). Animal Models in Orthopaedic Research. Boca Raton, FL: CRC Press, 1998:241–260.
12. Hollinger JO, Buck DC, Bruder S. Biology of bone healing: Its impact on clinical therapy. In: Lynch S, Gengo R, Marx R (eds). Tissue Engineering: Applications in Maxillofacial Surgery and Periodontics. Chicago: Quintessence, 1999:17–53.
13. Barnes G, Kostenuik P, Geerstenfeld L, Einhorn T. Growth factor regulation of fracture repair. J Bone Miner Res 1999;14:1805–1815.
14. Einhorn T, Lee CA. Bone regeneration: New findings and potential clinical applications. J Am Acad Orthop Surg 2001;9:157–165.
15. Gerstenfeld L, Cullilane D, Barnes G, Graves D, Einhorn T. Fracture healing as a post-natal developmental process: Molecular, spatial, and temporal aspects of its regulation. J Cell Biochem 2003;88:873–884.
16. Gerstenfeld LC, Wronski TJ, Hollinger JO, Einhorn TA. Application of histomorphometric methods to the study of bone repair. J Bone Miner Res 2005;20:1715–1722.
17. Schmitz JP, Schwarts Z, Hollinger JO, Boyan BD. Characterization of rat calvarial nonunion defects. Acta Anat 1990;138:185–192.
18. Aalami OO, Nacamuli RP, Lenton KA, et al. Applications of a mouse model of calvarial healing: Differences in regenerative abilities of juveniles and adults. Plast Reconstr Surg 2004;114:713–720.
19. Lu C, Miclau T, Hu D, et al. Cellular basis for age-related changes in fracture repair. J Orthop Res 2005;23:1300–1307.

20. Xiao Y, Fu H, Prasadam I, Yang YC, Hollinger JO. Gene expression profiling of bone marrow stromal cells from juvenile, adult, aged and osteoporotic rats: With an emphasis on osteoporosis. Bone 2007;40:700–715.

21. Hollinger JO. Bone dynamics: Morphogenesis, growth modeling, and remodeling. In: Lieberman J, Friedlaender G (eds). Bone Regeneration and Repair: Biology and Clinical Applications. Totowa, NJ: Humana Press, 2005:1–20.

22. Raisz L. Physiology and pathophysiology of bone remodeling. Clin Chem 1999; 45(8B):1353–1358.

23. Parfitt MA. The physiologic and clinical significance of bone histomorphometric data. In: Recker RR (ed). Bone Histomorphometry: Techniques and Interpretation. Boca Raton, FL: CRC Press, 1983:143–224.

24. Delmas PD, Malaval L. The proteins of bone. In: Mundy GR, Martin TJ (ed). Physiology and Pharmacology of Bone. New York: Springer-Verlag, 1993:673–724.

25. Frost HM. Bone histomorphometry: Analysis of trabecular bone dynamics. In: Recker RR (ed). Bone Histomorphometry: Techniques and Interpretation. Boca Raton, FL: CRC Press, 1983:109–132.

26. Boyce B, Xing L. Osteoclasts, no longer osteoblast slaves. Nature Med 2006; 12:1356–1358.

27. Wong ME. The biology of alveolar healing following removal of impacted teeth. In: Helfrick JF, Alling CC, Alling RD (eds). Impacted Teeth. Philadelphia: Saunders,1993:25–45.

28. Malizos K, Papatheodorou L. The healing potential of the periosteum. Molecular aspects. Injury 2005;36(suppl 3):S13–S19.

29. Taba M, Jin Q, Giannobile WV. Current concepts in periodontal bioengineering. Orthod Craniofac Res 2005;8:292–306.

30. Singer AJ, Clark RA. Cutaneous wound healing. N Engl J Med 1999;341:738–746.

31. Hammacher A, Hellman U, Johnsson A, et al. A major part of platelet-derived growth factor purified from human platelets is a heterodimer of one A and one B chain. J Biol Chem 1988;263:16493–16498.

32. Hart CE, Bailey M, Curtis DA, et al. Purification of PDGF-AB and PDGF-BB from human platelet extracts and identification of all three PDGF dimers in human platelets. Biochemistry 1990;29:166–172.

33. Fang L, Yan Y, Komuves LG, et al. PDGF C is a selective α platelet-derived growth factor receptor agonist that is highly expressed in platelet alpha granules and vascular smooth muscle. Arterioscler Thromb Vasc Biol 2004;24:787–792.

34. Deuel TF, Senior RM, Huang JS, Griffin GL. Chemotaxis of monocytes and neutrophils to platelet-derived growth factor. J Clin Invest 1982;69:1046–1049.

35. Tzeng DY, Deuel TF, Huang JS, Senior RM, Boxer LA, Baehner RL. Platelet-derived growth factor promotes polymorphonuclear leukocyte activation. Blood 1984; 64:1123–1128.

36. Tzeng DY, Deuel TF, Huang JS, Baehner RL. Platelet-derived growth factor promotes human peripheral monocyte activation. Blood 1985;66:179–183.

37. Siegbahn A, Hammacher A, Westermark B, Heldin CH. Differential effects of the various isoforms of platelet-derived growth factor on chemotaxis of fibroblasts, monocytes, and granulocytes. J Clin Invest 1990;85:916–920.

38. Inaba T, Shimano H, Gotoda T, et al. Expression of platelet-derived growth factor β receptor on human monocyte-derived macrophages and effects of platelet-derived growth factor BB dimer on the cellular function. J Biol Chem 1993;268:24353–24360.

39. Berglundh T, Abrahamsson I, Lang NP, Lindhe J. De novo alveolar bone formation adjacent to endosseous implants. Clin Oral Implants Res 2003;14:251–262.

40. Cardaropoli G, Araujo M, Lindhe J. Dynamics of bone tissue formation in tooth extraction sites. An experimental study in dogs. J Clin Periodontol 2003;30: 809–818.

41. Nagai MK, Embil JM. Becaplermin: Recombinant platelet derived growth factor, a new treatment for healing diabetic foot ulcers. Expert Opin Biol Ther 2002;2: 211–218.

42. Tyndall WA, Beam HA, Zarro C, O'Connor JP, Lin SS. Decreased platelet derived growth factor expression during fracture healing in diabetic animals. Clin Orthop 2003(408):319–330.

43. Pietrzak WS, Eppley B. Platelet rich plasma: Biology and new technology. J Craniofac Surg 2005;16:1043–1054.

44. Alvarez R, Kantarjian H, Cortes JE. Biology of platelet-derived growth factor and its involvement in disease. Mayo Clin Proc 2006;81:1241–1257.

45. Fredriksson L, Li H, Eriksson U. The PDGF family: Four gene products form five dimeric isoforms. Cytokine Growth Factor Rev 2004;15:197–204.

46. Heldin CH, Westermark B. Mechanism of action and in vivo role of platelet-derived growth factor. Physiol Rev 1999;79:1283–1316.

47. Betsholtz C. Insight into the physiological functions of PDGF through genetic studies in mice. Cytokine Growth Factor Rev 2004;15:215–228.

48. Tallquist M, Kazlauskas A. PDGF signaling in cells and mice. Cytokine Growth Factor Rev 2004;15:205–213.

49. Missbach M, Jeschke M, Feyen J, et al. A novel inhibitor of the tyrosine kinase Src suppresses phosphorylation of its major cellular substrates and reduces bone resorption in vitro and in rodent models in vivo. Bone 1999;24:437–449.

50. Martelli AM, Borgatti P, Bortul R, et al. Phosphatidylinositol 3-kinase translocates to the nucleus of osteoblast-like MC3T3-E1 cells in response to insulin-like growth factor I and platelet-derived growth factor but not to the proapoptotic cytokine tumor necrosis factor α. J Bone Miner Res 2000;15:1716–1730.

51. Chaudhary LR, Hruska KA. The cell survival signal Akt is differentially activated by PDGF-BB, EGF, and FGF-2 in osteoblastic cells. J Cell Biochem 2001;81:304–311.

52. Sowa H, Kaji H, Yamaguchi T, Sugimoto T, Chihara K. Activations of ERK1/2 and JNK by transforming growth factor β negatively regulate Smad3-induced alkaline phosphatase activity and mineralization in mouse osteoblastic cells. J Biol Chem 2002;277:36024–36031.

53. Suzuki A, Guicheux J, Palmer G, et al. Evidence for a role of p38 MAP kinase in expression of alkaline phosphatase during osteoblastic cell differentiation. Bone 2002;30:91–98.

54. Guicheux J, Lemonnier J, Ghayor C, Suzuki A, Palmer G, Caverzasio J. Activation of p38 mitogen-activated protein kinase and c-Jun-NH2-terminal kinase by BMP-2 and their implication in the stimulation of osteoblastic cell differentiation. J Bone Miner Res 2003;18:2060–2068.

55. Centrella M, McCarthy TL, Kusmik WF, Canalis E. Isoform-specific regulation of platelet-derived growth factor activity and binding in osteoblast-enriched cultures from fetal rat bone. J Clin Invest 1992;89:1076–1084.

56. Centrella M, Casinghino S, Ignotz R, McCarthy TL. Multiple regulatory effects by transforming growth factor-β on type I collagen levels in osteoblast-enriched cultures from fetal rat bone. Endocrinology 1992;131:2863–2872.

57. Yu X, Hsieh SC, Bao W, Graves DT. Temporal expression of PDGF receptors and PDGF regulatory effects on osteoblastic cells in mineralizing cultures. Am J Physiol 1997;272(5 pt 1):C1709–C1716.

58. Gruber R, Karreth F, Frommlet F, Fischer MB, Watzek G. Platelets are mitogenic for periosteum-derived cells. J Orthop Res 2003;21:941–948.

59. Piche JE, Graves DT. Study of the growth factor requirements of human bone-derived cells: A comparison with human fibroblasts. Bone 1989;10:131–138.

60. Pfeilschifter J, Diel I, Pilz U, Brunotte K, Naumann A, Ziegler R. Mitogenic responsiveness of human bone cells in vitro to hormones and growth factors decreases with age. J Bone Miner Res 1993;8:707–717.

61. Tanaka H, Liang CT. Effect of platelet-derived growth factor on DNA synthesis and gene expression in bone marrow stromal cells derived from adult and old rats. J Cell Physiol 1995;164:367–375.

62. Satomura K, Derubeis AR, Fedarko NS, et al. Receptor tyrosine kinase expression in human bone marrow stromal cells. J Cell Physiol 1998;177:426–338.

63. Fiedler J, Roderer G, Gunther KP, Brenner RE. BMP-2, BMP-4, and PDGF-bb stimulate chemotactic migration of primary human mesenchymal progenitor cells. J Cell Biochem 2002;87:305–312.

64. Kubota K, Sakikawa C, Katsumata M, Nakamura T, Wakabayashi K. Platelet-derived growth factor BB secreted from osteoclasts acts as an osteoblastogenesis inhibitory factor. J Bone Miner Res 2002;17:257–265.

65. Cassiede P, Dennis JE, Ma F, Caplan AI. Osteochondrogenic potential of marrow mesenchymal progenitor cells exposed to TGF-β 1 or PDGF-BB as assayed in vivo and in vitro. J Bone Miner Res 1996;11:1264–1273.

66. Hsieh SC, Graves DT. Pulse application of platelet-derived growth factor enhances formation of a mineralizing matrix while continuous application is inhibitory. J Cell Biochem 1998;69:169–180.

67. Cho TJ, Gerstenfeld LC, Einhorn TA. Differential temporal expression of members of the transforming growth factor β superfamily during murine fracture healing. J Bone Miner Res 2002;17:513–520.

68. Kugimiya F, Kawaguchi H, Kamekura S, et al. Involvement of endogenous bone morphogenetic protein (BMP) 2 and BMP6 in bone formation. J Biol Chem 2005;280:35704–35712.

69. Murakami S, Noda M. Expression of Indian hedgehog during fracture healing in adult rat femora. Calcif Tissue Int 2000;66:272–276.

70. Hadjiargyrou M, Lombardo F, Zhao S, et al. Transcriptional profiling of bone regeneration. Insight into the molecular complexity of wound repair. J Biol Chem 2002;277:30177–30182.

71. Bouletreau PJ, Warren SM, Spector JA, Steinbrech DS, Mehrara BJ, Longaker MT. Factors in the fracture microenvironment induce primary osteoblast angiogenic cytokine production. Plast Reconstr Surg 2002;110:139–148.

72. Blanquaert F, Pereira RC, Canalis E. Cortisol inhibits hepatocyte growth factor/scatter factor expression and induces c-met transcripts in osteoblasts. Am J Physiol Endocrinol Metab 2000;278:E509–E515.

73. Franchimont N, Durant D, Rydziel S, Canalis E. Platelet-derived growth factor induces interleukin-6 transcription in osteoblasts through the activator protein-1 complex and activating transcription factor-2. J Biol Chem 1999;274:6783–6789.

74. Carano RA, Filvaroff EH. Angiogenesis and bone repair. Drug Discov Today 2003;8:980–989.

75. Gazzerro E, Gangji V, Canalis E. Bone morphogenetic proteins induce the expression of noggin, which limits their activity in cultured rat osteoblasts. J Clin Invest 1998;102:2106–2114.

76. Pereira RC, Economides AN, Canalis E. Bone morphogenetic proteins induce gremlin, a protein that limits their activity in osteoblasts. Endocrinology 2000;141:4558–4563.

77. Canalis E. PDGF—Review. Ann NY Acad Sci 2002;22:678–688.

78. Yeh YL, Kang YM, Chaibi MS, Xie JF, Graves DT. IL-1 and transforming growth factor-β inhibit platelet-derived growth factor-AA binding to osteoblastic cells by reducing platelet-derived growth factor-α receptor expression. J Immunol 1993;150:5625–5632.

79. Xie JF, Stroumza J, Graves DT. IL-1 down-regulates platelet-derived growth factor-α receptor gene expression at the transcriptional level in human osteoblastic cells. J Immunol 1994;153:378–383.

80. Afink G, Westermark UK, Lammerts E, Nister M. C/EBP is an essential component of PDGFRA transcription in MG-63 cells. Biochem Biophys Res Commun 2004;315:313–318.

81. Kose KN, Xie JF, Carnes DL, Graves DT. Pro-inflammatory cytokines down regulate platelet derived growth factor-α receptor gene expression in human osteoblastic cells. J Cell Physiol 1996;166:188–197.

82. Tsukamoto T, Matsui T, Nakata H, et al. Interleukin-1 enhances the response of osteoblasts to platelet-derived growth factor through the α receptor-specific up-regulation. J Biol Chem 1991;266:10143–10147.

83. Carmeliet P. Mechanisms of angiogenesis and arteriogenesis. Nat Med 2000; 6:389–395.

84. Hirschi KK, Rohovsky SA, Beck LH, Smith SR, D'Amore PA. Endothelial cells modulate the proliferation of mural cell precursors via platelet-derived growth factor-BB and heterotypic cell contact. Circ Res 1999;84:298–305.

85. Hellstrom M, Gerhardt H, Kalen M, et al. Lack of pericytes leads to endothelial hyperplasia and abnormal vascular morphogenesis. J Cell Biol 2001;153:543–553.

86. Armulik A, Abramsson A, Betsholtz C. Endothelial/pericyte interactions. Circ Res 2005;97:512–523.

87. Benjamin LE, Hemo I, Keshet E. A plasticity window for blood vessel remodelling is defined by pericyte coverage of the preformed endothelial network and is regulated by PDGF-B and VEGF. Development 1998;125:1591–1598.

88. Richardson TP, Peters MC, Ennett AB, Mooney DJ. Polymeric system for dual growth factor delivery. Nat Biotechnol 2001;19:1029–1034.

89. Cao R, Brakenhielm E, Pawliuk R, et al. Angiogenic synergism, vascular stability and improvement of hind-limb ischemia by a combination of PDGF-BB and FGF-2. Nat Med 2003;9:604–613.

90. Sato N, Beitz JG, Kato J, et al. Platelet-derived growth factor indirectly stimulates angiogenesis in vitro. Am J Pathol 1993;142:1119–1130.

91. Guo P, Hu B, Gu W, et al. Platelet-derived growth factor-B enhances glioma angiogenesis by stimulating vascular endothelial growth factor expression in tumor endothelia and by promoting pericyte recruitment. Am J Pathol 2003;162:1083–1093.

92. Lee YM, Park YJ, Lee SJ, et al. Tissue engineered bone formation using chitosan/tricalcium phosphate sponges. J Periodontol 2000;71:410–417.

93. Lee YM, Park YJ, Lee SJ, et al. The bone regenerative effect of platelet-derived growth factor-BB delivered with a chitosan/tricalcium phosphate sponge carrier. J Periodontol 2000;71:418–424.

94. Vikjaer D, Blom S, Hjorting-Hansen E, Pinholt EM. Effect of platelet-derived growth factor-BB on bone formation in calvarial defects: an experimental study in rabbits. Eur J Oral Sci 1997;105:59–66.

95. Marden LJ, Fan RS, Pierce GF, Reddi AH, Hollinger JO. Platelet-derived growth factor inhibits bone regeneration induced by osteogenin, a bone morphogenetic protein, in rat craniotomy defects. J Clin Invest 1993;92:2897–2905.

96. Marden L, Quigley N, Reddi AH, Hollinger JO. Temporal changes during bone formation in the calvarium induced by osteogenin. Calcif Tissue Int 1993;53: 262–268.

97. Ranly DM, McMillan J, Keller T, et al. Platelet-derived growth factor inhibits demineralized bone matrix–induced intramuscular cartilage and bone formation. A study of immunocompromised mice. J Bone Joint Surg Am 2005;87:2052–2064.

98. Howes R, Bowness J, Grotendorst G, Martin G, Reddi A. Platelet-derived growth factor enhances demineralized bone matrix-induced cartilage and bone formation. Calcif Tissue Int 1988;42:34–38.

99. Quarto R, Thomas D, Liang CT. Bone progenitor cell deficits and the age-associated decline in bone repair capacity. Calcif Tissue Int 1995;56:123–129.

100. Albandar JM, Kingman A. Gingival recession, gingival bleeding, and dental calculus in adults 30 years of age and older in the United States, 1988–1994. J Periodontol 1999;70:30–43.

101. American Dental Association. The 1999 Survey of Dental Services Rendered. 1990. Chicago: American Dental Association, 2002:47–49.

102. Hammerle CH, Jung RE. Bone augmentation by means of barrier membranes. Periodontol 2000, 2003;33:36–53.

103. Selvig KA, Sorensen RG, Wozney JM, Wikesjö UME. Bone repair following recombinant human bone morphogenetic protein-2 stimulated periodontal regeneration. J Periodontol 2002;73:1020–1029.

104. Green RJ, Usui ML, Hart CE, Ammons WF, Narayanan AS. Immunolocalization of platelet-derived growth factor A and B chains and PDGF-α and β receptors in human gingival wounds. J Periodontal Res 1997;32:209–214.

105. Pinheiro ML, Feres-Filho, EJ, Graves DT, et al. Quantification and localization of platelet-derived growth factor in gingiva of periodontitis patients. J Periodontol 2003;74:323–328.

106. Doxey DL, Cutler CW, Iacopino AM. Diabetes prevents periodontitis-induced increases in gingival platelet derived growth factor-B and interleukin 1-β in a rat model. J Periodontol 1998;69:113–119.

107. Wang HL, Pappert TD, Castelli WA, Chiego DJ Jr, Shyr Y, Smith BA. The effect of platelet-derived growth factor on the cellular response of the periodontium: An autoradiographic study on dogs. J Periodontol 1994;65:429–436.

108. Lynch SE. Bone regeneration techniques in the orofacial region. In: Lieberman J, Friedlaender G (eds). Bone Regeneration and Repair: Biology and Clinical Applications. Totowa, NJ: Humana Press, 2005:359–390.

109. Lynch SE, Buser D, Hernandez RA, et al. Effects of the platelet-derived growth factor/insulin like growth factor-1 combination on bone regeneration around titanium dental implants. Results of a pilot study in beagle dogs. J Periodontol 1991;62:710–716.

110. Lynch SE, de Castilla GR, Williams RC, et al. The effects of short-term application of a combination of platelet-derived and insulin-like growth factors on periodontal wound healing. J Periodontol 1991;62:458–467.

111. Bowen-Pope DF, Malpass T, Foster DW, Ross R. Platelet-derived growth factor in vivo: Levels, activity, and rate of clearance. Blood 1984;64:458–965.

112. Hollinger JO, Wong MEK. The integrated processes of hard tissue regeneration with special emphasis on fracture healing. Oral Surg Oral Med Oral Pathol 1996;82:594–606.

113. Becker W, Lynch SE, Lekholm U, et al. Comparison of ePTFE membranes alone or in combination with platelet-derived growth factors and insulin-like growth factor-1 or demineralized freeze-dried bone in promoting bone formation around immediate extraction socket implants. J Periodontol 1992;63:929–940.

114. Giannobile WV, Hernandez RA, Finkelman RD, et al. Comparative effects of platelet-derived growth factor-BB and insulin-like growth factor-1, individually and in combination, on periodontal regeneration in Macaca fascicularis. J Periodontal Res 1996;31:301–312.

115. Park JB, Matsuura M, Han KY, et al. Periodontal regeneration in class III furcation defects of beagle dogs using guided tissue regenerative therapy with platelet-derived growth factor. J Periodontol 1995;66:462–477.

116. Giannobile WV. Periodontal tissue engineering by growth factors. Bone 1996; 19(suppl):23–37.

117. Howell TH, Fiorellini J, Jones A, et al. A feasibility study evaluating rhBMP-2/absorbable collagen sponge device for local alveolar ridge preservation or augmentation. Int J Periodontics Restorative Dent 1997;17:124–139.

118. Howell TH, Fiorellini JP, Paquette DW, Offenbacher S, Giannobile WV, Lynch SE. A phase I/II clinical trial to evaluate a combination of recombinant human platelet-derived growth factor-BB and recombinant human insulin-like growth factor-1 in patients with periodontal disease. J Periodontol 1997;68:1186–1193.

119. Camelo M, Nevins M, Schanck R, Lynch S, Nevins ML. Periodontal regeneration can be achieved in human class II furcations using purified recombinant human platelet-derived growth factor-BB (rhPDGF-BB) with bone allograft. Int J Periodontics Restorative Dent 2003;23:213–225.

120. Nevins M, Camelo M, Nevins ML, Schenck R, Lynch S. Periodontal regeneration in humans using recombinant human platelet-derived growth factor BB (rhPDGF-BB) and allogeneic bone. J Periodontol 2003;74:1282–1292.

121. Bateman J, Intini G, Margarone J, et al. Platelet-derived growth factor enhancement of two alloplastic bone matrices. J Periodontol 2005;76:1833–1841.

122. Nevins M, Giannobile WV, McGuire MH, et al. Platelet derived growth factor stimulates bone fill and rate of attachment level gain: Results of a large multicenter randomized controlled trial. J Periodontol 2005;76:2205–2215.

123. Smiell JM. Clinical safety of becaplermin (rhPDGF-BB) gel. Becaplermin Studies Group. Am J Surg 1998;176(2A suppl):68S–73S.

124. Klinger MH, Jelkmann W. Role of blood platelets in infection and inflammation. J Interferon Cytokine Res 2002;22:913–922.

125. Schmitz JP, Hollinger JO. The biology of platelet-rich plasma. J Oral Maxillofac Surg 2001;59:1119–1121.

126. Freymiller EG, Aghaloo TL. Platelet-rich plasma: Ready or not? J Oral Maxillofac Surg 2004;62:484–488.

127. Marx RE. Platelet-rich plasma: Evidence to support its use. J Oral Maxillofac Surg 2004;62:489–496.

128. Frechette J, Martineau I, Gagnon G. Platelet-rich plasmas: Growth factor content and roles in wound healing. J Dent Res 2005;84:434–439.

129. Hollinger JO, Onikepe A, Mackrell J, et al. Accelerated fracture healing in the geriatric, osteoporotic rat with recombinant human platelet-derived growth factor-BB and an injectable beta-tricalcium phosphate/collagen matrix. J Orthop Res 2007 (in press).

130. Mitlak B, Finkelman R, Hill E, et al. The effect of systematically administered PDGF-BB on the rodent skeleton. J Bone Miner Res 1996;11:238–247.

131. Nash TJ, Howlett CR, Martin C, Steele J, Johnson KA, Hicklin DJ. Effect of platelet-derived growth factor on tibial osteotomies in rabbits. Bone 1994;15: 203–208.

132. Reddi AH. Bone and cartilage morphogenesis: Cell biology to clinical applications. Curr Opin Genet Dev 1994;4:737–744.

133. Reddi AH. Morphogenetic messages are in the extracellular matrix: Biotechnology from bench to bedside. Biochem Soc Trans 2000;28:345–349.

134. Hoffmann A, Weich G, Gross G, Hillman G. Perspectives in the biological function, the technical and therapeutic application of bone morphogenetic proteins. Appl Microbiol Biotechnol 2001;57:294–308.

135. Li R, Wozney J. Delivering on the promise of bone morphogenetic proteins. Trends Biotech 2001;19:255–265.

136. von Bubnoff A, Cho KS. Intracellular BMP signalling regulation in vertebrates: Pathway or network. Dev Biol 2001;239:1–14.

137. Lieberman J, Daluiski A, Einhorn T. Current concepts review: The role of growth factors in the repair of bone. J Bone Joint Surg Am 2002;84-A:1032–1044.

138. Schliephake H. Bone growth factors in maxillofacial skeletal reconstruction. Int J Oral Maxillofac Surg 2002;31:469–484.

139. Wozney J. Overview of bone morphogenetic proteins. Spine 2002;27(16 suppl 1):S2–S8.

140. Ten Dijke P, Fu J, Schaap P, Roelen B. Signal transduction of bone morphogenetic proteins in osteoblast differentiation. J Bone Joint Surg Am 2003;85-A(suppl 3):34–38.

141. Hing K. Bone repair in the twenty-first century: Biology, chemistry or tissue engineering? Philos Transact A Math Phys Eng Sci 2004;362:2821–2850.

142. Oreffo R. Growth factors for skeletal reconstruction and fracture repair. Curr Opin Invest Drugs 2004;5:419–423.

143. Wozney J, Seeherman H. Protein-based tissue engineering in bone and cartilage repair. Curr Opin Cell Biol 2004;15:392–398.

144. Celil A, Hollinger JO, Campbell P. Osx transcriptional regulations is mediated by additional pathways to BMP2/Smad signaling. J Cell Biol 2005;95:518–528.

145. Cheng H, Feldman EL, Jiang W, et al. Osteogenic activity of the fourteen types of human bone morphogenetic proteins (BMPs). J Bone Joint Surg Am 2003; 85-A:1544–1552.

146. Reddi AH. Role of morphogenetic proteins in skeletal tissue engineering and regeneration. Nat Biotechnol 1998;16:247–252.

147. Ray RD, Holloway JA. Bone implants. Preliminary report of an experimental study. J Bone Joint Surg Am 1957;39-A:1119–1128.

148. Urist MR. Bone: Formation by autoinduction. Science 1965;150:893–899.

149. Urist MR, Strates BS. Bone morphogenetic protein. J Dent Res 1971;50: 1392–1406.

150. Reddi AH, Huggins CB. Influence of geometry of transplanted tooth and bone on transformation of fibroblasts. Proc Soc Exp Biol Med 1973;143:634–637.

151. Reddi AH, Huggins CB. Formation of bone marrow in fibroblast-transformation ossicles. Proc Natl Acad Sci U S A 1975;72:2212–2216.

152. Reddi AH, Anderson WA. Collagenous bone matrix-induced endochondral ossification and hemopoiesis. J Cell Biol 1976;69:557–572.

153. Muthukumaran N, Ma S, Reddi AH. Dose-dependence of and threshold for optimal bone induction by collagenous bone matrix and osteogenin-enriched fraction. Coll Relat Res 1988;8:433–441.

154. Lacroix P. Organizers and the growth of bone. J Bone Joint Surg 1947;29: 292–296.

155. Bahamonde ME, Lyons K. BMP3: To be or not to be a BMP? J Bone Joint Surg Am 2001;83-A(suppl 1):S56–S62.

156. Reddi AH. Morphogenesis and tissue engineering of bone and cartilage: Inductive signals, stem cells, and biomimetic biomaterials. Tissue Eng 2000;6:351–359.

157. Wozney JM, Rosen V, Celeste AJ, et al. Novel regulators of bone formation: Molecular clones and activities. Science 1988;242:1528–1534.

158. Özkaynak E, Rueger DC, Drier EA, et al. OP-1 cDNA encodes an osteogenic protein in the TGF-ß family. EMBO J 1990;9:2085–2093.

159. Kingsley D. What do BMPs do in mammals? Clues from the mouse short-ear mutation. Trends Genet 1994;10:16–21.

160. Kingsley DM. The TGF-β superfamily: New members, new receptors, and new genetic tests of function in different organisms. Genes Dev 1994;8:133–146.

161. Kingsley DM. Genes that define the number and shape of bones in the mouse skeleton. Presented at the Portland Bone Symposium, Portland, OR, 19–21 July 1995.

162. Hogan BL. Bone morphogenetic proteins: Multifunctional regulators of vertebrate development. Genes Dev 1996;10:1580–1594.

163. Hogan BL. Bone morphogenetic proteins in development. Curr Opin Gen Develop 1996;6:432–438.

164. Hogan BL. Morphogenesis. Cell 1999;96:225–233.

165. Schmitt JM, Hwang K, Winn SR, Hollinger JO. Bone morphogenetic proteins: An update on basic biology and clinical relevance. J Orthop Res 1999;17:269–278.

166. Hoffmann A, Gross G. BMP signaling pathways in cartilage and bone formation. Critical Rev Eukaryot Gene Expr 2001;11:23–45.

167. Jadlowiec J, Celil A, Hollinger JO. Bone tissue engineering: Recent advances and promising therapeutic agents. Exp Opin Biol Ther 2004;3:409–423.

168. Nohe A, Hassel S, Ehrlich M, et al. The mode of bone morphogenetic protein (BMP) receptor oligomerization determines different BMP-2 signaling pathways. J Biol Chem 2002;277:5330–5338.

169. Dimitriou R, Tsiridis EE, Carr I, Simpson H, Giannoudis P. The role of inhibitory molecules in fracture healing. Injury Int J Care Injured 2006;375:S20–S29.

170. Wozney J. The bone morphogenetic family: Multifunctional cellular regulators in the embryo and adult. Eur J Oral Sci 1998;106(suppl 1):160–166.

171. Kaneko H, Arakawa T, Mano H, et al. Direct stimulation of osteoclastic bone resorption by bone morphogenetic protein (BMP)-2 and expression of BMP receptors in mature osteoclasts. Bone 2000;27:479–486.

172. Wan M, Cao X. BMP signaling in skeletal development. Biochem Biophys Res Commun 2005;328:651–657.

173. Chen X, Kidder L, Schmidt A, Lew W. Osteogenic protein-1 induces bone formation in the presence of bacterial infection in a rat intramuscular osteoinduction model. J Orthop Trauma 2004;18:436–442.

174. Seifert R, Hart C, Phillips P, et al. Two different subunits associate to create isoform-specific platelet-derived growth factor receptors. J Biol Chem 1989; 264:8771–8778.

175. Ross R. Platelets: Cell proliferation and atherosclerosis. Metabolism 1979;28: 410–414.

176. Hirschi K, Rohovsky S, D'Amore P. TGF-β and heterotypic cell-cell interactions mediate endothelial cell-induced recruitment of 10T1/2 cells and their differentiation to a smooth muscle fate. J Cell Biol 1998;141:805–814.

177. Alexander D, Hesson T, Mannarino A, Cable M, Dalie B. Isolation and purification of a biologically active human platelet-derived growth factor BB expressed in Escherichia coli. Protcin Expr Purif 1992;3:204–211.

178. Giese N, May-Siroff M, LaRochelle W, van Wyke Coelingh K, Aaronson S. Expression and purification of biologically active v-sis/platelet-derived growth factor B protein by using a baculovirus vector system. J Virol 1989;63: 3080–3086.

179. Ostman A, Backstrom G, Fong N, et al. Expression of three recombinant homodimeric isoforms of PDGF in Saccharomyces cerevisiae: Evidence for difference in receptor binding and functional activities. Growth Factors 1989;1: 271–281.

180. Hammonds RG, Schwall R, Dudley A, et al. Bone-inducing activity of mature BMP-2b produced from a hybrid BMP-2a/2b precursor. Mol Endocrinol 1991; 5:149–155.

181. Maruoka Y, Oida S, Iimura T, et al. Production of functional human bone morphogenetic protein-2 using a baculovirus/Sf-9 insect cell system. Biochem Mol Biol Int 1995;35:957–963.

182. Klosch B, Furst W, Kneidinger R, et al. Expression and purification of biologically active rat bone morphogenetic protein-4 produced as inclusion bodies in recombinant Escherichia coli. Biotechnol Lett 2005;27:1559–1564.

183. Long S, Truong L, Bennett K, Phillips A, Wong-Staal F, Ma H. Expression, purification, and renaturation of bone morphogenetic protein-2 from Escherichia coli. Protein Expr Purif 2006;46:374–378.

184. Tiesman J, Hart C. Identification of a soluble receptor for platelet-derived growth factor in cell-conditioned medium and human plasma. J Biol Chem 1993;268:9621–9628.

185. Dahlfors G, Chen Y, Wasteson M, Arnqvist H. PDGF-BB-induced DNA synthesis is delayed by angiotensin II in vascular smooth muscle cells. Am J Physiol 1998;274:H1742–H1748.

186. Yang Z, Krasnici N, Luscher T. Endothelin-1 potentiates human smooth muscle cell growth to PDGF: Effects of ETA and ETB receptor blockade. Circulation 1999;100:5–8.

187. Leppanen O, Rutanen J, Hiltunen M, et al. Oral imatinib mesylate (STI571/gleevec) improves the efficacy of local intravascular vascular endothelial growth factor-C gene transfer in reducing neointimal growth in hypercholesterolemic rabbits. Circulation 2004;109:1140–1146.

188. Lotinun S, Sibonga J, Turner R. Triazolopyrimidine (trapidil), a platelet-derived growth factor antagonist, inhibits parathyroid bone disease in an animal model for chronic hyperparathyroidism. Endocrinology 2003;35:957–963.

189. Schermuly R, Dony E, Ghofrani, H, et al. Reversal of experimental pulmonary hypertension by PDGF inhibition. J Clin Invest 2005;115:2811–2821.

190. Skovseth D, Veuger M, Sorensen D, De Angelis P, Haraldsen G. Endostatin dramatically inhibits endothelial cell migration, vascular morphogenesis, and perivascular cell recruitment in vivo. Blood 2005;105:1044–1051.

191. Demetriou M, Binkert C, Sukhu B, Tenenbaum H, Dennis J. Fetuin/alpha2-HS glycoprotein is a transforming growth factor-β type II receptor mimic and cytokine antagonist. J Biol Chem 1996;274:12755–12761.

192. Canalis E, Economides A, Gazzerro E. Bone morphogenetic proteins, their antagonists, and the skeleton. Endocr Rev 2003;24:218–235.

193. Yanagita M. BMP antagonists: their roles in development and involvement in pathophysiology. Cytokine Growth Factor Rev 2005;16:309–317.

194. Khokha M, Hsu D, Brunet L, Dionne M, Harland R. Gremlin is the BMP antagonist required for maintenance of Shh and Fgf signals during limb patterning. Nat Genet 2003;34:303–307.

195. Kassai Y, Munne P, Hotta Y, et al. Regulation of mammalian tooth cusp patterning by ectodin. Science 2005;309:2067–2070.

196. Stephenson D, Mercola M, Anderson E, et al. Platelet-derived growth factor receptor α-subunit gene (Pdgfra) is deleted in the mouse patch (Ph) mutation. Proc Natl Acad Sci U S A 1991;88:6–10.

197. Leveen P, Pekny M, Gebre-Medhin S, Swolin B, Larsson E, Betsholz C. Mice deficient for PDGF BB show renal, cardiovascular, and hematological abnormalities. Genes Dev 1994;8:1875–1887.

198. Schatteman G, Loushin C, Li T, Hart C. PDGF-AA is required for normal murine cardiovascular development. Dev Biol 1996;176:133–142.

199. Lindahl P, Johansson B, Leveen P, Betsholtz C. Pericyte loss and microaneurysm formation in PDGF-BB-deficient mice. Science 1997;277:242–245.

200. Karsenty G, Luo G, Hofmann C, Bradley A. BMP 7 is required for nephrogenesis, eye development, and skeletal patterning. Ann NY Acad Sci 1996;705: 98–107.

201. Salgado A, Coutinho O, Reis RL. Bone tissue engineering: State of the art and future trends. Macromol Biosci 2004;4:743–765.

202. Winn SR, Uludag H, Hollinger JO. Sustained release emphasizing recombinant human bone morphogenetic protein-2. Adv Drug Deliv Rev 1998;31:303–318.

203. Winn SR, Uludag H, Hollinger JO. Carrier systems for bone morphogenetic proteins. Clin Orthop Relat Res 1999;(367 suppl):S95–S106.

204. Kirker-Head C. Potential applications and delivery strategies for bone morphogenetic proteins. Adv Drug Deliv Rev 2000;43:65–92.

205. Seeherman H, Li R, Wozney J. A review on preclinical program development of evaluating injectable carriers for osteogenic factors. J Bone Joint Surg Am 2003; 85-A(suppl 3):96–108.

206. Seeherman H, Wozney JM. Delivery of bone morphogenetic proteins for orthopaedic tissue regeneration. Cytokine Growth Factor Rev 2005;16: 329–345.

207. Friedlaender GE, Perry CR, Cole JD, et al. Osteogenic protein-1 (bone morphogenetic protein-7) in the treatment of tibial nonunions. J Bone Joint Surg Am 2001;83-A(suppl 1, pt 2):S151–S158.

208. Govender S, Csimma C, Genant H, et al. Recombinant human bone morphogenetic protein-2 for treatment of open tibial fractures: A prospective, controlled, randomized study of four hundred and fifty patients. J Bone Joint Surg Am 2002;84-A:2123–2134.

209. Boden S, Zdeblick TA, Sandhu HS. The use of rhBMP-2 in interbody fusion cages. Definitive evidence of osteoinduction in humans: A preliminary report. Spine 2000;25:376–381.

210. Burkus JK, Gornet MF, Dickman CA, Zdeblick TA. Anterior lumbar interbody fusion using rhBMP-2 with tapered interbody cages. J Spinal Disord Tech 2002;15:337–349.

211. Hollinger JO, Doll BA, Sfeir C, Mu Y, Azari K. Therapeutic potential of bone morphogenetic proteins. Expert Opin Investig Drugs 2001;10:1677–1686.

212. Vaccaro AR, Patel T, Firschgrund J, et al. A 2 year follow up pilot study evaluation of the safety and efficacy of OP-1 putty as an adjunct to iliac crest autograft in posterior lateral lumbar fusions. Eur Spine J 2005;14:623–629.

213. Jeppsson C, Saveland H, Rydholm U, Aspenberg P. OP-1 for cervical spine fusion: Bridging bone in only 1 of 4 rheumatoid patients but prednisolone did not inhibit bone induction in rats. Acta Orthop Scand 1999;70:559–563.

214. Boyne PJ, Marx RE, Nevins M, et al. A feasibility study evaluation rhBMP-2/absorbable collagen sponge for maxillary sinus augmentation. Int J Periodontics Restorative Dent 1997;17:11–15.

215. Boyne PJ, Lilly LC, Marx RE, et al. De novo bone induction by recombinant human bone morphogenetic protein-2 (rhBMP-2) in maxillary sinus floor augmentation. J Oral Maxillofac Surg 2005;63:1693–1707.

216. Cochran DL, Schenk R, Buser D, Wozney JM, Jones AA. Recombinant human bone morphogenetic protein-2 stimulation of bone formation around endosseous dental implants. J Periodontol 1999;70:139–150.

217. Cochran DL, Jones AA, Lilly L, Fiorellini JP, Howell H. Evaluation of recombinant human bone morphogenetic protein-2 in oral applications including the use of endosseous implants: 3 year results of a pilot study in humans. J Periodontol 2000;71:1241–1257.

218. Howell TH, Fiorellini JP, Paquette DW, Offenbacher S, Antoniades HN, Lynch SE. Evaluation of a combination of recombinant human platelet-derived growth factor-BB and recombinant human insulin-like growth factor-I in patients with periodontal disease [abstract]. J Dent Res 1995;74:253.

219. Fiorellini J, Howell TH, Cochran D, et al. Randomized study evaluating recombinant human bone morphogenetic protein-2 for extraction socket augmentation. J Periodontol 2005;76:605–613.

2

Basic Principles of Scaffolds in Tissue Engineering

Myron Spector, PhD

As with any engineering discipline, the working goal of tissue engineering is the implementation of existing knowledge for the creation of a product—tissue.[1] In addition, the engineering process often provides opportunities for the discovery of new knowledge, that is, the process of science. The unique circumstances related to the growth of cells in three-dimensional (3-D) scaffolds in vitro in the course of tissue engineering reveal aspects of the phenotypes of a wide variety of cells and insights into cell behaviors that would have otherwise escaped view.[1] In this regard, tissue engineering is likely to contribute important knowledge to the study of cell and molecular biology while adding to the fund of knowledge that can be drawn from for the advancement of health care. This chapter discusses the historical development of in vitro tissue engineering and in vivo tissue regeneration strategies and the evolving role of scaffolds in tissue engineering procedures, including cell delivery and gene transfer. The use of scaffolds for the delivery of exogenous factors, such as recombinant human platelet-derived growth factors (rhPDGFs) and bone morphogenetic proteins (rhBMPs), is covered in several other chapters in this book.

Scientific Basis of Tissue Engineering

One unique aspect of tissue engineering science is the investigation of the interactions of cells with absorbable matrices and environmental factors (eg, mechanical loading) that relate to the formation of tissue. Cellular responses to these interactions include cellular proliferation and biosynthesis of matrix molecules. Cell contraction is another important aspect of the cellular response to scaffolds employed for tissue engineering.[1] As more knowledge about the interaction of cells with matrices is acquired, researchers will be better able to prepare new scaffolds to more specifically elicit the responses from cells that best suit a tissue engineering application.

The challenging aspect of tissue engineering is, as with any engineering endeavor, the judicious use of existing knowledge for the production of a useful product, in this case, tissue. There are so many physical and biologic issues related to the production of tissue in vivo or in vitro, and so few hard facts to guide the engineering process, that tissue engineering is a much more demanding field than other engineering disciplines. Moreover, the stakes of tissue engineering pursuits are higher, because the risks of failure include death.

Tissue engineering can now be pursued because of advances in enabling technologies related to the tissue engineering triad of cells, matrices, and regulators. It is only relatively recently that technologies have been developed for the proliferation of cells in vitro under conditions that allow the maintenance or recovery of the cell phenotype. A critical aspect of most tissue engineering strategies is the expansion of cell number in culture to generate the requisite number of cells for the production of tissue in vitro or the implantation of cells alone or seeded in matrices for the regeneration of tissue in vivo. Many cell types lose critical phenotypic traits with increasing time in culture. Advances in cellular biology have allowed the creation of culture conditions that favor the proliferation of cells that maintain their phenotype or recover lost phenotypic gene expression postexpansion.

One of the most important technologic advances enabling tissue engineering is the means of production of the porous, absorbable scaffolds that are required to contain the cells for the production of tissue in vitro and in vivo. Synthetic and natural polymers and calcium phosphates have been developed as scaffolds for the engineering of soft and hard tissues. Control of the pore characteristics, including volume fraction, diameter, and orientation, as well as the chemical composition of the matrix, has played a critical role in the advances of tissue engineering.

Another important enabling technology that has impacted tissue engineering is the recombinant technology for the production of large quantities of selected cytokines, such as rhPDGFs and rhBMPs. These growth and differentiation factors and agents stimulate biosynthetic activity and are playing important roles in efforts to form tissue in vitro and to facilitate regeneration in vivo. Many regulatory molecules have already been shown to greatly enhance the regenerative process. In addition, a number of physical stimuli (eg, mechanical loading and shock wave therapy) are also proving to be promising adjunctive therapies to facilitate tissue engineering.

Clinicians now have a rather complete "technology toolbox" (Box 2-1) that can be employed to engineer a wide array of tissues. The challenges that lay ahead involve the determination of which combinations of tools are necessary, and the timing of their use, for the regeneration of specific tissues and organs (ie, a structure comprising two or more tissues).

Box 2-1 Technology toolbox for tissue engineering

Scaffolds (matrices)
- Porous, absorbable, spongelike biomaterials; membranes; tubes
- Nanoparticles

Cells (autologous or allogeneic)
- Differentiated cells of the tissue type
- Stem cells: adult, fetal, and embryonic
- Other cell types

Regulators
- Growth factors
- Genes for growth factors
- Antagonists of growth inhibitors
- Mechanical loading
- Hydrostatic pressure
- Fluid flow
- Shock waves and ultrasound
- Electromagnetic radiation

Historical perspective

Many investigations have served as the antecedents of tissue engineering; the following discussion provides a brief summary of a few of these studies.[2] Perhaps the earliest successful application of principles that now fall under the heading of tissue engineering was the implementation of porous collagen-glycosaminoglycan (GAG) matrices (Fig 2-1) for the in vivo regeneration of dermis.[3] This work, which led to the term *artificial skin*, served as the basis for the subsequent use of these matrices in tubular form for the regeneration of peripheral nerves.[4] The underlying concept was to develop analogs of the extracellular matrix (ECM) of the tissue to be regenerated. In addition to demonstrating that selected analogs could facilitate the regeneration of tissues that did not have the capability to spontaneously regenerate, these studies showed that tis-

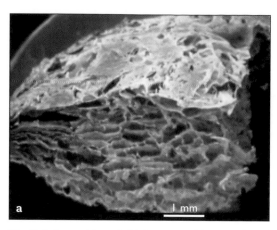
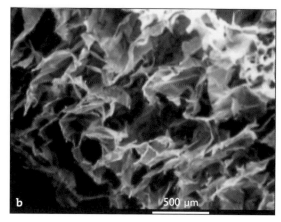

Fig 2-1 Low- *(a)* and high-power *(b)* scanning electron micrographs of a porous collagen-GAG scaffold employed for tissue engineering. The spongelike scaffold was produced using a freeze-drying procedure.

sue-specific pore characteristics (eg, pore diameter and orientation) were required for optimal performance.

The use of these regeneration templates also demonstrated the importance of having degradation rates for the matrix, controlled through cross-linking, which matched the regeneration rate of the tissue being regenerated in a process referred to as *isomorphous replacement*. Later work following this line of investigation[5] showed that an off-the-shelf scaffold used for treating peripheral nerve gaps in a rat model was more effective than autograft in regenerating these gaps.

Other early tissue engineering studies[6] investigated the endothelium-like cell layer that formed on polymethyl methacrylate implants used in the eye. Subsequent work demonstrated the ability of cell-seeded matrices, made from a synthetic polymer, to form and maintain a viable cartilaginous tissue of a selected shape when implanted in an animal model.[7] These and other studies formed the basis of a review article[8] that established tissue engineering as a distinct discipline.

Tissue engineering versus regenerative medicine

The term *tissue engineering* was initially introduced to describe the technology for producing tissue in vitro.[8] More recently, the term *regenerative medicine* has been used to describe the development of technology and sur-

gical procedures for the regeneration of tissue in vivo. There are advantages and disadvantages to both in vitro and in vivo strategies. One advantage of the synthesis of tissue in vitro is the ability to examine the tissue as it forms and to make certain nondestructive measurements to establish its functions prior to implantation.

A disadvantage of in vitro methods, particularly in the production of musculoskeletal tissue that must play a load-bearing role, is the absence of a physiologic mechanical environment during the formation of the tissue. It is now well established that mechanical force serves as a critical regulator of cell function and can profoundly influence the architecture of tissue as it is forming. Because the mechanical environment present during the formation of most musculoskeletal tissue in vivo is not well understood, it is not yet possible to re-create such an environment in vitro during the engineering of most tissues.

Another disadvantage of the formation of musculoskeletal tissue outside of the body is the necessary incorporation of the tissues after implantation. This incorporation requires that the engineered tissue be mechanically coupled to the surrounding structures. Union of the implanted tissue with the host organ requires remodeling—degradation and new tissue formation—at the interfaces of the implant with the host tissues. That remodeling of the implanted tissue is essential for its functional incorporation.

Thus, for certain tissues (eg, musculoskeletal), an effective strategy may be to facilitate tissue formation in vivo, under the influence of the physiologic mechanical environment. However, one disadvantage of this approach is that the regenerating tissue may be dislodged or degraded by the mechanical forces normally acting at the site before it is fully formed and incorporated.

In most cases a distinction is not made between tissue engineering and regenerative medicine, and both are considered to fall under the general heading of tissue engineering. Regardless of whether the process of tissue engineering occurs in vitro or in vivo, successful outcomes depend upon the strategic employment of tissue elements (cells, matrix, and soluble regulators). Decisions as to which elements might be required for regeneration of tissue in vivo are often guided by an understanding of the deficits of the natural (ie, spontaneous) healing processes that prevent regeneration.

Scaffolds for Tissue Engineering and Regenerative Medicine

For most of the decades of the 20th century, biomaterials played a critical role in enabling the fabrication of a large number and wide variety of medical implants. Except for a few examples, however, these were permanent devices meant to fix or replace the function of tissues and organs. Stainless steel devices were developed for the fixation of fractures and to fix allografts to host bone. Implants fashioned from metallic, ceramic, and polymeric materials facilitated life-saving procedures in many patients (eg, vascular prostheses and artificial heart valves) and profoundly improved the quality of the lives of other individuals (eg, joint replacement prostheses).

Despite these remarkable successes, the new roles for biomaterials in medicine will likely exceed these achievements. The new roles include the use of porous, absorbable (spongelike) biomaterial scaffolds in tissue engineering, regenerative medicine, and gene therapy. Scaffolds for engineering bone and the soft tissues have been synthesized from an array of synthetic and natural calcium phosphates and myriad synthetic (eg, polylactic acid and polyglycolic acid) and natural (eg, collagen and fibrin) polymers. These scaffolds, regardless of their composition, must be chosen based on a number of considerations:

• Scaffolds for engineering tissue in vitro, or to be used as implants to facilitate regeneration in vivo, must have a microstructure capable of accommodating cells and their functions. A porous structure is generally necessary. The required porosity and pore diameter, pore distribution, and pore orientation may be expected to vary with tissue type.
• The chemical composition of the matrix is important with respect to its influence on cellular adhesion and the phenotypic expression of the infiltrating cells.
• Because the objective is the regeneration of the original tissue, the scaffold has to be absorbable. The degradation rate of the material generally may be determined based on the rate of new tissue formation and the normal period for remodeling of the tissue at the site of implantation. It is important to consider the effects of moieties released during degradation of the matrix on the host and regenerating tissue.
• The mechanical properties of the biomaterial employed as a scaffold for tissue engineering are important for providing temporary support of applied loads in vivo during the regeneration process and for resisting the contractile forces that may be exerted by the seeded cells prior to implantation and by cells infiltrating the scaffold in vivo. The stiffness of the scaffold also is important because it affects the strain in the ingrown and surrounding tissue.

With regard to mechanical properties, design specifications for several bone graft substitute materials have emphasized the strength of the matrix material, with the principal objective of employing high-strength substances for immediate load bearing. Synthetic calcium phosphate ceramics were developed in this way as matrix materials for facilitating bone regeneration in vivo.[9,10] In addition to possessing high strength, however, these materials also have a high modulus of elasticity, making them very stiff structures. The presence of the stiff material greatly alters the distribution of mechanical forces in surrounding tissue and thereby adversely affects the stress-induced remodeling of neighboring bone.[11]

Because this class of matrix is essentially nonresorbable, the adverse effects on remodeling will persist indefinitely. This nonphysiologic remodeling can result in osteopenic regions around the implanted site, increasing the risk of fracture. Moreover, conventional methods for treatment of such fractures are likely to be difficult because the high density of the implanted biomaterial precludes drilling and cutting procedures. Revision surgical procedures at sites implanted with these substances may require their complete removal.

For these reasons, the use of high modulus biomaterials for reconstruction of bone in which implants are to be placed (eg, endosseous dental implants) is problematic. It may be judicious to employ materials that match the modulus of elasticity of the tissue at the implant site and thus to consider the composition and properties of the ECM when a scaffold for tissue engineering is designed or selected.

There have been numerous reviews of the characteristics of the biomaterial scaffolds generally used for tissue engineering.[12,13] A comprehensive review of biomaterial scaffolds is outside the scope of this chapter. Rather, the author will draw from his personal experience employing natural bone mineral and collagen-based biomaterials to discuss the use of scaffolds for specific tissue engineering applications.

Roles of a scaffold

A scaffold can play many roles in the tissue regeneration process:

- The scaffold can serve as a framework to support cellular migration into the defect from surrounding tissues; this is especially important when a fibrin clot is absent.
- Before it is absorbed, a scaffold can serve as a matrix for endogenous or exogenous cell adhesion and can facilitate and regulate certain cellular processes, including mitosis, synthesis, and migration. This may be mediated by ligands for cell receptors (integrins) on the biomaterial, and/or the biomaterial may selectively adsorb cell adhesion proteins.
- The scaffold may serve as a delivery vehicle for exogenous cells, growth factors, and genes. This activity is enabled by large surface area for attachment and the possible control of the density of the agents (ie, agents-per-unit volume).
- The scaffold may structurally reinforce the defect to maintain the shape of the defect and prevent distortion of surrounding tissue.
- The scaffold can serve as a barrier to prevent the infiltration of surrounding tissue that may impede the process of regeneration.

Design and production of scaffolds

Many methods have been used to produce porous materials to be used as scaffolds for tissue engineering and regenerative medicine:

- Manipulation of fibers into nonwoven and woven structures[8]
- Incorporation of sacrificial pore-forming agents including ice (through freeze-drying[3]; see Fig 2-1) and soluble particles (eg, sodium chloride and sucrose)
- Use of self-assembling molecules (eg, certain peptides[14] and collagen-hydroxyapatite composites[15])
- Use of solid free-form fabrication[16] (Fig 2-2)

The underlying concepts guiding the development of scaffolds can be predicated on the selected biomaterial or on the method of production of the scaffold. Examples of biomaterials-based approaches include:

- Biomaterials that have been frequently used for other implant applications (eg, polylactic acid–polyglycolic acid)[8]
- Treated natural extracellular matrix materials (eg, anorganic bone[17])
- Biomimetics and analogs of extracellular matrix (eg, collagen-GAG[3] and collagen-hydroxyapatite scaffolds[15])
- Biopolymers for nanoscale matrix (eg, self-assembling peptides[14])
- New types of biomaterials designed specifically for tissue engineering scaffolds

Alternatively, the driving force on the design of scaffolds may be the precision (computer) multiscale control of material, architecture, and cells: solid free-form fabrication technologies. This has become possible with the introduction of a wide array of solid free-form fabrication techniques and apparatuses.[16]

One design approach already mentioned has been the use of materials that can serve as analogs of the ECM of the tissue to be engineered.[3] This concept recognizes that the molecular composition and architecture of the ECM display chemical and mechanical properties required by the parenchymal cells and the physiologic demands of the tissue. For scaffolds for bone regeneration, this approach has led to the use of natural bone mineral produced by removal of the organic matter of bovine bone[11,17–24] (see Fig 2-2). The calcium-deficient carbonated apatite, which constitutes the mineral phase of bone, and the unique microstructure of the ECM of bone are determined by

tage of this approach is the lower efficiency of transfection. However, for some reparative processes (eg, articular cartilage) even relatively small amounts of the cytokine produced by a few transfected cells may be of significant value. This approach has provided promising results in studies directed toward enhancing bone regeneration using a collagen matrix as a carrier for selected genes.[44,45]

Prolonged release (over several weeks or months) of DNA from an implant is necessary when there is a benefit in transfecting selected cells that only appear at the implant site days or weeks postoperatively, when there is a rapid loss of expression in transfected cells, or when transfected cells migrate from the defect site.

In one study, porous gene-supplemented collagen-GAG (GSCG) matrices were loaded with plasmid DNA coding for the luciferase reporter gene, and the effects of cross-linking and pH (during gene loading) on release kinetics and DNA integrity were determined.[40] The optimal conditions produced luciferase expression in chondrocyte-seeded GSCG constructs for up to 28 days, demonstrating continuous transfection of articular chondrocytes throughout the culture period. More than 30% of the plasmid remained in selected scaffolds after 28 days in a buffer solution. In a prior study investigating release of plasmid DNA from copolymers of D,L-lactide and glycolide, less than 10% of the DNA remained in the synthetic polymer construct after 28 days in leaching studies performed using Tris ethylenediaminetetraacetic acid buffer.[46] Other matrix materials may lend themselves to modification for gene supplementation for more prolonged release of genes.

Rationale for gene transfer

Growth factors can make significant contributions to repair procedures and tissue engineering by stimulating cell proliferation, migration, differentiation, and matrix synthesis. There are, however, major challenges faced in the direct application of human recombinant proteins in a clinical setting. Proteins are difficult to administer exogenously in accurate, sustained, and therapeutically useful amounts. Single-bolus doses of growth factors alone in vivo have short half-lives as a result of degradation or diffusion from the defect site. Various delivery vehicles, including polymers, pumps, and heparin, have been investigated as possible methods by which to achieve constant levels of growth factors at a given injured site. One

notable clinical success is rhBMP-2 incorporated into an absorbable type I collagen sponge (ACS) used for spinal fusions.[47]

Delivery of a gene that could be expressed within the wound is an attractive alternative to application of the recombinant protein. Gene transfer provides the DNA that encodes for the desired protein, so that infected cells can create higher and more sustained levels of the growth factor over extended periods of time, a likely requirement for effective regeneration of many tissues. More than one gene can be transferred and independently regulated to supply multiple growth factors to the defect site. Some studies have suggested that endogenously expressed proteins induced by gene transfer may have a more positive and more potent effect than exogenous recombinant proteins on matrix synthesis and biologic activity.[42]

Approaches to gene transfer

A promising approach for enhancing gene transfer and retention of genes or expressed proteins within a defect site employs 3-D scaffolds as the delivery vehicle for the genes. The combination of gene therapy and tissue engineering could provide the ultimate treatment for defects in tissues because it involves a supporting scaffold that can serve as a carrier for gene vectors or infected cells, resulting in a sustained, prolonged, and localized delivery of therapeutic proteins in vivo. It has also been demonstrated that cells first seeded in 3-D scaffolds and then transfected show higher gene expression levels and longer expression times than do those administered by two-dimensional transfection.[48] This observation is important in demonstrating how the 3-D matrix environment can influence cellular behavior and processes.

Most studies that employ gene therapy and tissue engineering concepts for the regeneration of tissue such as articular cartilage involve ex vivo infection of cells that are transduced[49,50] or transfected[51] in vitro and then subsequently seeded into 3-D scaffolds (eg, fibrin or polymer scaffolds). Several investigations of various cell types and genes have been carried out for this application, including transfection of articular chondrocytes with the insulin-like growth factor I gene[51]; transduction of periosteal stem cells with the osteogenic protein I gene[49]; and transduction of mesenchymal cells from rib perichondrium with the BMP-2 and insulin-like growth factor I genes.[50] In all of these cases, chondrogenesis and matrix synthesis were significantly enhanced in vivo.

The disadvantage of methods that involve implantation of cells tranfected or transduced ex vivo is that there may be a decrease in expressed protein over time as the infected cells undergo apoptosis or migrate. It would be ideal if the scaffold could serve as a vehicle to immobilize gene vectors so that, when implanted, cells migrating to the scaffold and proliferating could take up the gene, and/or surrounding cells could take up the genes released as the scaffold degrades. The DNA vector as well as the transiently expressed therapeutic protein would be retained within the defect site, thereby increasing the opportunity for a maximal therapeutic response and decreasing the likelihood of vector dissemination to surrounding tissue.[52] With time, more endogenous cells could become infected and a prolonged release thus could be maintained over the full duration of tissue regeneration.

These gene-supplemented scaffolds could be particularly beneficial in regenerative medicine applications, because in vitro culture would not be required. A non–cell-seeded gene-supplemented scaffold could be implanted to induce regeneration in vivo.

Several studies have synthesized gene-supplemented scaffolds for treatment of defects in tissues, including bone[44,45] and skin.[46] Matrices loaded with naked DNA encoding for PDGF were shown to provide better transfection for enhancement of tissue formation and vascularization when implanted subcutaneously in Lewis rats, compared with direct injection of plasmid.[46] High initial loading of plasmid DNA within the scaffolds, however, was needed to obtain sufficient transfection.

Although direct loading of either naked plasmid DNA or adenoviral vectors into the scaffold by simple immersion in or injection of a vector solution is the simplest method for gene incorporation within 3-D matrices, a major problem is still rapid vector diffusion from the scaffold, where the majority of the vector is expelled from the matrix within the first 24 hours. Tissue engineering of cutaneous wound repairs may benefit more from these types of matrices, because the healing time for these defects is on the order of weeks.[40,46,52,53] While certain cartilage defects may also benefit from such scaffolds, in other cases a longer period of gene delivery (eg, months) may be required.

One method of gene incorporation that has succeeded in retaining vectors within matrices is by assembly and subsequent fusion of plasmid DNA–loaded polymer microspheres using a gas foaming, particulate leaching process.[54] These scaffolds maintained DNA integrity and

exhibited sustained and gradual controlled release for at least 21 days.

Another method of gene retention within tissue engineering matrices involves mixing adenoviral vectors within collagen gels and injecting the gene-gel complex into a 3-D scaffold.[55] In one study,[55] an adenovirus containing the gene encoding for PDGF-B (AdPDGF-B) was mixed with a collagen gel and injected into a polyvinyl alcohol (PVA) sponge. This construct was compared with injection of an aqueous solution of the gene or injection(s) of the recombinant protein PDGF-B within a PVA sponge for in vivo studies in ischemic excisional wounds. The collagen-immobilized AdPDGF-B/PVA complexes were shown to retain both vector and transgene products within delivery sites for as long as 28 days. In contrast, the aqueous formulations allowed vector seepage from application sites, leading to PDGF-induced hyperplasia in surrounding tissues but not in wound beds. Furthermore, repeated applications of PDGF-B recombinant protein were required for neotissue induction approaching equivalence to a single application of collagen-immobilized AdPDGF-B, confirming the effectiveness and advantage of using gene transfer methods as a means to deliver therapeutic proteins.

The creation of scaffolds that more effectively control and retain gene vectors in a localized area would be very beneficial for tissue repair. For nonviral transfection with naked plasmid DNA, gene retention within a scaffold could increase the opportunity for the plasmid to be taken up by seeded or surrounding cells over time. For viral transduction using scaffolds, undesirable diffusion of viral vectors to surrounding tissues or other parts of the body could be reduced or prevented.

Conclusion

Tissue engineering holds the promise of solutions to a number of compelling clinical problems in dentistry that have not been adequately addressed through the use of permanent replacement devices. The challenge will be to select the optimal combination of biomaterial scaffold, cells, and soluble regulators for a particular clinical problem. For many connective tissues of the musculoskeletal system (including dental tissues), with microstructures that reflect the mechanical environment, it may be more advantageous to regenerate the tissue in vivo than to fully engineer the tissue in vitro for subsequent implantation. The porous materials that serve as the matrices to facilitate this regeneration must have certain pore characteristics, chemical compositions, and mechanical properties. One approach has been to employ substances that serve as analogs of the extracellular matrix of the tissue to be regenerated. In the case of bone, natural bone mineral—anorganic bone—has been shown to be efficacious in several experimental animal and clinical studies. For selected indications in which the supply of endogenous precursor cells has been compromised by disease or prior surgical procedures, it may be necessary to seed the matrix, before implantation, with exogenous cells or to have the matrix serve as a delivery vehicle for growth or differentiation factors or their genes.

Acknowledgments

The author would like to acknowledge the support of the US Departments of Veterans Affairs and Defense for work from which he has drawn this review.

References

1. Spector M. Novel cell-scaffold interactions encountered in tissue engineering: Contractile behavior of musculoskeletal connective tissue cells. Tissue Eng 2002;18:351–357.
2. Bonassar LJ, Vacanti CA. Tissue engineering: The first decade and beyond. J Cell Biochem Suppl 1998;30–31:297–303.
3. Yannas IV, Lee E, Orgill DP, Skrabut EM, Murphy GF. Synthesis and characterization of a model extracellular matrix that induces partial regeneration of adult mammalian skin. Proc Natl Acad Sci U S A 1989;86:933–937.
4. Yannas IV. Biologically active analogues of the extracellular matrix: Artificial skin and nerves. Angew Chem Int Ed Eng 1990;29:20–35.
5. Chamberlain LJ, Yannas IV, Hsu HP, Strichartz GR, Spector M. Near-terminus axonal structure and function following rat sciatic nerve regeneration through a collagen-GAG matrix in a ten-millimeter gap. J Neurosci Res 2000;60:666–677.
6. Wolter JR, Meyer RF. Sessile macrophages forming clear endothelium-like membrane on inside of successful keratoprosthesis. Trans Am Ophthalmol Soc 1984; 82:187–202.
7. Cima LG, Vacanti JP, Vacanti C, Ingber D, Mooney D, Langer R. Tissue engineering by cell transplantation using degradable polymer substrates. J Biomech Eng 1991; 113:143–151.
8. Langer R, Vacanti JP. Tissue engineering. Science 1993;260:920–926.
9. Damien CJ, Parsons JR. Bone graft and bone graft substitutes: A review of current technology and applications. J Appl Biomater 1991;2:187–208.
10. Bucholz RW, Carlton A, Holmes RE. Hydroxyapatite and tricalcium phosphate bone graft substitutes. Orthop Clin North Am 1987;30:19–67.
11. Orr TE, Villars PA, Mitchell SL, Hsu HP, Spector M. Compressive properties of cancellous bone defects in a rabbit model treated with particles of natural bone mineral and synthetic hydroxyapatite. Biomaterials 2001;22:1953–1959.
12. Agrawal CM, Ray RB. Biodegradable polymeric scaffolds for musculoskeletal tissue engineering. J Biomed Mater Res 2001;55:141–150.
13. Hutmacher DW. Scaffold design and fabrication technologies for engineering tissues—State of the art and future perspectives. J Biomater Sci Polym Ed 2001;12:107–124.
14. Zhang S. Fabrication of novel biomaterials through molecular self-assembly. Nat Biotechnol 2003;21:1171–1178.
15. Liao SS, Cui FZ, Zhang W, Feng QL. Hierarchically biomimetic bone scaffold materials: Nano-HA/collagen/PLA composite. J Biomed Mater Res 2004;69B: 158–165.
16. Sun W, Yan Y, Lin F, Spector M. Biomanufacturing: A US-China National Science Foundation-Sponsored Workshop. Tissue Eng 2006;12:1169–1181.
17. Nentwig GH, Gassner A. 2.5 years of clinical experience in the therapy of cystic alveolar defects with a spongious bovine hydroxyapatite material. In: Heimke G (ed). Bioceramics. Cologne, Germany: German Ceramic Society, 1990:383–390.
18. Spector M. Anorganic bovine bone and ceramic analogs of bone mineral as implants to facilitate bone regeneration. Clin Plastic Surg 1994;21:437–444.
19. Jensen SS, Aaboe M, Pinholt EM, Hjørting-Hansen E, Melsen F, Ruyter IE. Tissue reaction and material characteristics of four bone substitutes. Int J Oral Maxillofac Implants 1996;11:55–66.
20. Rosen VB, Hobbs LW, Spector M. The ultrastructure of anorganic bovine bone and selected hydroxyapatites used as bone graft substitute materials. Biomaterials 2002;23:921–928.
21. Clergeau L, Danan M, Clergeau-Guerithault S, Brion M. Healing response to anorganic bone implantation in periodontal intrabony defects in dogs. I. Bone regeneration. A microradiographic study. J Periodontol 1996;67:140–149.
22. Wetzel AC, Stich H, Caffesse RG. Bone apposition onto oral implants in the sinus area filled with different grafting materials. Clin Oral Implants Res 1995;6: 155–163.
23. Klinge B, Alberius P, Isaksson S, Johsson J. Osseous response to implanted natural bone mineral and synthetic hydroxylapatite ceramic in the repair of experimental skull defects. J Oral Maxillofac Surg 1992;50:241–249.
24. Berglundh T, Lindhe J. Healing around implants placed in bone defects treated with Bio-Oss. An experimental study in the dog. Clin Oral Implants Res 1997; 8:117–124.
25. Chu CR, Coutts RD, Yoshioka M, Harwood FL, Monosov AZ, Amiel D. Articular cartilage repair using allogeneic perichondrocyte-seeded biodegradable porous polylactic acid (PLA): A tissue-engineering study. J Biomed Mater Res 1995; 29:1147–1154.
26. Hendrickson DA, Nixon AJ, Grande DA, et al. Chondrocyte-fibrin matrix transplants for resurfacing extensive articular cartilage defects. J Orthop Res 1994;12: 485–497.
27. Wakitani S, Goto T, Pineda SJ, et al. Mesenchymal cell-based repair of large, full-thickness defects of articular cartilage. J Bone Joint Surg Am 1994;76A:579–592.
28. Speer DP, Chvapil M, Volz RG, Holmes MD. Enhancement of healing in osteochondral defects by collagen sponge implantation. Clin Orthop 1979;144: 326–335.
29. Larsen NE, Lombard KM, Parent EG, Balazs EA. Effect of Hylan on cartilage and chondrocyte cultures. J Orthop Res 1992;10:23–32.
30. Burke JF, Yannas IV, Quinby WC, Bondoc CC, Jung WK. Successful use of a physiologically acceptable artificial skin in the treatment of extensive burn injury. Ann Surg 1981;194:413–428.
31. Chang AS, Yannas IV, Perutz S, et al. Electrophysiological study of recovery of peripheral nerves regenerated by a collagen-glycosaminoglycan copolymer matrix. In: Gebelein CG (ed). Progress in Biomedical Polymers. New York: Plenum Press, 1990:107–120.
32. Stone KR, Rodkey WR, Webber RJ, McKinney L, Steadman JR. Future directions. Collagen-based prostheses for meniscal regeneration. Clin Orthop 1990;252: 129–135.
33. Louie LK, Yannas IV, Spector M. Development of a collagen-GAG copolymer implant for the study of tendon regeneration. In: Mikos AG, Murphy RM, Bernstein H, Peppas NA (eds). Biomaterials for Drug and Cell Delivery. Pittsburgh: MRS, 1994:19–24.
34. Brittberg M, Lindahl A, Nilsson A, Ohlsson C, Isaksson O, Peterson L. Treatment of deep cartilage defects in the knee with autologous chondrocyte transplantation. N Engl J Med 1994;331:889–894.
35. Ganey T, Libera J, Moos V, et al. Disc chondrocyte transplantation in a canine model: A treatment for degenerated or damaged intervertebral disc. Spine 2003;28:2609–2620.

36. Cummings BJ, Uchida N, Tamaki SJ, et al. Human neural stem cells differentiate and promote locomotor recovery in spinal cord-injured mice. Proc Nat Acad Sci U S A 2005;102:14069–14074.

37. Stamm C, Westphal B, Kleine HD, et al. Autologous bone-marrow stem-cell transplantation for myocardial regeneration. Lancet 2003;361:45–46.

38. Tomita M, Adachi Y, Yamada H, et al. Bone marrow-derived stem cells can differentiate into retinal cells in injured rat retina. Stem Cells 2002;20:279–283.

39. Caplan AI, Dink DJ, Goto T, et al. Mesenchymal stem cells and tissue repair. In: Jackson DW, Arnoczky SP, Woo SLY, Frank CB, Simon TM (eds). The Anterior Cruciate Ligament: Current and Future Concepts. New York: Raven Press, 1993: 405–417.

40. Samuel RE, Lee CR, Ghivizzani S, et al. Delivery of plasmid DNA to articular chondrocytes via novel collagen-glycosaminoglycan matrices. Hum Gene Ther 2002;13:791–802.

41. O'Connor WJ, Botti T, Khan SN, Lane JM. The use of growth factors in cartilage repair. Orthop Clin North Am 2000;31:399–410.

42. Smith P, Shuler FD, Georgescu HI, et al. Genetic enhancement of matrix synthesis by articular chondrocytes: Comparison of different growth factor genes in the presence and absence of interleukin-1. Arthritis Rheum 2000;43:1156–1164.

43. Cohen H, Levy RJ, Gao J, et al. Sustained delivery and expression of DNA encapsulated in polymeric nanoparticles. Gene Ther 2000;7:1896–1905.

44. Fang J, Zhu YY, Smiley E, et al. Stimulation of new bone formation by direct transfer of osteogenic plasmid genes. Proc Natl Acad Sci U S A 1996;93:5753–5758.

45. Bonadio J, Smiley E, Patil P, Goldstein S. Localized, direct plasmid gene delivery in vivo: Prolonged therapy results in reproducible tissue regeneration. Nat Med 1999;5:753–759.

46. Shea LD, Smiley E, Bonadio J, Mooney DJ. DNA delivery from polymer matrices for tissue engineering. Nat Biotech 1999;17:551–554.

47. Boden SD, Kang J, Sandhu H, Heller JG. Use of recombinant human bone morphogenetic protein-2 to achieve posterolateral lumbar spine fusion in humans: A prospective, randomized clinical pilot trial. Spine 2002;27:2662–2673.

48. Xie Y, Yang ST, Kniss DA. Three-dimensional cell-scaffold constructs promote efficient gene transfection: Implications for cell-based gene therapy. Tissue Eng 2001; 7:585–598.

49. Grande DA, Mason J, Light E, Dines D. Stem cells as platforms for delivery of genes to enhance cartilage repair. J Bone Joint Surg Am 2003;85A(suppl 2): 111–116.

50. Gelse K, von der Mark K, Aigner T, Park J, Schneider H. Articular cartilage repair by gene therapy using growth factor-producing mesenchymal cells. Arthritis Rheum 2003;48:430–441.

51. Madry H, Padera R, Seidel J, et al. Gene transfer of a human insulin-like growth factor I cDNA enhances tissue engineering of cartilage. Hum Gene Ther 2002; 13:1621–1630.

52. Chandler LA, Gu DL, Ma C, et al. Matrix-enabled gene transfer for cutaneous wound repair. Wound Repair Regen 2000;8:473–479.

53. Chandler LA, Doukas J, Gonzalez AM, et al. FGF2-Targeted adenovirus encoding platelet-derived growth factor-B enhances de novo tissue formation. Mol Ther 2000;2:153–160.

54. Jang JH, Shea LD. Controllable delivery of non-viral DNA from porous scaffolds. J Control Release 2003;86:157–168.

55. Doukas J, Chandler LA, Gonzalez AM, et al. Matrix immobilization enhances the tissue repair activity of growth factor gene therapy vectors. Hum Gene Ther 2001;12:783–798.

Advances in Gene Therapy for Periodontal Bioengineering

William V. Giannobile, DDS, DMSc

Periodontal disease is characterized by microbially induced chronic inflammation of tissues that leads to destruction of tooth-supporting structures, including alveolar bone, cementum, and periodontal ligament (PDL). A challenge in the management of periodontitis is the predictable regeneration of tissues lost as a consequence of disease. The application of periodontal regenerative biomaterials, such as bone autografts, allografts, guided tissue regeneration procedures, enamel matrix proteins, and most recently growth factors has been pursued with varying degrees of success to regenerate lost tooth support.[1] Examples of currently available regenerative biomaterials are shown in Box 3-1.

These therapeutic measures demonstrate some success as regenerative biomaterials in clinical practice. Thus far, however, the ability to completely and predictably regenerate damaged periodontal supporting structures has not been achieved in humans. Several key complicating factors that represent challenges to predictable periodontal regeneration are the contamination of periodontal wounds with tooth-associated biofilms of anaerobic bacteria; the nature of the transmucosal hard and soft tissue environment, which allows entry of pathogens into wounds; the existence of multiple junctional complexes and stromal-cellular interactions, creating difficulty in rebuilding tissue interfaces (eg, tooth-PDL-bone and

epithelial tissue–connective tissue–bone); and the effects of occlusal forces that deliver intermittent loads in axial and transverse dimensions.[57,58]

Wound-healing approaches that use growth factors to target restoration of tooth-supporting bone, PDL, and cementum can greatly advance the field of periodontal regenerative medicine. A major focus of periodontal research has evaluated the impact of applied growth factors on periodontal tissue regeneration.[59–61] These reviews describe various delivery systems and applications of growth factors, which are highlighted throughout this book.

Advances in molecular cloning have made available unlimited quantities of recombinant growth factors for applications in tissue engineering. Recombinant growth factors known to promote skin and bone wound healing, such as PDGFs,[42,53,62–64] fibroblast growth factors,[34,65–68] and BMPs,[69–73] have been used in preclinical and human clinical trials for the treatment of large periodontal or intrabony defects as well as around dental implants.[54–56]

The success of these techniques is well documented, but the results are not always predictable, because of limitations imposed by the delivery systems. This chapter discusses the general effects of local delivery of growth factors as well as recent developments in gene therapy to stimulate periodontal engineering.

Local Application of Growth Factors

Therapeutic application of growth factors to restore damaged tissues aims at regeneration through biomimetic processes that occur during embryonic and postnatal development.[74] The complexity of these events suggests that creating an optimal regenerative environment requires a combination of different growth factors found in natural reparative processes. The use of a single recombinant growth factor may also induce several molecular, biochemical, and morphologic cascades that will result in tissue regeneration.

In the periodontium, regenerative treatment has been a challenge because of the morphologic and functional specificities of each component of tooth-supporting tissues. The growth factors most thoroughly studied for periodontal regeneration have been PDGF, insulin-like growth factor I (IGF-I), fibroblast growth factor 2, transforming growth factor β, and different BMPs.

PDGF has been evaluated in both preclinical periodontal and peri-implant regenerative studies. Proliferation, migration, and matrix synthesis were observed on cultures of periodontal cells stimulated by PDGF, including gingival and PDL fibroblasts, cementoblasts, preosteoblasts, and osteoblastic cells.[64,75–79] These effects were shown to be time and dose dependent.[64]

The PDGF family is composed of four growth factors: PDGF-A, PDGF-B, PDGF-C, and PDGF-D. All of them participate in the wound-healing process. The signal transduction pathway of PDGF binding and the elicitation of intracellular effects is shown in Fig 3-1. PDGF-BB is the most effective isoform, and its effect on PDL cell mitogenesis and matrix biosynthesis is well studied.[80,81] Several preclinical studies have been performed using the combination of PDGF-BB and IGF-I for periodontal and peri-implant bone regeneration.[40,41,43,62,82–84] In a human phase I and phase II clinical trial, a combination of PDGF and IGF-I was considered safe when applied topically to periodontal osseous lesions, resulting in a significant improvement in bone growth and fill of periodontal defects compared with open flap debridement.[40]

The use of PDGF-BB combined with various delivery systems has been studied in several case series and in a randomized, controlled trial.[53,63,85] In a multicenter phase III clinical trial of 180 patients possessing periodontal intrabony defects, the effectiveness of rhPDGF-BB associated with synthetic β-tricalcium phosphate was evaluated.[53] The results demonstrated that the use of rhPDGF-BB is safe and improves bone fill and the rate of clinical attachment level gain.

To better determine the mechanisms of PDGF-induced periodontal regeneration, an investigation was performed to examine the effects of rhPDGF-BB on the release of the bone turnover biomarker, the C-terminal telopeptide of type I collagen (ICTP).[86] Periodontal wound fluid was harvested from sites treated by rhPDGF-BB in a subgroup of 47 patients. Defects receiving local delivery of rhPDGF-BB demonstrated greater bone turnover, as measured by early, elevated levels of ICTP emanating from the wounds during healing.

In another substudy, 16 patients were evaluated for fluid levels of the angiogenic factor vascular endothelial growth factor (VEGF) released from periodontal wound sites following rhPDGF-BB delivery.[87] Levels of VEGF were potently increased during the first 2 weeks after rhPDGF-BB application. Taken together, these two studies

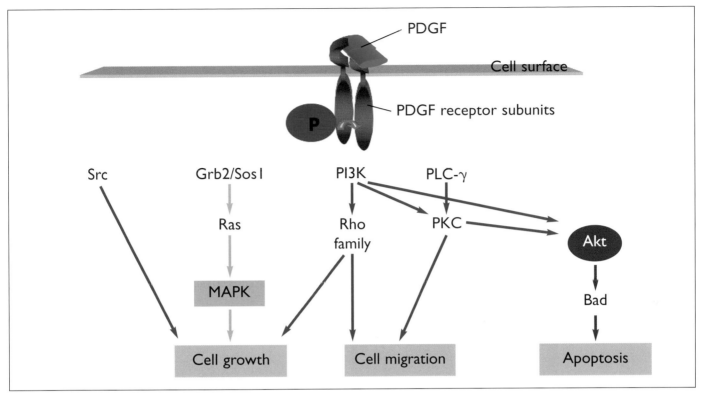

Fig 3-1 PDGF signal transduction. Dimeric extracellular PDGF receptors bind PDGF dimers and transduce intracellular tyrosine kinase phosphorylation with subsequent targeting of cellular activities, including cell growth, chemotaxis, or blocking cell death (apoptosis). (P) Phospho-protein activation sites; (Grb2) growth factor receptor-bound protein 2; (Sos1) son of sevenless 1; (MAPK) mitogen-activated protein kinase, (PI3K) phosphoinositol 3 kinase; (PLC-γ) phospholipase C gamma; (PKC) protein kinase C; (Bad) Bcl-2-associated death promoter protein.

aid in the better understanding of PDGF-mediated peri-odontal regeneration by demonstrating the ability of rhPDGF-BB to (1) stimulate angiogenesis by increasing local VEGF production; and (2) stimulate bone turnover via ICTP release at the early stage of periodontal wound repair.

Application of Gene Therapy

Rationale and delivery strategies

In general, topical delivery of growth factors to periodon-tal wounds has been shown to have promising impact, yet some limitations for the promotion of predictable peri-odontal tissue engineering.[59,63] Growth factor proteins, once delivered to the target lesion, tend to suffer from

instability and quick dilution, presumably because of pro-teolytic breakdown, receptor-mediated endocytosis, and solubility of the carrier matrix.[58] Because the half-lives of locally applied growth factors are significantly reduced in vivo, the period of exposure may not be sufficient to act on osteoblasts, cementoblasts, or PDL cells. Therefore, dif-ferent methods of growth factor delivery have been con-sidered[88] (Fig 3-2).

Investigations have examined a variety of approaches combining scaffolds with growth factors to target the defect site in order to optimize bioavailability.[90] The scaf-folds are designed to optimize the dosage of the growth factor and to control its release pattern, which may be pulsatile, constant, or time programmed.[91] Additionally, the kinetics of the release and the duration of the expo-sure of the growth factor may be better controlled.[92]

To address the transient bioactivity of growth factor peptides in vivo, gene therapy approaches using gene transfer vectors that encode growth factors have been used to stimulate periodontal engineering (see Fig 3-2).

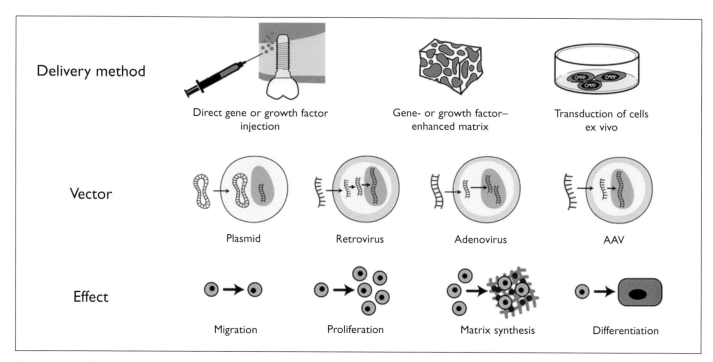

Fig 3-2 Gene therapy approaches. *(top)* DNA and growth factors can be delivered to cells through different mechanisms, including direct injection to an in vivo site, transport to a site via a carrier matrix, or introduction ex vivo prior to cell transplantation. *(middle)* Genetic material can be transferred to cells through different vectors, the most common of which are plasmids, retroviruses, adenoviruses, and adeno-associated viruses (AAV). *(bottom)* Gene therapy strategies aim to modulate cellular proliferation, migration, matrix synthesis, and differentiation. (Adapted from Kaigler et al.[89] Used with permission.)

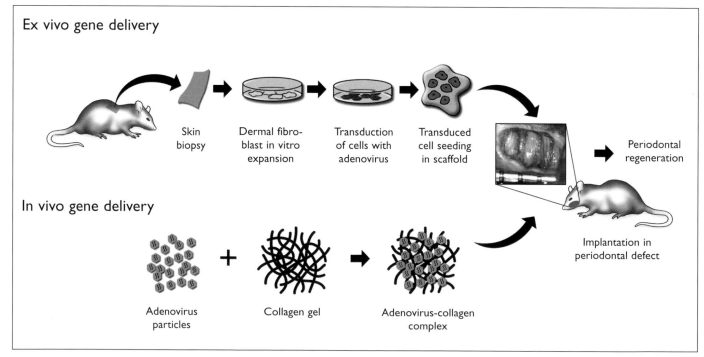

Fig 3-3 Gene delivery approaches for periodontal tissue engineering. Ex vivo gene delivery involves the harvesting of tissue biopsies, expansion of cell populations, genetic manipulations of cells, and subsequent transplantation to periodontal osseous defects. The in vivo gene transfer approach involves the direct delivery of growth factor transgenes to the periodontal osseous defects. (From Ramseier et al.[61] Reprinted with permission.)

Fig 3-4 PDGF-B gene transfer stimulates ex vivo gingival defect fill. Standardized digital images show human gingival fibroblasts filling in the wound area 10 days after no treatment (a); or after treatment with a control gene therapy vector, ie, green fluorescent protein (b); adenovirus encoding PDGF-A (c); or adenovirus vector encoding PDGF B (d). N = 4 defects per group (original magnification ×20). (From Anusaksathien et al.[102] Reprinted with permission.)

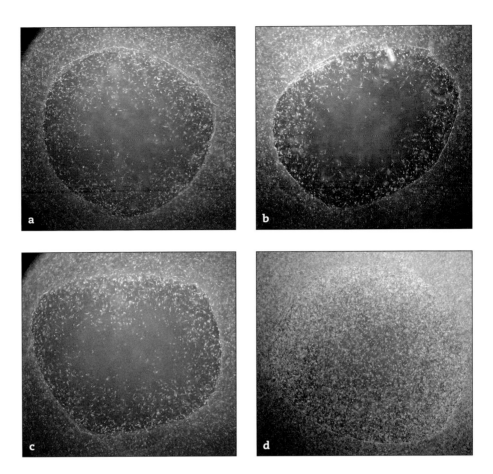

Thus far, two main strategies of gene vector delivery have been applied to periodontal regenerative medicine. Gene vectors can be introduced directly to the target site (in vivo approach)[93] or selected cells can be harvested, expanded, genetically transduced, and then reimplanted (ex vivo technique)[36] (Fig 3-3). In vivo gene transfer involves the insertion of the gene of interest directly into the defect, promoting genetic modification of the target cell. Ex vivo gene transfer includes the incorporation of genetic material into cells exposed from a tissue biopsy and subsequent transplantation into the recipient.

Results

Gene transfer strategies for tissue engineering have demonstrated success in healing soft tissues such as skin wounds.[94,95] Both PDGF plasmid[96] and PDGF adenoviral[97] vectors have been evaluated in preclinical and human trials. However, the latter has exhibited more robust results favorable for clinical use.[98]

Early studies in dental applications using recombinant adenoviral vectors encoding PDGF showed that vector constructs can transduce cells derived from the periodontium (osteoblasts, cementoblasts, PDL cells, and gingival fibroblasts).[99,100] Additionally, Chen and Giannobile[101] were able to demonstrate the sustained effects of adenoviral delivery of PDGF for the better understanding of extended PDGF signaling. In an ex vivo investigation, it was shown that the expression of PDGF genes was prolonged for up to 10 days in gingival wounds (Fig 3-4). An adenovirus encoding PDGF-B (AdPDGF-B) transduced gingival fibroblasts and enhanced defect fill by induction of human gingival fibroblast migration and proliferation.[102]

However, in another study, continuous exposure of cementoblasts to PDGF-A had an inhibitory effect on cementum mineralization, possibly via the upregulation of osteopontin and subsequent enhancement of multinucleated giant cells in cementum-engineered scaffolds. Furthermore, an adenovirus encoding PDGF-1308 (a dominant-negative mutant of PDGF-A) inhibited mineral-

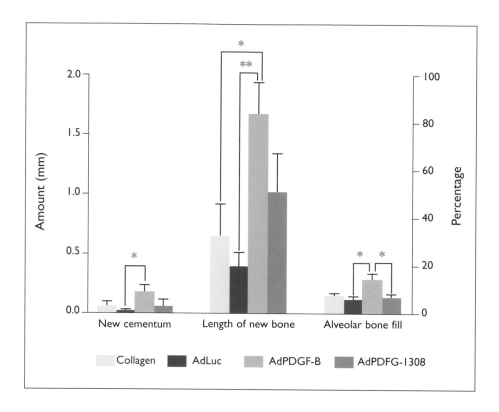

Fig 3-5 PDGF gene delivery promotes periodontal tissue engineering. Histomorphometric analysis of specimens was carried out 14 days after surgery and gene delivery. Treatment with AdPDGF-B increased cementum formation when compared to treatment with adenovirus-encoding luciferase (AdLuc) (*P < .05). Furthermore, AdPDGF-B treatment not only improved the bridging length of newly formed alveolar bone when compared to treatment with AdLuc (**P < .01) and collagen matrix alone (*P < .05) but also enhanced the percentage of alveolar bone fill when compared to treatment with AdLuc and treatment with adenovirus encoding a dominant negative mutant of PDGF-A (AdPDGF-1308) (*P < .05). N = 6 to 8 specimens per group. (From Jin et al.[93] Reprinted with permission.)

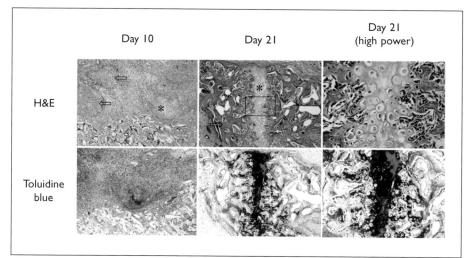

Fig 3-6 Gene transfer of BMP-7 leads to bone regeneration through a cartilage intermediate. Periodontal osseous defects were treated with syngeneic dermal fibroblasts transduced by adenovirus encoding BMP-7 delivered in gelatin scaffolds. Specimens demonstrate evidence of islands of cartilage and chrondroblast-like cells (day 10) or bone-like tissue (day 21). Note the presence of immature woven bone (*arrows*) and an island of cartilage (*) at day 10. At day 21, more mature cartilage (*) is associated intimately with newly formed bone (*arrow*) that is consistent with chondroblasts and a cartilaginous matrix (*right*) (hematoxylin-eosin [H&E] and toluidine blue stain; original magnification ×10, left and center columns; original magnification ×20, right column). (From Jin et al.[36] Reprinted with permission.)

ization of tissue-engineered cementum possibly due to downregulation of bone sialoprotein and osteocalcin and persistent stimulation of multinucleated giant cells. These findings suggest that continuous exogenous delivery of PDGF-A may delay mineral formation induced by cementoblasts, while PDGF is clearly required for mineral neogenesis.[39]

Jin et al[93] demonstrated that direct in vivo gene transfer of PDGF-B stimulated tissue regeneration in large periodontal defects. Descriptive histology and histomorphometry revealed that human PDGF-B gene delivery promotes the regeneration of both cementum and alveolar bone, while PDGF-1308 has minimal effects on periodontal tissue regeneration (Fig 3-5).

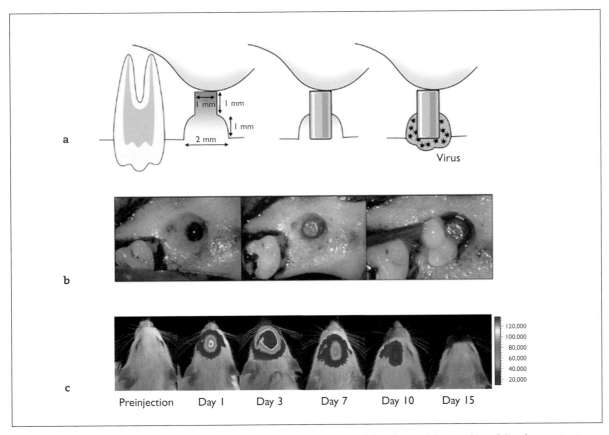

Fig 3-7 Gene targeting model to evaluate osseointegration of dental implants. (*a*) In a dental implant osteotomy defect model for gene delivery, well-type osteotomy defects that measured 1 mm in depth and 2 mm coronally were created (*left*). The titanium dental implant was press fitted into position (*center*), and the 2.6% collagen matrix containing either adenovirus/BMP-7 or adenovirus/luciferase was delivered (*right*). (*b*) Corresponding photographs from the surgical operation, including defect creation (*left*), dental implant placement (*center*), and gene delivery (*right*). (*c*) In vivo bioluminescence images of a luciferase-treated rat. Dorsal images were taken from 15 to 25 minutes postinjection. To localize the signal, color images of the photon emissions were superimposed on grayscale images of the animals, and signals were quantified in relative light unit. Distribution of gene delivery is shown beginning at day 1; the peak expression is at day 3. In this case, transgene expression was sustained at measurable levels for 10 days. (From Dunn et al.[103] Reprinted with permission.)

The ex vivo delivery of BMP-7–transduced fibroblasts in a gelatin matrix promoted periodontal tissue repair in large mandibular osseous defects.[36] BMP-7 gene transfer not only enhanced alveolar bone repair but also stimulated cementogenesis and PDL fiber formation. The alveolar bone formation was found to occur via a cartilage intermediate (Fig 3-6). However, when genes encoding the BMP antagonist, noggin, were delivered, periodontal tissue formation was inhibited.[36,38] Dunn et al[103] recently demonstrated that direct in vivo gene delivery of BMP-7 in a collagen matrix promoted regeneration of extraction socket bone defects around dental implants (Fig 3-7). These experiments provide promising evidence showing the feasibility of both in vivo and ex vivo gene therapy for periodontal tissue regeneration and peri-implant osseointegration.

Application of Cell Therapy

The transplantation of periodontal stem cells or more mature cell populations has been examined for the potential to reconstruct periodontal tooth support.[104–106] Certainly there is significant potential for the use of stem cells in periodontal repair, and this is reviewed elsewhere.[1] Transplantation of cells derived from the periodontal ligament have shown potential to regenerate periodontal attachment structures in vivo.[107–111] Cementoblasts or tooth-lining cells have a marked ability to induce mineralization in an ex vivo model to tissue engineer cementum[37] and in vivo in periodontal wounds.[112] However, when less differentiated dental follicle cells are delivered in a similar delivery system, these cells inhibit periodontal healing.[112] Of significant interest, periodontal stem cells have been shown to be able to promote the formation of cementum-like mineralized tissue ex vivo.[113,114]

In terms of soft tissue regeneration, the use of allogeneic foreskin fibroblasts has been recently demonstrated to promote clinical new attachment of recessed gingival[115] and furcation[116] defects.

Conclusion

Significant progress has been made over the past decade in the reconstruction of complex periodontal and alveolar bone wounds resulting from periodontal or peri-implant disease. Developments in scaffolding matrices for cell, protein, and gene delivery have demonstrated significant potential to provide biomaterials that can interact with the matrix, cells, and bioactive factors. The targeting of growth factors to the periodontium and peri-implant structures has led to significant new knowledge of the factors that promote cellular replication, differentiation, matrix biosynthesis, and angiogenesis.

A major challenge that has been less studied is the modulation of the exuberant host response to microbial infection that contaminates and complicates the periodontal and oral wound microenvironment. In addition, in the future, clinical researchers will have to consider the following areas to advance tissue engineering of the periodontium: improved delivery methods[117]; dual and multifactor release of regenerative and anti-inflammatory molecules; and three-dimensional reconstruction of anatomic defects.[118]

Acknowledgments

This work has been supported by NIH/NIDCR Grants DE 13397 and DE 16619 and the Swiss OA Foundation. The author would like to acknowledge Dr Joni Cirelli, Dr Qiming Jin, Dr Darnell Kaigler, Jr, and Dr Christoph Ramseier for their contributions to research cited in this article.

References

1. Slavkin HC, Bartold PM. Challenges and potential in tissue engineering. Periodontol 2000 2006;41:9–15.
2. Blumenthal NM, Koh-Kunst G, Alves ME, et al. Effect of surgical implantation of recombinant human bone morphogenetic protein-2 in a bioabsorbable collagen sponge or calcium phosphate putty carrier in intrabony periodontal defects in the baboon. J Periodontol 2002;73:1494–1506.
3. Russell JL. Grafton demineralized bone matrix: Performance consistency, utility, and value. Tissue Eng 2000;6:435–440.
4. Anderegg CR, Martin SJ, Gray JL, Mellonig JT, Gher ME. Clinical evaluation of the use of decalcified freeze-dried bone allograft with guided tissue regeneration in the treatment of molar furcation invasions. J Periodontol 1991;62:264–268.
5. Gager AH, Schultz AJ. Treatment of periodontal defects with an absorbable membrane (polyglactin 910) with and without osseous grafting: Case reports. J Periodontol 1991;62:276–283.
6. Rummelhart JM, Mellonig JT, Gray JL, Towle HJ. A comparison of freeze-dried bone allograft and demineralized freeze-dried bone allograft in human periodontal osseous defects. J Periodontol 1989;60:655–663.
7. Bowers GM, Chadroff B, Carnevale R, et al. Histologic evaluation of new attachment apparatus formation in humans. 3. J Periodontol 1989;60:683–693.
8. Mellonig JT. Human histologic evaluation of a bovine-derived bone xenograft in the treatment of periodontal osseous defects. Int J Periodontics Restorative Dent 2000;20:19–29.
9. Richardson CR, Mellonig JT, Brunsvold MA, McDonnell HT, Cochran DL. Clinical evaluation of Bio-Oss: A bovine-derived xenograft for the treatment of periodontal osseous defects in humans. J Clin Periodontol 1999;26:421–428.
10. Camelo M, Nevins ML, Schenk RK, et al. Clinical, radiographic, and histologic evaluation of human periodontal defects treated with Bio-Oss and Bio-Gide. Int J Periodontics Restorative Dent 1998;18:321–331.
11. Camelo M, Nevins ML, Lynch SE, Schenk RK, Simion M, Nevins M. Periodontal regeneration with an autogenous bone-Bio-Oss composite graft and a Bio-Gide membrane. Int J Periodontics Restorative Dent 2001;21:109–119.
12. Nevins ML, Camelo M, Lynch SE, Schenk RK, Nevins M. Evaluation of periodontal regeneration following grafting intrabony defects with Bio-Oss collagen: A human histologic report. Int J Periodontics Restorative Dent 2003;23:9–17.
13. Yukna RA, Callan DP, Krauser JT, et al. Multi-center clinical evaluation of combination anorganic bovine-derived hydroxyapatite matrix (ABM)/cell binding peptide (P-15) as a bone replacement graft material in human periodontal osseous defects. 6-month results. J Periodontol 1998;69:655–663.
14. Yukna R, Salinas TJ, Carr RF. Periodontal regeneration following use of ABM/P-15: A case report. Int J Periodontics Restorative Dent 2002;22:146–155.
15. Yukna RA, Mayer ET, Amos SM. 5-year evaluation of durapatite ceramic alloplastic implants in periodontal osseous defects. J Periodontol 1989;60:544–551.
16. Stahl SS, Froum SJ. Histologic and clinical responses to porous hydroxylapatite implants in human periodontal defects. Three to twelve months postimplantation. J Periodontol 1987;58:689–695.
17. Yukna RA, Harrison BG, Caudill RF, Evans GH, Mayer ET, Miller S. Evaluation of durapatite ceramic as an alloplastic implant in periodontal osseous defects. 2. Twelve month reentry results. J Periodontol 1985;56:540–547.
18. Rabalais ML Jr, Yukna RA, Mayer ET. Evaluation of durapatite ceramic as an alloplastic implant in periodontal osseous defects. 1. Initial six-month results. J Periodontol 1981;52:680–689.
19. Saffar JL, Colombier ML, Detienville R. Bone formation in tricalcium phosphate-filled periodontal intrabony lesions. Histological observations in humans. J Periodontol 1990;61:209–216.
20. Stahl SS, Froum S. Histological evaluation of human intraosseous healing responses to the placement of tricalcium phosphate ceramic implants. 1. Three to eight months. J Periodontol 1986;57:211–217.
21. Trombelli L, Heitz-Mayfield LJ, Needleman I, Moles D, Scabbia A. A systematic review of graft materials and biological agents for periodontal intraosseous defects. J Clin Periodontol 2002;29(suppl 3):117–135; discussion 60–62.
22. Rafter M, Baker M, Alves M, Daniel J, Remeikis N. Evaluation of healing with use of an internal matrix to repair furcation perforations. Int Endod J 2002;35:775–783.
23. Wikesjö UM, Sorensen RG, Kinoshita A, Wozney JM. RhBMP-2/alphaBSM induces significant vertical alveolar ridge augmentation and dental implant osseointegration. Clin Implant Dent Relat Res 2002;4:174–182.

24. Stahl SS, Froum SJ, Tarnow D. Human clinical and histologic responses to the placement of HTR polymer particles in 11 intrabony lesions. J Periodontol 1990;61:269–274.

25. Yukna RA, Yukna CN. Six-year clinical evaluation of HTR synthetic bone grafts in human grade II molar furcations. J Periodontal Res 1997;32:627–633.

26. Yukna RA, Evans GH, Aichelmann-Reidy MB, Mayer ET. Clinical comparison of bioactive glass bone replacement graft material and expanded polytetrafluoroethylene barrier membrane in treating human mandibular molar class II furcations. J Periodontol 2001;72:125–133.

27. Nevins ML, Camelo M, Nevins M, et al. Human histologic evaluation of bioactive ceramic in the treatment of periodontal osseous defects. Int J Periodontics Restorative Dent 2000;20:458–467.

28. Yukna RA, Yukna CN. A 5-year follow-up of 16 patients treated with coralline calcium carbonate (Biocoral) bone replacement grafts in infrabony defects. J Clin Periodontol 1998;25:1036–1040.

29. Kim CK, Choi EJ, Cho KS, Chai JK, Wikesjö UM. Periodontal repair in intrabony defects treated with a calcium carbonate implant and guided tissue regeneration. J Periodontol 1996;67:1301–1306.

30. Mora F, Ouhayoun JP. Clinical evaluation of natural coral and porous hydroxyapatite implants in periodontal bone lesions: Results of a 1-year follow-up. J Clin Periodontol 1995;22:877–884.

31. Hanisch O, Sorensen RG, Kinoshita A, Spiekermann H, Wozney JM, Wikesjö UM. Effect of recombinant human bone morphogenetic protein-2 in dehiscence defects with non-submerged immediate implants: an experimental study in Cynomolgus monkeys. J Periodontol 2003;74:648–657.

32. Selvig KA, Sorensen RG, Wozney JM, Wikesjö UM. Bone repair following recombinant human bone morphogenetic protein-2 stimulated periodontal regeneration. J Periodontol 2002;73:1020–1029.

33. Choi SH, Kim CK, Cho KS, et al. Effect of recombinant human bone morphogenetic protein-2/absorbable collagen sponge (rhBMP-2/ACS) on healing in 3-wall intrabony defects in dogs. J Periodontol 2002;73:63–72.

34. Giannobile WV, Ryan S, Shih MS, Su DL, Kaplan PL, Chan TC. Recombinant human osteogenic protein-1 (OP-1) stimulates periodontal wound healing in class III furcation defects. J Periodontol 1998;69:129–137.

35. Ripamonti U, Heliotis M, Rueger DC, Sampath TK. Induction of cementogenesis by recombinant human osteogenic protein-1 (hop-1/bmp-7) in the baboon (Papio ursinus). Arch Oral Biol 1996;41:121–126.

36. Jin QM, Anusaksathien O, Webb SA, Rutherford RB, Giannobile WV. Gene therapy of bone morphogenetic protein for periodontal tissue engineering. J Periodontol 2003;74:202–213.

37. Jin Q, Zhao M, Webb SA, Berry JE, Somerman MJ, Giannobile WV. Cementum engineering with three-dimensional polymer scaffolds. J Biomed Mater Res A 2003;67:54–60.

38. Jin QM, Zhao M, Economides AN, Somerman MJ, Giannobile WV. Noggin gene delivery inhibits cementoblast-induced mineralization. Connect Tissue Res 2004;45:50–59.

39. Anusaksathien O, Jin QM, Zhao M, Somerman MJ, Giannobile WV. Effect of sustained delivery of platelet-derived growth factor (PDGF) or its antagonist (PDGF-1308) on tissue-engineered cementum. J Periodontol 2004;75:429–440.

40. Howell TH, Fiorellini JP, Paquette DW, Offenbacher S, Giannobile WV, Lynch SE. A phase I/II clinical trial to evaluate a combination of recombinant human platelet-derived growth factor-BB and recombinant human insulin-like growth factor-I in patients with periodontal disease. J Periodontol 1997;68:1186–1193.

41. Giannobile WV, Hernandez RA, Finkelman RD, et al. Comparative effects of platelet-derived growth factor-BB and insulin-like growth factor-I, individually and in combination, on periodontal regeneration in Macaca fascicularis. J Periodontal Res 1996;31:301–312.

42. Rutherford RB, Niekrash CE, Kennedy JE, Charette MF. Platelet-derived and insulin-like growth factors stimulate regeneration of periodontal attachment in monkeys. J Periodontal Res 1992;27(4 pt 1):285–290.

43. Lynch SE, Williams RC, Polson AM, et al. A combination of platelet-derived and insulin-like growth factors enhances periodontal regeneration. J Clin Periodontol 1989;16:545–548.

44. Wikesjö UM, Lim WH, Thomson RC, Cook AD, Wozney JM, Hardwick WR. Periodontal repair in dogs: Evaluation of a bioabsorbable space-providing macroporous membrane with recombinant human bone morphogenetic protein-2. J Periodontol 2003;74:635–647.

45. Park YJ, Lee YM, Park SN, Sheen SY, Chung CP, Lee SJ. Platelet derived growth factor releasing chitosan sponge for periodontal bone regeneration. Biomaterials 2000;21:153–159.

46. Scheyer ET, Velasquez-Plata D, Brunsvold MA, Lasho DJ, Mellonig JT. A clinical comparison of a bovine-derived xenograft used alone and in combination with enamel matrix derivative for the treatment of periodontal osseous defects in humans. J Periodontol 2002;73:423–432.

47. Okuda K, Momose M, Miyazaki A, et al. Enamel matrix derivative in the treatment of human intrabony osseous defects. J Periodontol 2000;71:1821–1828.

48. Parashis A, Tsiklakis K. Clinical and radiographic findings following application of enamel matrix derivative in the treatment of intrabony defects. A series of case reports. J Clin Periodontol 2000;27:705–713.

49. Parodi R, Liuzzo G, Patrucco P, et al. Use of Emdogain in the treatment of deep intrabony defects: 12-month clinical results. Histologic and radiographic evaluation. Int J Periodontics Restorative Dent 2000;20:584–595.

50. Rasperini G, Silvestri M, Schenk RK, Nevins ML. Clinical and histologic evaluation of human gingival recession treated with a subepithelial connective tissue graft and enamel matrix derivative (Emdogain): A case report. Int J Periodontics Restorative Dent 2000;20:269–275.

51. Sculean A, Chiantella GC, Windisch P, Donos N. Clinical and histologic evaluation of human intrabony defects treated with an enamel matrix protein derivative (Emdogain). Int J Periodontics Restorative Dent 2000;20:374–381.

52. Pontoriero R, Wennstrom J, Lindhe J. The use of barrier membranes and enamel matrix proteins in the treatment of angular bone defects. A prospective controlled clinical study. J Clin Periodontol 1999;26:833–840.

53. Nevins M, Giannobile WV, McGuire MK, et al. Platelet-derived growth factor stimulates bone fill and rate of attachment level gain: Results of a large multicenter randomized controlled trial. J Periodontol 2005;76:2205–2215.

54. Cochran DL, Jones AA, Lilly LC, Fiorellini JP, Howell H. Evaluation of recombinant human bone morphogenetic protein-2 in oral applications including the use of endosseous implants: 3-year results of a pilot study in humans. J Periodontol 2000;71:1241–1257.

55. Fiorellini JP, Howell TH, Cochran D, et al. Randomized study evaluating recombinant human bone morphogenetic protein-2 for extraction socket augmentation. J Periodontol 2005;76:605–613.

56. Howell TH, Fiorellini J, Jones A, et al. A feasibility study evaluating rhBMP-2/absorbable collagen sponge device for local alveolar ridge preservation or augmentation. Int J Periodontics Restorative Dent 1997;17:124–139.

57. McCulloch CA. Basic considerations in periodontal wound healing to achieve regeneration. Periodontol 2000 1993;1:16–25.

58. Anusaksathien O, Giannobile WV. Growth factor delivery to re-engineer periodontal tissues. Curr Pharm Biotechnol 2002;3:129–139.

59. Cochran DL, Wozney JM. Biological mediators for periodontal regeneration. Periodontol 2000 1999;19:40–58.

60. Nakashima M, Reddi AH. The application of bone morphogenetic proteins to dental tissue engineering. Nat Biotechnol 2003;21:1025–1032.

61. Ramseier CA, Abramson ZR, Jin Q, Giannobile WV. Gene therapeutics for periodontal regenerative medicine. Dent Clin North Am 2006;50:245–263.

62. Giannobile WV, Finkelman RD, Lynch SE. Comparison of canine and non-human primate animal models for periodontal regenerative therapy: results following a single administration of PDGF/IGF-I. J Periodontol 1994;65:1158–1168.

63. Camelo M, Nevins ML, Schenk RK, Lynch SE, Nevins M. Periodontal regeneration in human Class II furcations using purified recombinant human platelet-derived growth factor-BB (rhPDGF-BB) with bone allograft. Int J Periodontics Restorative Dent 2003;23:213–225.

64. Ojima Y, Mizuno M, Kuboki Y, Komori T. In vitro effect of platelet-derived growth factor-BB on collagen synthesis and proliferation of human periodontal ligament cells. Oral Dis 2003;9:144–151.

65. Murakami S, Takayama S, Kitamura M, Shimabukuro Y, Yanagi K, Ikezawa K, et al. Recombinant human basic fibroblast growth factor (bFGF) stimulates periodontal regeneration in class II furcation defects created in beagle dogs. J Periodontal Res 2003;38:97–103.

66. Sigurdsson TJ, Lee MB, Kubota K, Turek TJ, Wozney JM, Wikesjö UM. Periodontal repair in dogs: Recombinant human bone morphogenetic protein-2 significantly enhances periodontal regeneration. J Periodontol 1995;66:131–138.

67. Takayama S, Murakami S, Shimabukuro Y, Kitamura M, Okada H. Periodontal regeneration by FGF-2 (bFGF) in primate models. J Dent Res 2001;80:2075–2079.

68. Terranova VP, Odziemiec C, Tweden KS, Spadone DP. Repopulation of dentin surfaces by periodontal ligament cells and endothelial cells. Effect of basic fibroblast growth factor. J Periodontol 1989;60:293–301.

69. Huang KK, Shen C, Chiang CY, Hsieh YD, Fu E. Effects of bone morphogenetic protein-6 on periodontal wound healing in a fenestration defect of rats. J Periodontal Res 2005;40:1–10.

70. Wikesjö UM, Qahash M, Thomson RC, et al. rhBMP-2 significantly enhances guided bone regeneration. Clin Oral Implants Res 2004;15:194–204.

71. Wikesjö UM, Sorensen RG, Kinoshita A, Jian Li X, Wozney JM. Periodontal repair in dogs: Effect of recombinant human bone morphogenetic protein-12 (rhBMP-12) on regeneration of alveolar bone and periodontal attachment. J Clin Periodontol 2004;31:662–670.

72. Sorensen RG, Wikesjo UM, Kinoshita A, Wozney JM. Periodontal repair in dogs: Evaluation of a bioresorbable calcium phosphate cement (Ceredex) as a carrier for rhBMP-2. J Clin Periodontol 2004;31:796–804.

73. Gao Y, Yang L, Fang YR, Mori M, Kawahara K, Tanaka A. The inductive effect of bone morphogenetic protein (BMP) on human periodontal fibroblast-like cells in vitro. J Osaka Dent Univ 1995;29:9–17.

74. Schilephake H. Bone growth factors in maxillofacial skeletal reconstruction. Int J Oral Maxillofac Surg 2002;31:469–484.

75. Nishimura F, Terranova VP. Comparative study of the chemotactic responses of periodontal ligament cells and gingival fibroblasts to polypeptide growth factors. J Dent Res 1996;75:986–992.

76. Saygin NE, Tokiyasu Y, Giannobile WV, Somerman MJ. Growth factors regulate expression of mineral associated genes in cementoblasts. J Periodontol 2000;71:1591–1600.

77. Strayhorn CL, Garrett JS, Dunn RL, Benedict JJ, Somerman MJ. Growth factors regulate expression of osteoblast-associated genes. J Periodontol 1999;70:1345–1354.

78. Canalis E. Effect of platelet-derived growth factor on DNA and protein synthesis in cultured rat calvaria. Metabolism 1981;30:970–975.

79. Bartold PM, Raben A. Growth factor modulation of fibroblasts in simulated wound healing. J Periodontal Res 1996;31:205–216.

80. Boyan LA, Bhargava G, Nishimura F, Orman R, Price R, Terranova VP. Mitogenic and chemotactic responses of human periodontal ligament cells to the different isoforms of platelet-derived growth factor. J Dent Res 1994;73:1593–1600.

81. Matsuda N, Lin WL, Kumar NM, Cho MI, Genco RJ. Mitogenic, chemotactic, and synthetic responses of rat periodontal ligament fibroblastic cells to polypeptide growth factors in vitro. J Periodontol 1992;63:515–525.

82. Lynch SE, Buser D, Hernandez RA, et al. Effects of the platelet-derived growth factor/insulin-like growth factor-I combination on bone regeneration around titanium dental implants. Results of a pilot study in beagle dogs. J Periodontol 1991;62:710–716.

83. Lynch SE, de Castilla GR, Williams RC, et al. The effects of short-term application of a combination of platelet-derived and insulin-like growth factors on periodontal wound healing. J Periodontol 1991;62:458–467.

84. Stefani CM, Machado MA, Sallum EA, Sallum AW, Toledo S, Nociti FH Jr. Platelet-derived growth factor/insulin-like growth factor-I combination and bone regeneration around implants placed into extraction sockets: A histometric study in dogs. Implant Dent 2000;9:126–131.

85. Nevins M, Camelo M, Nevins ML, Schenk RK, Lynch SE. Periodontal regeneration in humans using recombinant human platelet-derived growth factor-BB (rhPDGF-BB) and allogenic bone. J Periodontol 2003;74:1282–1292.

86. Sarment DP, Cooke JW, Miller SE, et al. Effect of rhPDGF-BB on bone turnover during periodontal repair. J Clin Periodontol 2006;33:135–140.

87. Cooke JW, Sarment DP, Whitesman LA, et al. Effect of rhPDGF-BB delivery on mediators of periodontal wound repair. Tissue Eng 2006;12:1–7.

88. Anusaksathien O, Jin Q, Ma PX, Giannobile WV. Scaffolding in periodontal engineering. In: Ma PX, Elisseeff J (eds). Scaffolding in Tissue Engineering. Boca Raton, FL: CRC Press, 2006:437–454.

89. Kaigler D, Cirelli JA, Giannobile WV. Growth factor delivery for oral and periodontal tissue engineering. Expert Opin Drug Del 2006;3:647–662.

90. Lutolf MP, Hubbell JA. Synthetic biomaterials as instructive extracellular microenvironments for morphogenesis in tissue engineering. Nat Biotechnol 2005;23:47–55.

91. Babensee JE, McIntire LV, Mikos AG. Growth factor delivery for tissue engineering. Pharm Res 2000;17:497–504.

92. Hutmacher DW, Teoh SH, Zein I, Ranawake M, Lau S. Tissue engineering research: The engineer's role. Med Device Technol 2000;11:33–39.

93. Jin Q, Anusaksathien O, Webb SA, Printz MA, Giannobile WV. Engineering of tooth-supporting structures by delivery of PDGF gene therapy vectors. Mol Ther 2004;9:519–526.

94. Eming SA, Whitsitt JS, He L, Krieg T, Morgan JR, Davidson JM. Particle-mediated gene transfer of PDGF isoforms promotes wound repair. J Invest Dermatol 1999;112:297–302.

95. Erdag G, Medalie DA, Rakhorst H, Krueger GG, Morgan JR. FGF-7 expression enhances the performance of bioengineered skin. Mol Ther 2004;10:76–85.

96. Hijjawi J, Mogford JE, Chandler LA, et al. Platelet-derived growth factor B, but not fibroblast growth factor 2, plasmid DNA improves survival of ischemic myocutaneous flaps. Arch Surg 2004;139:142–147.

97. Printz MA, Gonzalez AM, Cunningham M, et al. Fibroblast growth factor 2-retargeted adenoviral vectors exhibit a modified biolocalization pattern and display reduced toxicity relative to native adenoviral vectors. Hum Gene Ther 2000;11:191–204.

98. Gu DL, Nguyen T, Gonzalez AM, et al. Adenovirus encoding human platelet-derived growth factor-B delivered in collagen exhibits safety, biodistribution, and immunogenicity profiles favorable for clinical use. Mol Ther 2004;9:699–711.

99. Giannobile WV, Lee CS, Tomala MP, Tejeda KM, Zhu Z. Platelet-derived growth factor (PDGF) gene delivery for application in periodontal tissue engineering. J Periodontol 2001;72:815–823.

100. Zhu Z, Lee CS, Tejeda KM, Giannobile WV. Gene transfer and expression of platelet-derived growth factors modulate periodontal cellular activity. J Dent Res 2001;80:892–897.

101. Chen QP, Giannobile WV. Adenoviral gene transfer of PDGF downregulates gas gene product PDGFαR and prolongs ERK and Akt/PKB activation. Am J Physiol Cell Physiol 2002;282:C538–C544.

102. Anusaksathien O, Webb SA, Jin QM, Giannobile WV. Platelet-derived growth factor gene delivery stimulates ex vivo gingival repair. Tissue Eng 2003;9:745–756.

103. Dunn CA, Jin Q, Taba M Jr, Franceschi RT, Rutherford BR, Giannobile WV. BMP gene delivery for alveolar bone engineering at dental implant defects. Mol Ther 2005;11:294–299.

104. Bartold PM, Shi S, Gronthos S. Stem cells and periodontal regeneration. Periodontol 2000 2006;40:164–172.

105. Mao JJ, Giannobile WV, Helms JA, et al. Craniofacial tissue engineering by stem cells. J Dent Res 2006;85:966–979.

106. Risbud MV, Shapiro IM. Stem cells in craniofacial and dental tissue engineering. Orthod Craniofac Res 2005;8:54–59.

107. Akizuki T, Oda S, Komaki M, et al. Application of periodontal ligament cell sheet for periodontal regeneration: a pilot study in beagle dogs. J Periodontal Res 2005;40:245–251.

108. Hasegawa M, Yamato M, Kikuchi A, Okano T, Ishikawa I. Human periodontal ligament cell sheets can regenerate periodontal ligament tissue in an athymic rat model. Tissue Eng 2005;11:469–478.

109. Lekic PC, Rajshankar D, Chen H, Tenenbaum H, McCulloch CA. Transplantation of labeled periodontal ligament cells promotes regeneration of alveolar bone. Anat Rec 2001;262:193–202.

110. Nakahara T, Nakamura T, Kobayashi E, et al. In situ tissue engineering of periodontal tissues by seeding with periodontal ligament-derived cells. Tissue Eng 2004;10:537–544.

111. Dogan A, Ozdemir A, Kubar A, Oygur T. Healing of artificial fenestration defects by seeding of fibroblast-like cells derived from regenerated periodontal ligament in a dog: A preliminary study. Tissue Eng 2003;9:1189–1196.

112. Zhao M, Jin Q, Berry JE, Nociti FH Jr, Giannobile WV, Somerman MJ. Cementoblast delivery for periodontal tissue engineering. J Periodontol 2004;75:154–161.

113. Seo BM, Miura M, Gronthos S, et al. Investigation of multipotent postnatal stem cells from human periodontal ligament. Lancet 2004;364:149–155.

114. Trubiani O, Di Primio R, Traini T, et al. Morphological and cytofluorimetric analysis of adult mesenchymal stem cells expanded ex vivo from periodontal ligament. Int J Immunopathol Pharmacol 2005;18:213–221.

115. McGuire MK, Nunn ME. Evaluation of the safety and efficacy of periodontal applications of a living tissue-engineered human fibroblast-derived dermal substitute. 1. Comparison to the gingival autograft: A randomized controlled pilot study. J Periodontol 2005;76:867–880.

116. Hovey LR, Jones AA, McGuire M, Mellonig JT, Schoolfield J, Cochran DL. application of periodontal tissue engineering using enamel matrix derivative and a human fibroblast-derived dermal substitute to stimulate periodontal wound healing in class III furcation defects. J Periodontol 2006;77:790–799.

117. Hollister SJ. Porous scaffold design for tissue engineering. Nat Mater 2005;4:518–524.

118. Chen VJ, Smith LA, Ma PX. Bone regeneration on computer-designed nanofibrous scaffolds. Biomaterials 2006;27:3973–3979.

Application of Tissue Engineering Principles to Clinical Practice

Robert E. Marx, DDS

Clinicians may not have been aware that they were practicing tissue engineering but have indeed done so for many years. Tissue engineering is too often thought of as a sophisticated laboratory procedure in which cells, a tissue composite, or an organ is grown in tissue culture and then transplanted into a patient. Actually, tissue engineering may simply be directing or accelerating natural tissue healing by the clinician. Such tissue engineering may therefore be accomplished in vivo as well as in vitro. Examples of tissue engineering include many commonplace adjuncts in use today, such as hyperbaric oxygen, guided bone regeneration via the use of barrier membranes, demineralized bone matrix, enamel matrix derivative, and freeze-dried allogeneic bone. Although none of these involves all three elements of the tissue engineering triangle described in this chapter, they all either contain or direct one or more of these elements.

Recombinant human platelet-derived growth factor BB (rhPDGF-BB), recombinant human bone morphogenetic protein (rhBMP) on an absorbable collagen sponge (ACS), and platelet-rich plasma (PRP) actually contain all three elements of the tissue engineering triangle and thus are the most reliable techniques. This chapter will briefly explore the clinical applications of many of these methods, describing how they can be used effectively to enhance clinical outcomes as well as their limitations.

Tissue Engineering Principles

The basic principle of tissue engineering is a plagiarism of natural tissue regeneration and healing. That is, both require three elements that must be present and work together: cells, a signal, and a matrix. This concept is often represented as a triangle (Fig 4-1), indicating that an absence or dysfunction of one element will halt tissue regeneration.

Cells

The cells are thought to be pluripotential stem cells or cells that have only partially differentiated along their lineage. In bone regeneration, the cells range from CD34[+] marrow cells or colony-forming unit (CFU) cells at their earliest stages all the way to the preosteoblast CBFA-1[+] cells and even the endosteal or periosteal osteoblasts.[2]

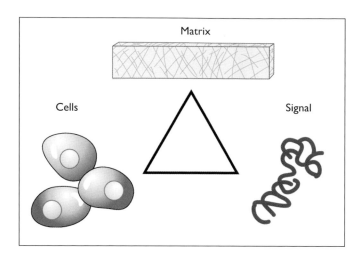

Fig 4-1 Natural tissue healing and tissue engineering require three fundamental elements: cells, a signal, and a matrix. (Modified from Marx.[1] Reprinted with permission.)

Signal

The signals are the growth and differentiation factors (cytokines), such as the three PDGFs (PDGF-AA, PDGF-AB, and PDGF-BB); several forms of transforming growth factor β (TGF-β), among which numerous BMPs are included; vascular endothelial growth factor; and epidermal growth factor, among many more.[3] These growth factors act on the external cell membrane receptors of a target cell to stimulate an expression of a normal gene[4] (Fig 4-2). Because these growth factors act on the external membrane receptors, cause normal gene function to be expressed, and are not mutagens, they do not pose a risk for hyperplasia or neoplasia.[5] These cytokines have pleotropic effects, some of which will overlap and may include new capillary ingrowth (angiogenesis), target cell proliferation (mitogenesis), cellular specification (differentiation), and upregulation of normal cellular functions.

Matrix

Although most clinicians focus on the cells (stem cells) and the signal (PRP and recombinant growth factors), another important and poorly understood component is the matrix. The matrix is a scaffold or latticework on which tissue is grown and over which cells migrate. Although most clinicians believe that they use allogeneic bone, xenogeneic bone, hydroxyapatite preparations, and other nonviable graft materials as a scaffold or matrix, this is not exactly true. The actual biologic scaffolds are exposed collagen and the cell adhesion molecules fibrin and fibronectin from plasma and vitronectin secreted by platelets.[3,6] The value of allogeneic bone, commercial bone products such as Bio-Oss (Osteohealth), and hydroxyapatite preparations such as C-graft (ScionX) and Interpore-500 (Interpore Cross) is their ability to adhere these molecules to their surface.

In fact, the osseointegration of dental implants does not form bone directly on the titanium surface. Instead, bone forms on these cell adhesion molecules that are first deposited and become adherent onto the titanium surface. Osteoblasts then secrete not bone but a cementing line of sialoprotein and osteopontin into which actual bone becomes anchored.[7] Because osseointegration represents a good example of a clinical application of tissue engineering, the discussion will start there.

Osseointegration

When a drill site is prepared for the placement of a dental implant, bone marrow containing both stem cells and endosteal osteoblasts is exposed to the cylindrical cavity. In addition, the drill sites fill with blood that contains platelets (Fig 4-3). Once the implant is in place, the surface is surrounded by a blood clot in the microspace between bone and the implant surface. The sequence of events leading to osseointegration begins with platelet degranulation that releases PDGF-AA, PDGF-AB, PDGF-BB, TGF-β_1, TGF-β_2, vascular endothelial growth factor, epidermal growth factor, and vitronectin. In addition, the clotted plasma fraction of the blood deposits fibrin and

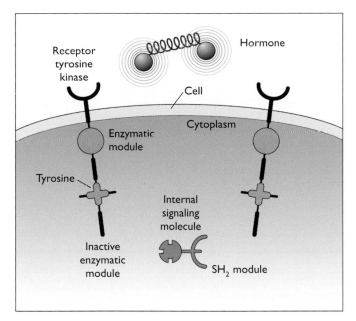

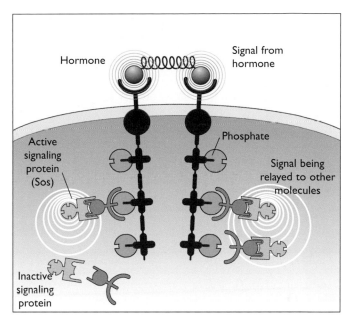

Fig 4-2a Most growth factors are dimers that activate dual transmembrane receptors on the external surface of target cell membranes.

Fig 4-2b Activated transmembrane receptors in turn activate and release a signaling protein that will float down to the cell nucleus.

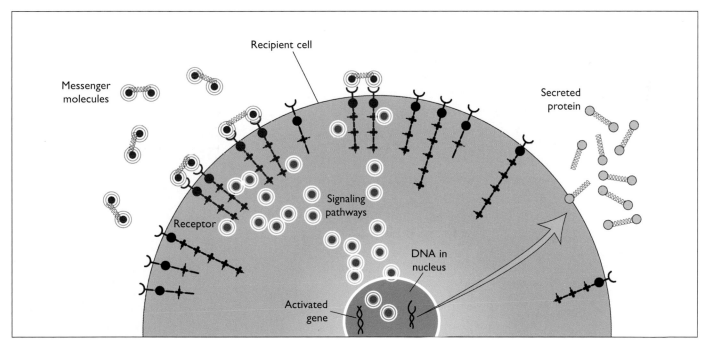

Fig 4-2c The activated signaling protein then causes expression of a gene related to tissue regeneration. (Figs 4-2a to 4-2c from Marx and Garg.[3] Reprinted with permission.)

fibronectin on the implant surface and forms a connection bridge between the bony wall and the implant surface (Fig 4-1).

The released growth factors act on the exposed marrow cells, endothelial cells, and endosteal osteoblasts to generate an angiogenic and mitogenic effect as well as migrations and cellular differentiation. The endosteal osteoblasts lay down osteoid on the strands of fibrin, fibronectin, and vitronectin and migrate toward the implant surface by pushing forward daughter cells on their surface

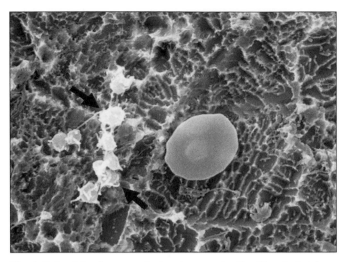

Fig 4-3 In this electron photomicrograph, the blood clot in a drill site for implant placement consists of a single red blood cell, several platelets (*arrows*), and numerous fibrin strands (original magnification ×10,000). (From Marx and Garg.[3] Reprinted with permission.)

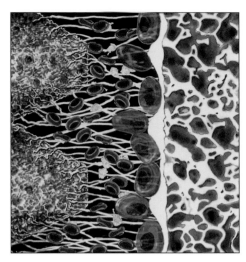

Fig 4-4 The electron photomicrograph in Fig 4-3 can be modeled to show thin fibrin strands connecting bone to the implant surface, exposed osteoblasts from the marrow, and the erythrocyte/blood/platelet clot between them. (From Marx and Garg.[3] Reprinted with permission.)

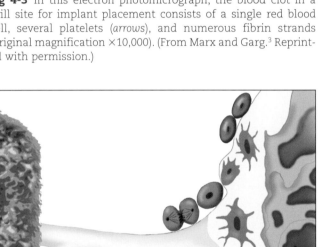

Fig 4-5a Growth factor activation of osteoblasts causes cellular division along the matrix of the fibrin/fibronectin strands.

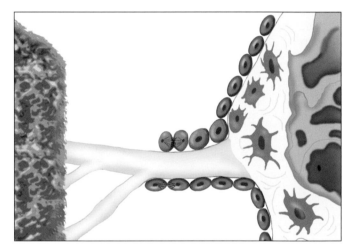

Fig 4-5b As cells divide, they push daughter cells forward in a "creeping substitution." The parent osteoblast then matures to secrete osteoid and becomes an osteocyte.

as they undergo mitosis (Figs 4-5a and 4-5b). These daughter cells (osteoblasts) become further differentiated and lay down bone on those strands of cell adhesion molecules (Fig 4-5c).

As this wave of cells, followed by osteoid, approaches the implant surface, it follows the cell adhesion molecule strands, which are adherent to the implant surface (Fig 4-5d). These now fully differentiated osteoblasts first secrete sialoprotein and osteopontin on and around the strands of cell adhesion molecules deposited on the implant surface, degrading them in the process but also

seeping into the valleys and undercuts of the implant surface. This sialoprotein-osteopontin composite is the same cementing substance found in the resting lines in normal bone, which function to cement (osseointegrate) two bone segments formed at different times (Fig 4-6).

Actual mature bone and therefore osseointegration of the implant comes when the osteoblasts insert collagen in the cementing substance and form bone attached to it; the collagen serves much the same role as steel rods do to help hold two cement blocks together in highway construction (Figs 4-7 and 4-8).

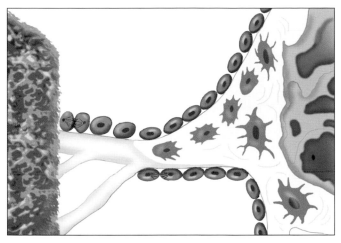

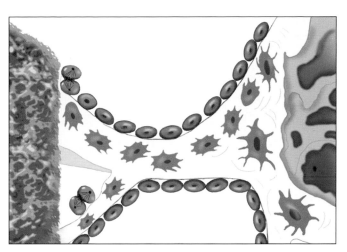

Fig 4-5c As continued cellular divisions and creeping substitution progress, bone bridges the space between the drill site wall and the implant surface.

Fig 4-5d Further cellular division and osteoid formation occurs along the implant surface to achieve osseointegration. (Figs 4-5a to 4-5d from Marx and Garg.[3] Reprinted with permission.)

Fig 4-6 Bone does not directly bond to a titanium implant surface. Instead, it bonds indirectly through the natural cementing substance of bone, as seen in resting lines, and is composed of sialoprotein and osteopontin. (From Marx and Garg.[3] Reprinted with permission.)

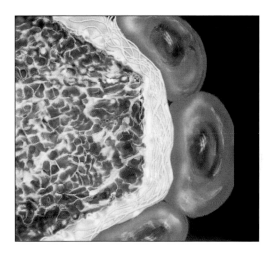

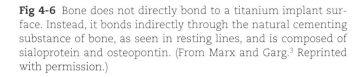

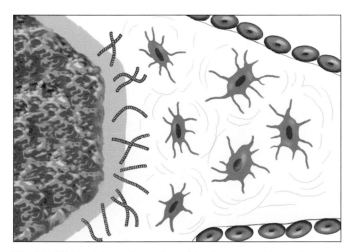

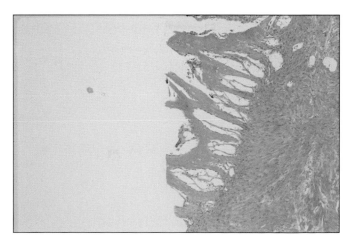

Fig 4-7 Distinct bone is anchored to the cementing substance on the implant surface via collagen fibrils that intimately connect the two together. (From Marx and Garg.[3] Reprinted with permission.)

Fig 4-8 This histology shows osteoblasts differentiating and migrating along strands of fibrin to form struts of trabecular bone with endosteal osteoblasts and osteocytes readily apparent. (From Marx and Garg.[3] Reprinted with permission.)

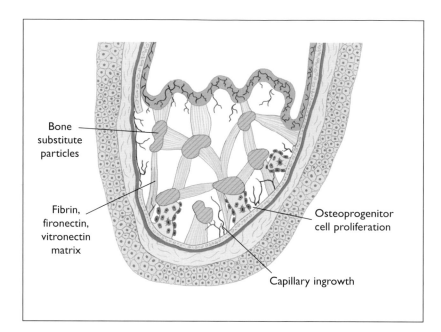

Bone
substitute
particles

Fibrin,
fironectin,
vitronectin
matrix

Osteoprogenitor
cell proliferation

Capillary ingrowth

Fig 4-9a Nonviable grafts develop bone via osteoconduction, which is dependent on the matrix formed by cell adhesion molecules that unite the graft particles together and to surrounding bony walls.

To date, the clinical application of tissue engineering to implant surgery has been accomplished mostly with PRP, although rhPDGF-BB and rhBMP-2 have also been suggested and are currently being explored. In this application, activated (clotted) PRP is placed in the drill site prior to implant placement. Because most dental implant surfaces are hydrophobic and will repel anticoagulated blood as well as water, it is not advisable either to use anticoagulated blood in the site or to place it on the implant. As the implant is placed, the PRP blood clot will come to occupy the microgap between the implant and the bone. The same biologic principles described earlier have been suggested to occur with PRP in the microgap but at a more accelerated rate and with greater bone regeneration by virtue of a five- to eightfold increase of the growth factors in this wound space.[6]

Augmentation with Nonviable Graft Materials

Ridge preservation

The clinical value of ridge preservation is the development of bone throughout the entire socket height and width so as to maintain ridge contour and provide suffi-

cient bone for the ideal positioning of dental implants. The clinical value of sinus augmentation with nonviable graft materials is to gain sufficient bone in the posterior maxilla so that implants can be placed without harvesting of autogenous bone.

If the socket or sinus augmentation site is grafted with nonviable graft systems such as hydroxyapatite, xenogeneic bone, or allogeneic bone, then all the bone that will eventually develop in this space will be the result of osteoconduction. None of these substances is osteoinductive; nor do any of them transplant viable cells capable of bone formation by independent osteogenesis.

Instead these materials represent the matrix on which the cell adhesion molecules from blood plasma (fibrin and fibronectin) and from blood platelets (vitronectin) will adhere, connecting the graft particles together and to the socket walls. The signals will come from the growth factors when platelets degranulate in the blood clot. The cells will come from open marrow spaces of the socket itself in ridge preservation or from the bony walls of the sinus cavity in sinus augmentations. Similarly to the mechanism of osseointegration, osteoprogenitor cells will divide and push their daughter cells along the strands of cell adhesion molecules, connecting the graft particles to the socket walls or sinus walls, and then along the strands connecting the graft particles (Fig 4-9a).

Because the cells-signal-matrix triangle is complete, this type of tissue engineering usually evolves into a fully regenerated socket or stable bone regeneration in a sinus cavity after 9 months to 1 year, depending on the patient's

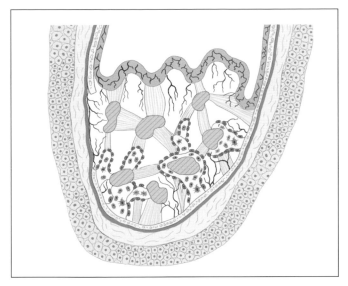

Fig 4-9b Osteoconduction begins as endosteal osteoblasts accomplish cellular divisions and differentiation along the strands of cell adhesion molecules. (Figs 4-9a and 4-9b from Marx and Garg.[3] Reprinted with permission.)

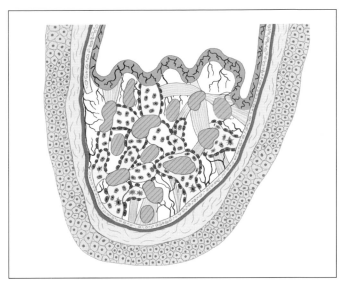

Fig 4-9c Osteoconduction will proceed as long as graft particles are connected by cell adhesion molecules and can often completely regenerate new bone in a graft site. (Modified from Marx and Garg[3] with permission.)

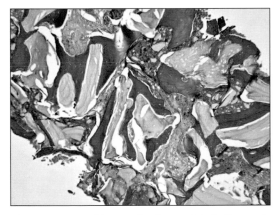

Fig 4-10 A core biopsy of a freeze-dried allogeneic graft in a sinus augmentation site reveals only 20% new viable bone and 80% residual mineralized graft particles, which will create a more radiodense appearance (hematoxylin-eosin [H&E] stain; original magnification ×4).

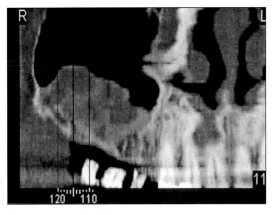

Fig 4-11 Despite little viable bone, this sinus augmentation graft shows an impressive radiodensity because of residual graft material.

age (Figs 4-9b and 4-9c). However, in sinus grafts where nonviable graft materials were used, only 12% to 28% of the graft represents viable bone.[8,9] The remaining volume is composed of a residual nonviable graft material (Fig 4-10), making radiographs appear to reveal more bone than is actually present (Fig 4-11).

If rhPDGF-BB or PRP were added to the socket or sinus cavity, they would not add another component to the triangle but would upregulate the signal component. Neither is osteoinductive, but each is known to enhance the local growth factor concentration, which would shorten the time needed to fully regenerate bone in

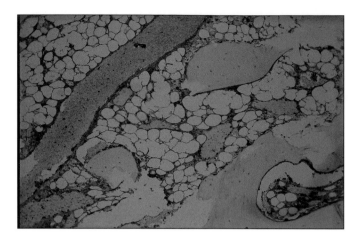

Fig 4-12 Osteoprogenitor cells are clustered around blood vessels as pericytes, as indicated by immunoperoxidase staining, which identifies cells with TGF-β1 receptors as staining brown (H&E stain; original magnification ×4). (From Marx and Garg.[3] Reprinted with permission.)

these applications and produce a denser bone. If rhBMP-2/ACS were added to this graft, it would likewise represent an upregulation of the signal. However, in this case, it also would represent a second signal, because rhBMP-2/ACS is actually osteoinductive. Therefore, in this clinical application, the native blood clot, rhPDGF-BB, or PRP would represent one signal, and rhBMP-2/ACS would represent both an upregulation of a native BMP signal as well as a second signal.

If a membrane were added to a socket graft or over the sinus entry window, it would also represent a form of tissue engineering. Although a membrane would not represent any of the components of the tissue engineering triangle, it would act to guide and promote the desired tissue regeneration in the wound space, in this instance bone regeneration in the socket or sinus rather than fibrous tissue ingrowth. The membrane is placed over the crestal opening of the socket or over the sinus entry window, stabilized, and covered. As a cell exclusion barrier, the membrane does not promote the cellular migration to the socket or sinus to regenerate bone but instead prevents the ingrowth of competing cells, namely fibroblasts that would fill the graft with fibrous tissue instead of bone.

This strategy may seem to be counterproductive, because it prevents ingrowth from the periosteum. Indeed, this would be true if the periosteum were osteogenic in the adult. However, most human adult periosteum around teeth that have been extracted or lateral sinus walls that have been altered by inflammation, previous reflections, or other surgeries is not osteogenic. This coupled with the advanced age of the majority of patients

requiring grafting renders adult periosteum in the jaws little more than scar tissue in most cases. In contrast, the cells in the bony walls are known to be osteogenic and are clustered around small blood vessels as pericytes[10] (Fig 4-12). The ingrowth of capillaries that originate in bone will provide a pathway for osteoprogenitor cells and therefore bone formation, whereas capillaries that originate from the nonosteogenic periosteum will provide a pathway for fibroblasts and therefore fibrous ingrowth. This is the basic biologic concept of barrier membranes.

Autogenous bone grafting

In sinus augmentations, continuity defects, and large horizontal or vertical ridge augmentations, a significant volume of regenerated bone is required. Therefore, autogenous bone is most commonly used. Autogenous bone represents the complete tissue engineering triangle; therefore its outcomes are more predictable, and it is regarded as the gold standard. The mineral component of the autogenous bone graft represents the matrix, the cancellous cellular marrow represents the cells, and the BMPs, PDGFs, and insulin-like growth factors 1 and 2 in the noncollagenous portion of the bone mineral matrix represent the signal. Although the tissue engineering triangle is complete, it is still possible to enhance one or more of these components. In fact, although autogenous bone represents the gold standard, improved and faster outcomes have

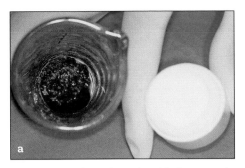

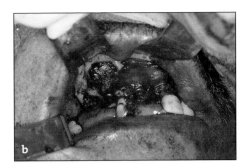

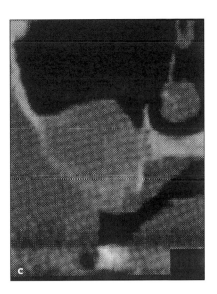

Fig 4-13a Activated PRP is added to a graft material before it is placed in a sinus augmentation site.

Fig 4-13b Activated PRP can also be placed directly on the graft site.

Fig 4-13c A more rapid and more mature bone forms when PRP is added to a graft. (Figs 4-13a to 4-13c from Marx and Garg.[13] Reprinted with permission.)

been documented after enhancement of one, two, or all three components of the tissue engineering triangle.[11,12]

The first type of enhancement is to upregulate the signal. This can be accomplished by adding growth factors directly to the graft. The most common and most studied method is to add activated PRP to the graft (Fig 4-13a). This is done by coagulating the PRP and applying it to the graft as the graft is placed. Then a coating of the coagulated PRP is placed over the graft, similar to a membrane (Fig 4-13b).

Studies have shown that the platelets in PRP degranulate and begin actively secreting their growth factors in 10 minutes and secrete 90% of their already synthesized growth factors in the first hour.[14] This burst of growth factors sends a more intense signal to the cells of the graft, resulting in faster and more complete bone formation (Fig 4-13c). After the wound is closed, the platelets synthesize and secrete more growth factors for their remaining time in the wound, which is about 1 week.

An additional method to upregulate the signal would be to add rhBMP-2 or rhPDGF-BB to the graft. Although neither of these two proteins is specifically cleared by the US Food and Drug Administration (FDA) for this application, and cost may be a deterrent in some cases, there has been off-label use of both for this indication. Mostly rhBMP-2 or rhPDGF-BB has been used to supplement the graft in larger defects when autogenous bone is the only option but the donor sites are limited because of previous harvesting or the patient's refusal.

In these instances, rhBMP-2/ACS is mixed into and draped over the graft (Fig 4-14a). The rhBMP-2 comes as a lyophilized white powder that is dissolved in sterile water (*not* saline) for 5 minutes. The solution is then squirted on the absorbable collagen sponge and allowed to soak in for 15 minutes, during which time 93% becomes bound to the sponge.

The rhPDGF-BB solution comes already prepared in a physiologic buffer. It is to be added to tricalcium phosphate, bone allograft, or another conductive matrix, and the fully saturated particulate is mixed with the particulate autograft.

The recombinant growth factors will act directly on the cells of the graft as well as any local stem cells to upregulate cellular proliferation and osseous differentiation. Outcomes using rhBMP-2/ACS in a limited number of cases—where it has been added to a smaller amount of autogenous graft material than has normally been required—have been acceptable, allowing reconstruction in some patients whose defects otherwise could not be corrected (Figs 4-14b and 4-14c).

The second way to enhance regeneration is to upregulate the matrix. This is seldom needed when autogenous bone grafts are used. They contain their own matrix by virtue of their cancellous bone and the natural blood clot, which contains the cell adhesion molecules fibrin, fibronectin, and vitronectin. However, the matrix can be enhanced with the addition of PRP, which adds cell adhesion molecules, or with the addition of demineralized or nondemineralized freeze-dried allogeneic bone or other nonviable graft materials.

Such nonviable graft materials are commonly combined with autogenous bone in sinus augmentation graft-

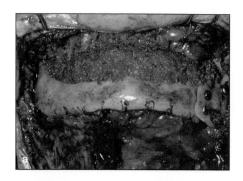
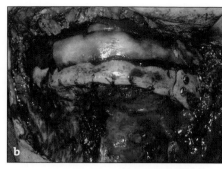

Fig 4-14a In a mandibular continuity defect, rhBMP-2/ACS has been added to increase the signal within the autogenous graft.

Fig 4-14b This large mandibular continuity graft regenerated sufficient bone with the increased signal from rhBMP-2/ACS.

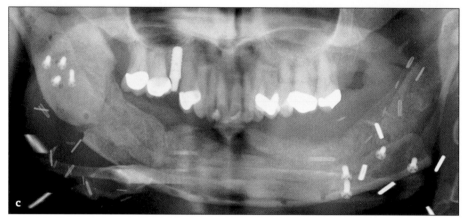

Fig 4-14c This rhBMP-2/ACS–enhanced graft regenerated sufficient bone to support dental restorations.

ing; these are referred to as *composite grafts*. In this use, the surgeon often rationalizes the use of the allogeneic bone or even xenogeneic bone or other graft materials as fillers or expanders. This concept is frequently employed when there is an oral harvest site and therefore less than sufficient autogenous bone to completely graft a maxillary sinus. In this type of use, the allogeneic bone or other graft material is serving as a matrix that will adhere the cell adhesion molecules to its surface and provide a framework across which the cells transplanted by the autogenous graft will migrate and deposit osteoid.

Various publications have conjectured about the percentage of autogenous bone required for successful bone regeneration in the maxillary sinus.[8,15,16] However, most publications do not account for age, local factors, or systemic disease factors that may compromise bone regeneration, each one of which, if present, would indicate the need for a higher percentage of autogenous bone. Table 4-1 presents guidelines for the percentage of autogenous bone required based on these factors as well as the need for further upregulation with PRP, rhPDGF, or rhBMP.

The third way to enhance bone regeneration is to increase the number of cells in the tissue engineering triangle. To some extent this is already done by the selection of autogenous cancellous marrow, but the number can be further improved by physical compression of the graft. This can be accomplished clinically with two techniques. One technique is to condense the autogenous cancellous marrow within a 3-mL syringe by introducing the graft into the barrel of the syringe with the plunger removed. If the plunger is sequentially replaced and activated to condense the graft material, and then more graft material is added before the maneuver is repeated, a syringe full of condensed, high-density graft cells is effectively created (Fig 4-15). The graft is then extruded into the regional site after the syringe tip is cut off.

A second technique is to physically compact the autogenous graft material with bone compactors (Fig 4-16). Penfield neurosurgical instruments are specially made for this purpose, but routine amalgam condensers can accomplish the same task.

Table 4-1 Guidelines for autogenous bone requirements and indications for recommended use of supplemental growth factors in various patient types*

Patient type	Percent autogenous bone required	Supplemental growth factors indicated?
Type Ia: Age less than 40 years, no systemic or local tissue compromise	0 to 20	No
Type Ib: Age less than 40 years, presence of either a systemic or a local tissue compromise	20 to 50	No
Type Ic: Age less than 40 years, presence of both a systemic and a local tissue compromise	20 to 50	Yes
Type IIa: Age 40 to 60 years, no systemic or local tissue compromise	20 to 50	No
Type IIb: Age 40 to 60 years, presence of either a systemic or a local tissue compromise	20 to 50	Yes
Type IIc: Age 40 to 60 years, presence of both a systemic and a local tissue compromise	50 to 80	Yes
Type IIIa: Age 60 to 75 years, no systemic or local tissue compromise	50 to 80	Yes
Type IIIb: Age 60 to 75 years, presence of either a systemic or a local tissue compromise	50 to 80	Yes
Type IIIc: Age 60 to 75 years, presence of both a systemic and a local tissue compromise	80 to 100	Yes
Type IV: All individuals 75 years and older	80 to 100	Yes

*Developed by the University of Miami Division of Oral and Maxillofacial Surgery.

Although condensation is recommended and beneficial for autogenous grafts by virtue of increasing the viable cellular density in the graft, it is counterproductive when nonviable graft materials that rely on osteoconduction for bone regeneration are used. Compaction of the nonviable graft materials reduces the surface area and the space between the particles needed for osteoconduction.

A fourth way under study to improve the outcome of bone regeneration is to increase the cell component of the tissue engineering triangle by actually increasing the number of stem cells in the graft. The author has explored this avenue by aspirating bone marrow in the coagulated state and then concentrating the bone marrow aspirate with a similar technology used to concentrate whole blood into PRP. In fact, because platelets are also present in bone marrow, differential centrifugations of bone marrow yield a bone marrow concentrate of stem cells and platelet-rich bone marrow at the same time.

The technique requires 60 mL of bone marrow aspirate, which is aspirated with specially designed trocar/needle devices that must be heparinized to prevent clotting (Fig 4-17a). In the harvesting procedure, 15 mL of bone marrow is aspirated from the ilium at each of four needle placement positions (Fig 4-17b). The resultant 60 mL of bone marrow aspirate has been documented to contain 4×10^6 to 7×10^6 CD34[+] cells or CFU cells per milliliter; these are the osteoprogenitor cells in bone marrow.[18]

This volume is then processed in a sterile fashion at the point of care with differential centrifugation programmed to separate the CD34[+] and CFU cells by density in 14 minutes (Fig 4-17c). This process can yield 7 to 10 mL of bone marrow concentrate with 30×10^6 to 50×10^6 CD34[+] or CFU cells per milliliter, a concentration six to eight times greater than that found in the original aspirate.

Early experience with this concept has been limited to continuity defect grafts. It has produced excellent radiographically identifiable bone in cases of radiated and scarred tissue beds and has allowed osseointegration of implants (Fig 4-18). Core biopsies also reveal an impressive amount of bone density, providing hope that this concept may be refined to be clinically applicable to more routine cases (Fig 4-19).

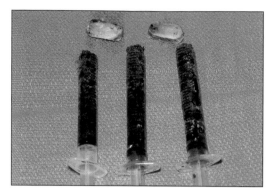

Fig 4-15 The cellular density of an autogenous graft can be increased technically by syringe condensation. (From Marx and Garg.[13] Reprinted with permission.)

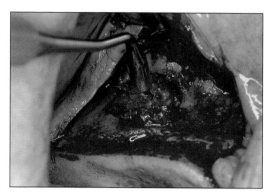

Fig 4-16 A second technical means of increasing the cellular density of an autogenous graft is compaction with a bone-compacting hand instrument. (From Garg.[17] Reprinted with permission.)

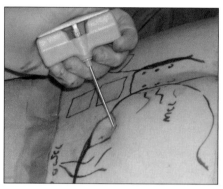

Fig 4-17a A bone trocar is used to aspirate stem cells containing autologous bone marrow.

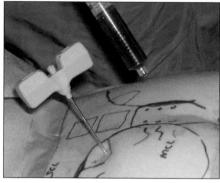

Fig 4-17b Aspiration of 15 mL of bone marrow is accomplished from four different locations within the same bone to gain a 60-mL total volume.

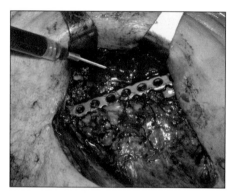

Fig 4-17c Concentrated bone marrow stem cells are obtained by differential centrifugation and added to the graft in a clotted state similar to that of PRP.

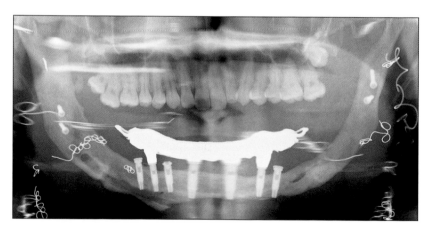

Fig 4-18 Excellent bone regeneration enhancement has been observed when bone marrow concentrates are added to grafts.

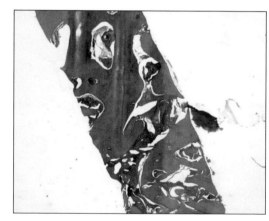

Fig 4-19 Bone marrow concentrates added to grafts have been observed to regenerate a greater amount of bone (H&E stain; original magnification ×4).

Tissue Regeneration with Growth Factors

The concept employed when growth factors are used alone as a grafted substance is one of significantly upregulating the signal; their carrier represents the matrix. The cellular component is expected to be recruited from the host. This is exemplified by the use of rhPDGF-BB (GEM 21S, BioMimetic Therapeutics) and rhBMP-2/ACS (InFuse, Medtronic Sofamor Danek).

rhPDGF-BB is a more than 98% pure recombinant protein developed using conventional recombinant expression techniques under highly controlled conditions. Like most commercially available recombinant proteins, rhPDGF-BB and rhBMP-2/ACS are first produced by removing the specific DNA sequence from a human cell and transfecting it into a bacterial plasmid. The bacterial plasmid is then transfected into host cells capable of large-scale growth. In the case of rhPDGF-BB, the host cells are yeast; in the case of rhBMP-2/ACS, the host cells are Chinese hamster ovary cells. These are essentially protein factories that synthesize and secrete many proteins, one of which is human rhPDGF-BB or rhBMP-2. The rhPDGF-BB or rhBMP-2 then is separated by sophisticated analytical protein chemistry techniques, sterile filtered, and formulated into a dose specified for clinical use.

The clinical indication for these proteins is de novo regeneration of bone and/or periodontal complex as well as an adjunct to local socket grafting and smaller ridge augmentation procedures. rhPDGF-BB has been shown to regenerate up to 10 mm of cementum, periodontal ligament, and alveolar bone, and rhBMP-2/ACS has been shown to regenerate greater than 10 mm of bone in maxillary sinus augmentations. Their mechanism of action is that of upregulation of cellular proliferation, chemotaxis, and angiogenesis in bone and periodontal ligament (see chapters 6 and 11 for additional information on application of rhPDGF-BB and rhBMP-2/ACS, respectively).

The use of rhBMP-2/ACS (InFuse) is currently cleared by the FDA for two orthopedic indications: lumbar interbody spinal fusions and fresh tibial fractures.[19,20] It was also cleared by the FDA for maxillary sinus augmentation and ridge preservations in February 2007. The combination of rhBMP-2 and ACS has the ability to regenerate viable bone in bony defects. However, the amount of bone regenerated is dose dependent and limited by the carrier. Therefore, experience has indicated that its effectiveness is limited to small defects such as socket grafting and sinus augmentation at this time.

A study that documented the efficacy of rhBMP-2/ACS in fresh extraction sockets with the buccal wall missing showed a superior bone regeneration in socket width and regeneration of bone at the crest compared with the results in an unfilled extraction socket and a socket filled with the ACS carrier alone; these findings essentially proved bone induction de novo.[21] The de novo bone formation was superior at all levels of the socket and translated to a better condition in which to place an implant (Figs 4-20 and 4-21). However, the increase in bone width was only 2.0 ± 0.2 mm greater than that in an unfilled socket or the sponge alone at the midsocket level, representing only a moderate degree of bone induction. The implant survival at 2 years was 67% for the rhBMP-2/ACS–treated socket and 38% and 50% for the unfilled socket and ACS-filled sockets, respectively (see chapter 7 for more details).

A sinus augmentation study was a more controlled study comparing rhBMP-2/ACS to autogenous bone grafts in a randomized prospective study involving 187 patients, of whom 98 received 18 to 24 mg of rhBMP-2/ACS and 89 received an autogenous bone graft.[22] When used in sinus augmentation, 24 mg of rhBMP-2/ACS regenerated varying amounts of bone in 97 of 99 (97.9%) procedures (Fig 4-22). When directly compared with an autogenous bone graft, rhBMP-2/ACS regenerated bone sufficient to place a dental implant in fewer patients—82.8% of patients for rhBMP-2 compared with 93.0% for autograft—and evidenced a slightly smaller increase in bone height (8.2 mm versus 9.7 mm). However, considering the absence of any donor site morbidity such as pain, swelling, blood loss, or bone harvesting, the rhBMP-2/ACS represents a reasonable alternative with a good benefit-risk ratio rather than an absolute replacement for autogenous grafting in this indication.

Of important clinical relevance is that the regenerated bone responded to functional loading with an increased bone density and a 1-year implant survival nearly identical to that of implants placed in an autogenous bone graft (Fig 4-23).

In addition, the author (Marx RE, unpublished data, 2007) has used 12-mg doses of rhBMP-2/ACS in 10 continuity defects, two maxillary vertical ridge augmentations, and one adult maxillary alveolar cleft, with disappointing outcomes (Fig 4-24). Only one (10%) of the continuity defects showed evidence of de novo bone generation at 1 year, and that was the smallest defect, at 3 × 1 × 2 cm

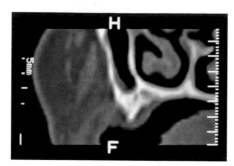

Fig 4-20 The remodeled extraction socket was not grafted and now has insufficient bone for implant placement.

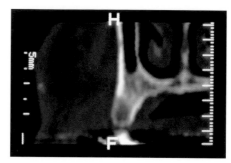

Fig 4-21 A 2-mg dose of rhBMP-2/ACS was placed in this extraction socket. The site shows bone regeneration and a ridge form capable of implant placement.

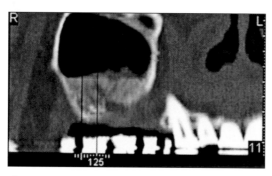

Fig 4-22 Bone regeneration 6 months after a sinus augmentation in which 24 mg of rhBMP-2/ACS was the only regenerative material placed.

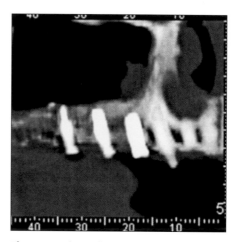

Fig 4-23 When placed under function, the bone regenerated with rhBMP-2/ACS exhibits increased bone density.

(6 cm³). Only one of the two (50%) vertical ridge augmentations has shown evidence of de novo bone generation (Fig 4-25). The adult alveolar cleft graft also showed no significant bone regeneration at 1 year, and two sinuses grafted with only 6 mg of rhBMP-2/ACS also failed to regenerate any bone.

The findings from the two rhBMP-2/ACS studies[21,22] and the clinical case experiences identify the limitations of rhBMP-2/ACS. At their current dose and with their current carriers, the amount of bone or other tissue that can be regenerated clinically is very limited. Therefore, clinicians should not expect outcomes that are unachievable at this time.

There is also little doubt that the more spectacular results achieved in animal models have not yet been duplicated in human clinical use (Fig 4-26). It has been observed that higher doses of rhBMP-2/ACS are required in each animal model as it ascends the evolutionary hierarchy toward humans. Because the doses currently being used in humans are either identical or similar to those used in animal trials, it is possible that these growth factors are underperforming because of species-specific underdosing.

The currently available growth factors may also be limited because they are single growth factors and are not native growth factors. Growth factors do not work singly in nature; they work together with a vast network of other growth factors, signals, and cell-to-cell interactions. It may be naive to think that adding a greater amount of a single growth factor such as rhPDGF-BB or rhBMP-2 can regenerate any more tissue than has been accomplished so far without upregulating other growth factors with which it works in concert, such as PDGF-AA, PDGF-AB, and TGF-β.

Fig 4-24a To encourage de novo bone growth, 12 mg of rhBMP-2/ACS was placed in a continuity defect of the mandible.

Fig 4-24b The continuity defect is shown immediately after placement of 12 mg of rhBMP-2/ACS.

Fig 4-24c Nine months after placement of 12 mg of rhBMP-2/ACS, there is no radiographic evidence of bone regeneration in the continuity defect.

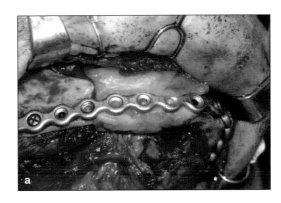

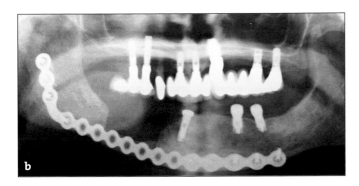

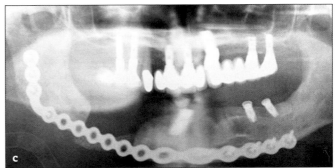

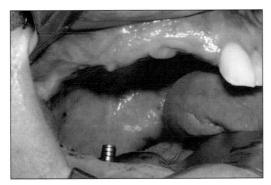

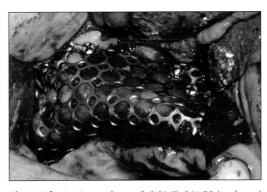

Fig 4-25a A vertical ridge defect of the maxilla is planned for bone regeneration with rhBMP-2/ACS.

Fig 4-25b A 12-mg dose of rhBMP-2/ACS is placed beneath titanium mesh used to maintain space for bone regeneration.

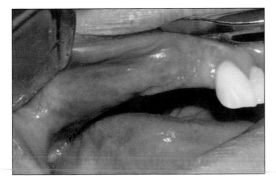

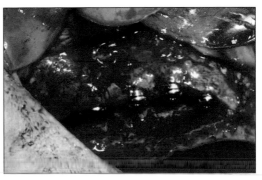

Fig 4-25c The vertical and horizontal ridge is improved after surgical placement of 12 mg of rhBMP-2/ACS within a titanium mesh.

Fig 4-25d Four dental implants have been placed in the bone induced by 12 mg of rhBMP-2/ACS.

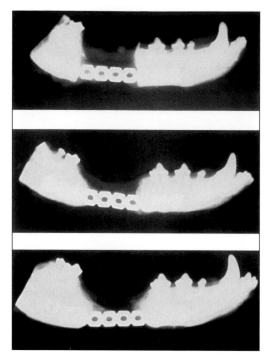

Fig 4-26a A dog model was used to examine the effectiveness of rhBMP-2/ACS in large continuity defects. This control specimen with 0 mg of rhBMP-2/ACS failed to regenerate bone.

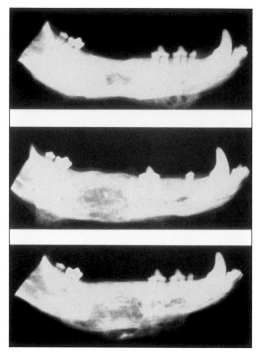

Fig 4-26b These treatment specimens from the same dog model described in Fig 4-26a exhibited an impressive amount of regenerated bone after application of only 10 mg of rhBMP-2/ACS. This experiment has not yet been duplicated in the human condition. (Figs 4-26a and 4-26b courtesy of Medtronics Sofamor Danek.)

It may also be naive to think that yeast or a Chinese hamster ovary cell can manufacture human recombinant growth factors that are as complete or biologically active as a human cell. Although the human recombinant growth factors are proteins with the exact amino acid sequence of their corresponding native proteins and should have the same tertiary structure, the glycosylation of the protein and histone additions required for biologic activity of each protein may not be efficiently accomplished by the yeast or Chinese hamster cells. This phase of the protein synthesis is not a part of the recombinant technology but rather relies on the inherent ability of the transfected cell. It is therefore possible that the yeast or Chinese hamster ovary cells can effectively complete the packaging of their own proteins but not human proteins, therefore producing a recombinant human growth factor of diminished biologic activity.

Research and clinical experience have also revealed that the carrier matrix is far more important than originally thought. Most of the commercial carriers that deliver these growth factors lack the ability to adhere cell adhesion molecules, resorb too quickly, and do not have the internal structure to control the soft tissue. They may be good carriers, but they are not necessarily a good matrix.

Conclusion

There is no doubt that tissue engineering is very much in its infancy and needs many more advances. The fact that many clinicians already apply tissue engineering principles in their clinical practice and achieve improved results is encouraging and counterbalances the limitations of the current clinically available products. Therefore, the clinician should not be discouraged but rather resolved to help basic science researchers identify these limitations and improve each component of the classic tissue engineering triangle.

References

1. Marx RE. PRP and BMP: A comparison of their use and efficacy in sinus grafting. In: Jensen OT (ed). The Sinus Bone Graft, ed 2. Chicago: Quintessence, 2006: 289–304.

2. Majors AK, Boehm CA, Nitto H, Midura RJ, Muschler GF. Characterization of human bone marrow stromal cells with respect to osteoblast differentiation. J Orthop Res 1997;15:546–547.

3. Marx RE, Garg AK. The biology of platelets and the mechanism of platelet-rich plasma. In: Dental and Craniofacial Applications of Platelet-Rich Plasma. Chicago: Quintessence, 2005:3–30.

4. Kratchmarova I, Blagoev B, Haack-Sorensen M, Kassem M, Mann M. Mechanism of divergent growth factor effects in mesenchymal stem cell differentiation. Science 2005;308:1472–1477.

5. Franceschi RT. Biologic approaches to bone regeneration by gene therapy. J Dent Res. 2005;84:1093–1103.

6. Marx RE. Platelet rich plasma: Evidence to support its use. J Oral Maxillofac Surg 2004;62:489–496.

7. Davies JE, Lowenberg B, Shiga A. The bone-titanium interface in vitro. J Biomed Mater Res 1990;24:1289–1306.

8. Froum S, Wallace S, Elian N, Cho S, Tarnow D. Comparison of mineralized cancellous bone allograft (Puros) and anorganic bovine bone matrix (Bio Oss) for sinus augmentation: Histomorphometry at 26 to 32 weeks after grafting. Int J Periodontics Restorative Dent 2006;26:543–551.

9. Landi L, Pretel RW Jr, Hakimi NM, Setayesh R. Maxillary sinus floor elevation using a combination of DFDBA and bovine-derived porous hydroxyapatite: A preliminary histologic and histomorphometric report. Int J Periodontics Restorative Dent 2000;20:574–583.

10. Canfield AE, Doherty MJ, Ashton BA. Osteogenic potential of vascular pericytes. In: Davies JE (ed). Bone Engineering. Toronto: EM Squared, 2000:143–152.

11. Burkus JK, Harvinder S, Girnet MF, Longley MC. Use of rhBMP-2 in combination with structural cortical allografts: Clinical and radiographic outcomes in anterior lumbar spinal surgery. J Bone Joint Surg Am 2005;87A:1205–1212.

12. Marx RE, Carlson ER, Eichstaedt RM, Schimmele SR, Strauss JE, Georgeff KR. Platelet rich plasma: Growth factor enhancement for bone grafts. Oral Surg Oral Med Oral Pathol Oral Radiol Endod 1998;85:638–646.

13. Marx RE, Garg AK. Acceleration of bone regeneration in dental procedures. In: Dental and Craniofacial Applications of Platelet-Rich Plasma. Chicago: Quintessence, 2005:53–86.

14. Kevy SV, Jacobson MS. Comparison of methods for point of care preparation of autologous platelet gel. J Extra Corpor Technol 2004;36:28–35.

15. Peleg M, Major Z, Garg AK. Augmentation grafting of the maxillary sinus floor and simultaneous implant placement in patients with 3 to 5 mm of residual alveolar bone height. Int J Oral Maxillofac Implants 1999;14:549–556.

16. Kassolis JD, Rosen PS, Reynolds MA. Alveolar ridge and sinus augmentation utilizing platelet rich plasma in combination with freeze dried bone allograft: Case series. J Periodontol 2000;71:1654–1661.

17. Garg AK. Augmentation grafting of the maxillary sinus for placement of dental implants. In: Bone Biology, Harvesting, and Grafting for Dental Implants: Rationale and Clinical Applications. Chicago: Quintessence, 2004:171–211.

18. Lataillade JJ, Clay D, David C, et al. Phenotypic and functional characteristics of CD34+ cells are related to their anatomic environment: Is their versatility a prerequisite for their bioavailability? J Leukocyte Biol 2005;77:634–643.

19. Burkus JK, Transfeldt EE, Kitchel SH, Watkins RG, Balderstin RA. Clinical and radiographic outcomes of anterior lumbar interbody fusion using recombinant human bone morphogenetic protein-2. Spine 2002;27:2396–2408.

20. Govender S, Csimma C, Genant HK, et al. Recombinant human bone morphogenetic protein-2 for treatment of open tibial fractures: A prospective, controlled randomized study of four hundred and fifty patients. J Bone Joint Surg Am 2002;84A:2123–2134.

21. Fiorellini JP, Howell TH, Cochran D, et al. Randomized study evaluating recombinant human bone morphogenetic protein-2 for extraction socket augmentation. J Periodontol 2005; 76:605–613.

22. Boyne PJ, Lilly LC, Marx RE, et al. De novo induction by recombinant human bone morphogenetic protein-2 (rhBMP-2) in maxillary sinus floor augmentation. J Oral Maxillofac Surg 2005;63:1693–1707.

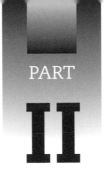

PART II

Periodontal Regeneration and Localized Implant Site Development

Treatment of Advanced Periodontal Defects Using Bioactive Therapies

Myron Nevins, DDS

Samuel E. Lynch, DMD, DMSc

Emil G. Cappetta, DMD

The loss of periodontium to inflammatory periodontal disease is frequently found in the form of an infrabony defect, for which there are three essential approaches to treatment. The first, and optimal, treatment is to regenerate the lost structures to the maximum degree; this is preferred to resective treatment, which is very predictable and useful for shallow defects. Because the angular bony defect is an indicator of further bone loss,[1] the third alternative, nonsurgical treatment, is inappropriate unless there are psychological or general health issues that preclude surgery. In any situation, some form of intervention is required; otherwise, the condition will likely worsen (Fig 5-1).

The predictability of regenerative approaches is guided by the defect morphology; the most contiguous envelope of bone provides the most protection for the blood clot to undergo organization. Classifications of such defects rely on the number of bony walls,[2] but most clinical defects consist of a combination of morphologies. There are few examples of pure three-wall defects, which offer the most likely success with the widest range of treatment modalities.[3–10]

This chapter discusses definitions of successful periodontal regeneration of infrabony defects and various approaches for achieving that success.

Definitions of Successful Regeneration

Periodontal regeneration includes the formation of new bone, new cementum, and new periodontal ligament (PDL) to form a new functional attachment apparatus over a root surface previously exposed to disease,[10] a histologic definition that can only be satisfied by human biopsy. Other criteria, such as reduced probing depth, attachment gain, radiographic observation, decreased tooth mobility, and surgical reopening (Fig 5-2) are meaningful indicators of treatment "success" but cannot prove the efficacy of a technique or material to accomplish the goal of regeneration.[11]

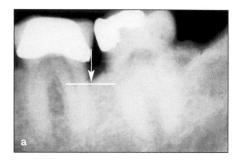

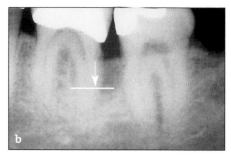

Fig 5-1a A 5-mm probing depth *(arrow)* on the distal surface of the mandibular left first molar is recorded at a routine hygiene visit. The patient rejected surgical treatment and decided to wait until reexamination at the next recall interval.

Fig 5-1b The defect *(arrow)* has worsened significantly at 3 months.

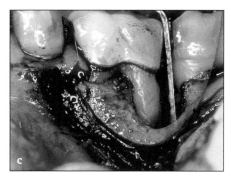

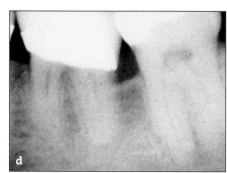

Fig 5-1c Surgery reveals the extensive bone loss.

Fig 5-1d Conditions are significantly improved 3 years later, after periodontal regeneration and placement of a new crown.

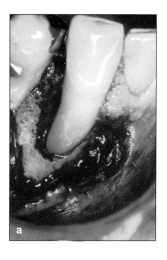

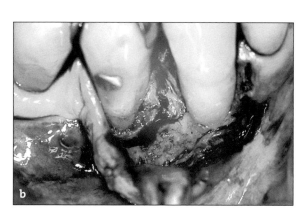

Fig 5-2a A deep, uncontained defect is located on the distal surface of the mandibular right canine. The treatment regimen included placement of mineralized allograft and a nonresorbable membrane.

Fig 5-2b The area, reopened after 6 years, demonstrates clinical regeneration.

It is necessary to distinguish between the endpoint goals of regeneration versus repair with a long junctional epithelium extending below the alveolar margin, as demonstrated by Caton and Zander[12] in a monkey model (Fig 5-3).

The histologic evaluation of new attachment in humans has been available in case report form for decades,[13-21] but not until a series of landmark studies by Bowers et al[22-24] in 1989 did histologic evaluation become a standard method of assessment. Biopsy specimens of teeth with infrabony defects were harvested 6 months after treatment with demineralized freeze-dried bone allograft in 12 patients. The grafted sites outperformed the nongrafted control sites by demonstrating new cementum, new alveolar bone, and new PDL, unlike the control sites, which healed with a long junctional epithelium. No evidence of root resorption or ankylosis accompanied the observed regeneration (Fig 5-4).

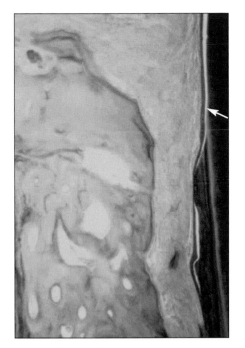

Fig 5-3 Histologic specimen from a monkey. The epithelium extends apical to the crestal bone (*arrow*), precluding any connective tissue attachment. This is not periodontal regeneration as defined at the World Workshop in Clinical Periodontics[10] in 1989 (H&E stain; original magnification ×10). (From Caton and Zander.[12] Reprinted with permission.)

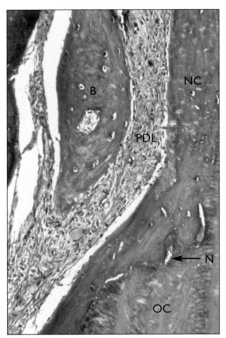

Fig 5-4a Periodontal regeneration after treatment of osseous deformities. Note new bone (B), cementum on dentin, acellular cementum, and periodontal ligament (PDL) with Sharpey fiber attachment (hematoxylin-eosin [H&E] stain; original magnification ×40). (NC) New cementum; (OC) old cementum; (N) notch.

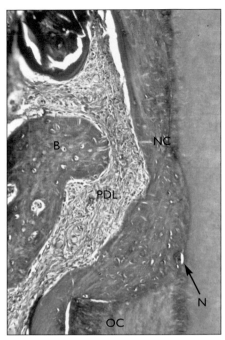

Fig 5-4b New cellular cementum (NC) covers the notch in the root (H&E stain; original magnification ×40). (B) Bone; (PDL) periodontal ligament; (OC) old cementum; (N) notch. (Figs 5-4a and 5-4b from Middleton and Bowers.[25] Reprinted with permission.)

The new cellular cementum formed on both old cementum and dentin, obviating the need to remove all existing cementum at the depth of the defect to gain regeneration.[25] This resolves a difficult clinical problem, because it is impossible to be sure that the acellular cementum is removed at the most apical aspect.

Because it defies logic to require histologic evidence for each and every procedure, the rational approach is to select methods and materials that have been subjected to such scrutiny and to evaluate therapeutic results less invasively.

Surgical Techniques

Deep, narrow bony defects seem to respond better than wide, shallow defects to regenerative techniques.[3–10,26–31] Whatever the shape and size of a defect, treatment regimens must adhere to basic surgical tenets:

- The surgical flap approach must result in clear access to and visibility of the defect (Fig 5-5).

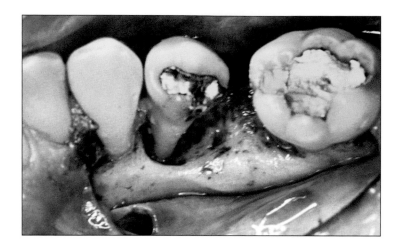

Fig 5-5 Clear access, visibility, degranulation, root conditioning, decortications, and primary closure of the wound are of paramount importance in attempts to achieve periodontal regeneration. The surgical procedure extends one tooth mesially beyond the circumferential intraosseous lesion. At that point there is a small cutback incision toward the procedure. The granulomatous tissue is removed and root instrumentation is completed. There are numerous decortications to allow communication of the regenerative elements in the marrow spaces.

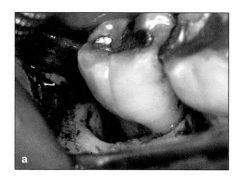

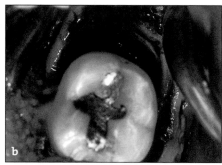

Figs 5-6a and 5-6b Three-wall defects located on the distal surfaces of the mandibular first and second molars extend to the buccal surface, approaching but not violating the furcation. The defects will be managed with a barrier membrane. The bone in the region is often very cancellous and thus decortications are unnecessary.

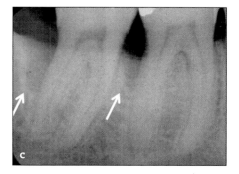

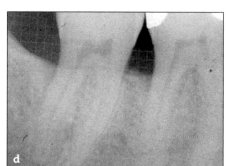

Fig 5-6c The preoperative radiograph reveals intraosseous defects (*arrows*) on the distal surfaces of both mandibular molars.

Fig 5-6d Radiograph of the area 4 years postoperatively. The defects have been resolved and there is minimal sulcus depth.

- The root surface must be decontaminated after the removal of all accretions.
- All granulation tissue must be removed from the infrabony defect, because its presence will interfere with clot formation and organization. Granulation tissue also will preclude the necessary space for new regenerative tissues.
- The infrabony surface must communicate with narrow spaces and the PDL space to account for the availabil-

ity of progenitor cells and capillary budding, resulting in angiogenesis.
- The flap must be completely coapted to cover the regenerative site to protect its integrity.

Three-wall defects have responded effectively to defect debridement with straight-line incisions to promote connective tissue attachment[3,4] (Fig 5-6). This approach has been confirmed and used successfully with an exclusion-

Fig 5-7a A clinical observation of the maxillary right canine and premolar area shows 5- to 6-mm probing depths after root planing. The gingiva is pink, and there is no bleeding on probing. Is this periodontal health?

Fig 5-7b The histologic appearance of the area shown in Fig 5-7a. Note the severe inflammatory infiltrate (I) and disorganized gingival corium with enlarged rete pegs (RP) and ulcerative epithelium. This histologic appearance is not consistent with periodontal health, although the gingiva is pink and no longer bleeding on probing after the root planing procedures. (AC) Alveolar crest; (JE) junctional epithelium; (CE) cementum; (SE) sulcular epithelium. (Figs 5-7a and 5-7b from Dragoo et al.[36] Reprinted with permission.)

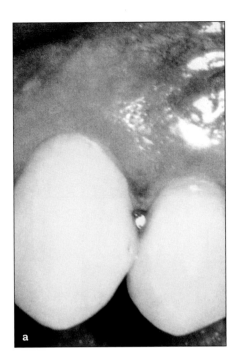

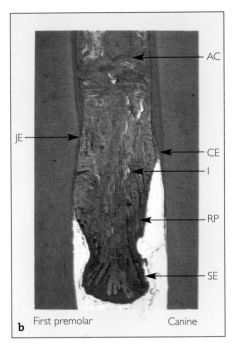

ary barrier membrane to promote hard tissue healing.[7,8] The use of a barrier membrane treatment for bone defects is dependent on space making for new hard tissue development. Its use in combination with grafting materials has been efficacious in clinical studies for both infrabony and some Class II furcation defects.[26–31]

Nonsurgical Techniques

There have been many products that claim to accomplish regeneration but offer inadequate histologic evidence of success. The hierarchy of evidence in periodontal wound healing suggests the human model as most significant, because animal models introduce morphologic, bacterial, and healing mechanisms that can be misleading but nevertheless, provide substantial observations in preclinical studies. It is necessary to continue the investigations in human trials to prove conclusively the ultimate goal of regeneration. These studies must be accomplished with a lucid protocol providing a satisfactory reconstruction of the biopsied area for the patient.

The selection of a nonsurgical approach to infrabony pockets is questionable when a probing depth greater than 5 mm is indicative of the presence of periodontal pathogens.[32,33] Because such defects are also indicative of the patient's susceptibility to disease, treatment that does not include surgical debridement and reduction of probing depth either by resection or regeneration is illogical. In such cases, the nonsurgical course is in discord with the overall approach to periodontal treatment, the goal of which is to create an environment that the hygienist and the patient can keep clean. There is no study to date that demonstrates histologic periodontal regeneration with a nonsurgical approach. In fact, the only study with such evidence demonstrates the connective tissue corium to be in disarray[34] (Fig 5-7).

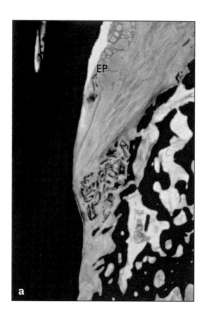

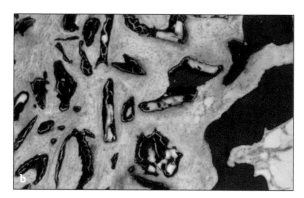

Fig 5-8a This infrabony defect was treated with bioactive ceramics. Although the material is biocompatible, epithelium (EP) is seen along the root surface to the base of the defect. Graft particles are evident within the defect, and there are limited signs of new bone formation. This is not the picture of periodontal regeneration (toluidine blue–basic fuschin stain).

Fig 5-8b The area grafted with bioactive ceramic material is invaded by dense connective tissue, and there are no signs of inflammation around the graft particles. There is minimal new bone formation (toluidine blue–basic fuschin stain).

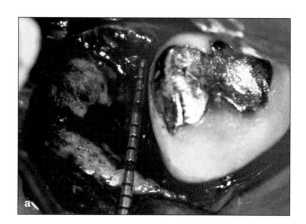

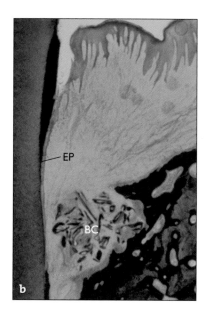

Fig 5-9a A three-wall defect is evident on the mesial surface of the molar. The defect is 10 mm in width but totally contained. It was treated with debridement, meticulous root planing, and placement of the bioactive ceramic graft material.

Fig 5-9b Bioactive ceramic graft material (BC) fills the defect, and epithelium (EP) extends apical to the mouth of the defect. There are no signs of periodontal regeneration, but the material is biocompatible (toluidine blue–basic fuschin stain; original magnification ×6.3). (Figs 5-9a and 5-9b from Nevins et al.[36] Reprinted with permission.)

Regenerative Techniques

The past decade has provided an opportunity to perform proof-of-principle research with an assortment of regenerative materials to demonstrate their efficacy and, in some instances, their limitations.[35]

Ceramics

Bioactive ceramics were used to treat six infrabony pockets, and the biopsy specimens were harvested at 6 months.[36] The base of the calculus was marked by the apical extent of the root planing, and the particulate graft material was placed in the debrided bone defect. The full flaps were coapted to cover the surgical site, and the patient returned frequently for debridement visits. The

Fig 5-10a A preoperative radiograph reveals a significant infrabony defect. The probe is placed to the base of the defect; there is 11 mm of clinical attachment loss.

Fig 5-10b The defect has three walls and is confined to the distal aspect of the canine.

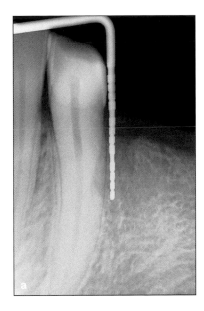
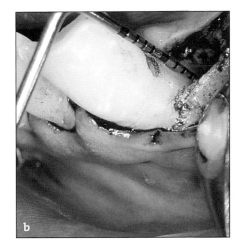

Fig 5-10c The infrabony defect is grafted with cancellous Bio-Oss.

Fig 5-10d The graft is then covered with a Bio-Gide membrane.

(Fig 5-10 continued on next page.)

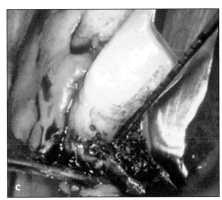
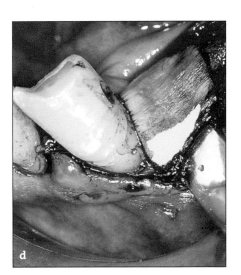

results demonstrate the material to be biocompatible, but there were no signs of periodontal regeneration. There was an absence of inflammatory infiltrate into the connective tissue corium, but the epithelium progressed apical to the level of bone, and there was almost no evidence of new bone formation even when a three-wall defect was treated (Figs 5-8 and 5-9).

Xenograft

A similar protocol was used to treat infrabony pockets with a deproteinized xenograft, Bio-Oss (Osteohealth),

which was used by itself and in combination with a resorbable collagen barrier membrane, Bio-Gide (Osteohealth).[37] The histologic biopsy specimens demonstrated approximately 5.0 mm of new cementum with the xenograft and 7.0 mm of new cementum with the xenograft and the collagen membrane (Fig 5-10). The epithelial downgrowth clearly stopped occlusal to the bone defect, at which point a dense insertion of Sharpey fibers into new cementum was observed.

This continued apically beyond the mouth of the bone defect, providing a true connective tissue seal. The xenograft particles were surrounded by new bone throughout the specimen to the area of root demarcation. The only shortcoming in this specimen was the inability of the osteoconductive materials to complete

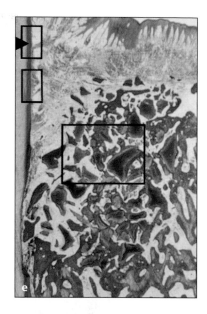

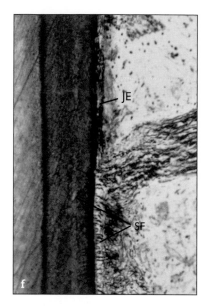

Fig 5-10e Histologic section 7 months after grafting with Bio-Oss and Bio-Gide. The grafted area is nearly completely invaded with new bone. New bone is present on the surface of the Bio-Oss granules apically. The apical extent of the epithelium (*arrowhead*) is coronal to the Sharpey fiber attachment. New cementum is present along the entire length of the root surface adjacent to the original defect. Collagen fibers are oriented perpendicular to the root surface. No graft particles were observed in direct contact with the root surface (H&E stain; original magnification ×3.2).

Fig 5-10f Top left box in Fig 5-10e. At higher magnification, the specimen reveals the apical extent of the junctional epithelium (JE), blocked by new cementum and Sharpey fiber (SF) attachment (H&E stain; original magnification ×50).

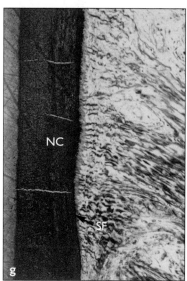

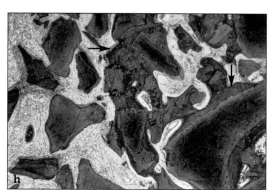

Fig 5-10g Bottom left box in Fig 5-10e. Higher magnification shows new cellular cementum (NC) with perpendicularly oriented inserting Sharpey fibers (SF) (H&E stain; original magnification ×50).

Fig 5-10h Increased magnification of the center box in Fig 5-10e reveals a dense growth of new bone (*arrowheads*) around and between the Bio-Oss particles (*). The new bone is densest on the Bio-Oss particles, suggesting that the graft performs as an osteoconductive material (H&E stain; original magnification ×12.5). (Figs 5-10a, 5-10b, and 5-10d to 5-10h from Camelo et al.[37] Reprinted with permission.)

bone regeneration at the occlusal (widest) portion of the defect, perhaps demonstrating the limits achieved with an osteoconductive material.

The search for an appropriate combination of material to further augment this result led to a composite graft of 50% autogenous bone and 50% Bio-Oss covered with a Bio-Gide membrane.[38] The composite graft provided an osteoconductive scaffold and, theoretically, some osteoinduction from the autograft. The bone defect was prepared for regeneration through meticulous surgical technique, including defect and root debridement to completely remove granulation tissue and subsequent

root decontamination using a wash of tetracycline (Figs 5-11a to 5-11d). The composite graft was then covered with the collagen barrier membrane, and the soft tissues were closed primarily to cover the entire surgical wound. The histologic observation of the biopsy specimens demonstrated periodontal regeneration; the defect was occupied by new cementum, new bone, and a functionally oriented PDL (Figs 5-11e and 5-11f).

This process was repeated with Bio-Oss Collagen, and results similar to those of Bio-Oss were achieved.[39] Significant new information was provided by the use of a microtomograph (Micro-CT, SkyScan) that demonstrated appar-

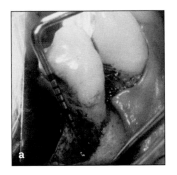
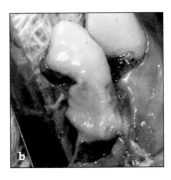
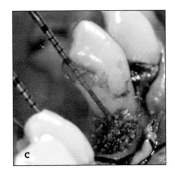
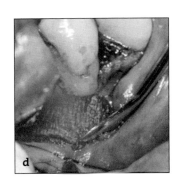

Fig 5-11a A periodontal defect is shown after removal of infected granulomatous tissue. Significant calculus accretions are present on the diseased root surface within the perimeters of the osseous defect and extend to the base of the defect.

Fig 5-11b Tetracycline paste is used to decontaminate and etch the root surface.

Fig 5-11c A composite of Bio-Oss and autogenous bone graft is placed in the defect.

Fig 5-11d A Bio-Guide membrane covers the graft. (Figs 5-11a to 5-11d from Camelo et al.[38] Reprinted with permission.)

Fig 5-11e Histologic block demonstrates periodontal regeneration to this previously diseased root surface. New bone (B), periodontal ligament (PDL), and cementum (NC) are visible above the notch (N) at the base of the defect (toluidine blue–basic fuschin stain; original magnification ×3.2).

Fig 5-11f A higher magnification of the coronal aspect of Fig 5-11e. There is bone (NB) surrounding the Bio-Oss and autogenous bone graft particles (toluidine blue–basic fuschin stain; original magnification ×63). (PDL) Periodontal ligament; (NC) new cementum.

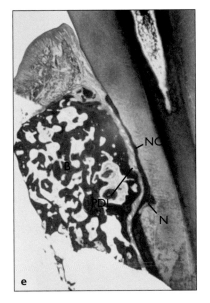
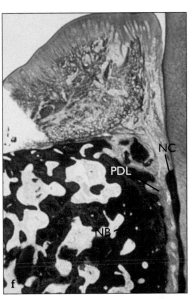

ent complete regeneration for the portion of the defects that were well contained (three-wall) and less organized tissues with granules of the graft in the portions of the defects that were less well contained (Fig 5-12). The interpretation appears to be that a more powerful product is necessary to predictably resolve poorly contained periodontal bone defects (one- and two-wall portions).

Recombinant growth factors

In recognition of the need for a more powerful regenerative agent, tissue engineering investigations have proceeded toward a biomimetic approach utilizing recombinant human platelet-derived growth factor (rhPDGF-BB).[40–42] This biomimetic approach to regeneration combines osteoconductive scaffolds, the patient's own progenitor cells for osteoblasts and fibroblasts in vivo, and potent signaling molecules that are capable of stimulating cellular events associated with periodontal regeneration.

Signaling molecules are factors capable of stimulating cellular events associated with tissue regeneration:

- Chemotaxis
- Proliferation
- Angiogenesis
- Cellular differentiation
- Production of extracellular matrix

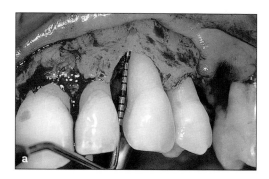

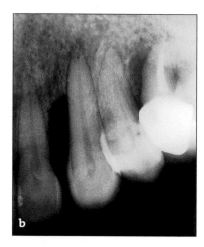

Fig 5-12a A 7-mm combination one-, two-, and three-wall infrabony defect is present on the mesial aspect of the maxillary left canine. In the defect, 4 mm are contained, and 4 mm provide one wall.

Fig 5-12b Preoperative radiograph of the one- and two-wall defect.

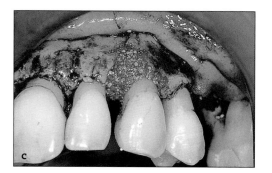

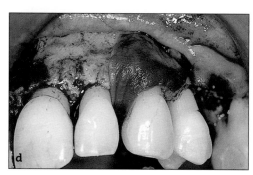

Fig 5-12c The bony defect is filled to the highest level of the retaining walls with the graft material.

Fig 5-12d Bio-Gide bilayer collagen membrane is fitted interproximally to cover the graft material.

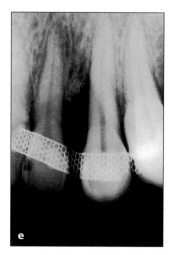

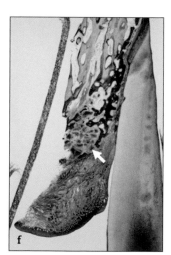

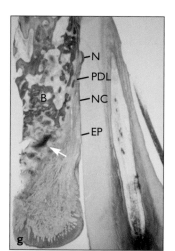

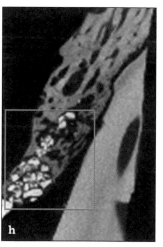

Fig 5-12e The partial recovery of the bony septum on the mesial aspect of the canine is suggested 6 months postoperatively. (Figs 5-12a to 5-12e from Nevins et al.[39] Reprinted with permission.)

Figs 5-12f and 5-12g Mesial aspect of the canine treated with Bio-Oss Collagen and Bio-Gide membrane. Some particles of graft material (*arrows*) have not resulted in regeneration, where the bone defect was uncontained (see Fig 5-12a) (toluidine blue–basic fuschin stain; original magnification ×10.5). (N) Notch; (PDL) periodontal ligament; (NC) new cementum; (B) bone; (EP) epithelium.

Fig 5-12h Particles of Bio-Oss Collagen are visible in the coronal portion of the microtomogram (*box*). This uncontained portion of the defect (one-wall) has not evidenced regeneration histologically or in the microtomogram, but the more apical portion of the defect meets the criteria of periodontal regeneration.

Recombinant PDGF has been studied extensively in relation to its contributions to wound healing and periodontal regeneration.[40–57] The naturally occurring form of the protein is contained in the alpha granules of blood platelets and bone matrix and has been shown to be both chemotactic and mitogenic for osteoblasts and periodontal ligament fibroblasts.[46–51,53,54] Although some early studies combined rhPDGF-BB with insulin-like growth factor I (IGF-I),[43–45,52–55,57] results from nonhuman primates have demonstrated significant regeneration of new attachment with rhPDGF-BB alone.[52,55,56] The results from phase I and II human clinical trials[50,51] demonstrated that the protein was safe and effective when applied locally to bone defects during periodontal surgery.[57] A single application resulted in statistically significant improvement in bone growth and fill of periodontal defects compared with open flap debridement alone.

A proof-of-principle trial measured the clinical, radiographic, and histologic effect of rhPDGF-BB delivered in an allograft matrix for the treatment of human periodontal defects.[41] Nine patients were selected; each had at least one stable tooth that had an infrabony defect and that was considered to be a candidate for extraction.[40] Full-thickness periodontal flaps were elevated, and notches were placed with a small carbide bur at the apical extent of the calculus to demarcate the extent of periodontal disease. Root planing was followed by decontamination with a slurry of tetracycline that was allowed to remain in place for 5 minutes and then eliminated with copious irrigation. Researchers cannot be selective with recruitment of patients for human histologic studies because not enough patients are available, regardless of the agreed on dental reconstructive benefits, so most osseous defects have compromised envelopes of bone. Three doses of rhPDGF-BB (0.5, 1.0, or 5.0 mg/mL) were tested to establish the most effective dose.

Presurgical findings were recorded, including clinical photographs, radiographs, probing depths, and attachment levels; the same parameters were recorded again 7 to 9 months after surgery. The three treatment groups resulted in no safety issues for any of the patients. Clinical measurements, including probing depth and clinical attachment level, were significantly improved compared with the baseline measurements. The radiographic appearance suggested bone fill in the defects and no abnormal changes in bone architecture or root configuration.

The histologic evaluation demonstrated robust regeneration of the periodontium, not only at the level of the notch but significantly occlusal to it. It is important to remember that the demarcation was placed at the apical extent of the calculus and that there was approximately a 1-mm plaque-free zone apical on the root surface with no bone. This must be taken into consideration with regard to the periodontal regeneration that was accomplished.

Two of the four specimens in that study are presented for observation. The first was a maxillary canine with extensive loss of periodontium and infrabony defects that were of the one- and two-wall varieties; only the base of 1 mm showed complete containment or protection of the blood clot (Figs 5-13a to 5-13c).

Comparison of the 9-month radiograph and the histologic image allows correlation of the notch and provides evidence of regeneration at the level of the notch and occlusal to it (Fig 5-13d). The periodontal ligament was mature, vascular, and demonstrated Sharpey fiber attachment into both the new cellular cementum and new bone with absolutely no root resorption or ankylosis (Figs 5-13e and 5-13f).

The second example was a mandibular anterior tooth with a probing depth of 8 mm (Fig 5-14a). Histologic evidence of regeneration included the notch area, an area occlusal to the notch, and the area of the mouth of the defect (Figs 5-14b to 5-14d). All three sites revealed new cellular cementum; a mature, functional, and vascular periodontal ligament; and new bone with little or no evidence of the allograft matrix. Previous testing of materials[36,37,39] revealed regenerative limitations at the mouth of noncontained defects except when osteoconductive material was mixed with autogenous bone, but the observed outcome of rhPDGF-BB with an allograft matrix was very positive. The apical migration of the junctional epithelium was easily identified at a level occlusal to the infrabony pocket, and the occlusal extent of the new cementum with Sharpey fiber attachment resulted in complete regeneration (Fig 5-14e). The new bone almost completely replaced the allograft matrix, with only two small pieces found above the new bone. Even these pieces appeared to demonstrate new bone on their surface.

The significance of this observation is obvious when translated into bone development for the purpose of implant placement. The suprabony connective tissue fiber apparatus was mature and dense, and the occlusal portion of the new periodontal ligament was as defined, vascular, and mature as the nonapical area of the notch.

The second phase of this proof-of-principle study was designed to test the capacity of rhPDGF-BB to promote regeneration in class II furcation defects in mandibular molars. Significant success has been reported previously with other clinical studies and different materials but has not been substantiated with histologic evidence.[7,26–31,58–75]

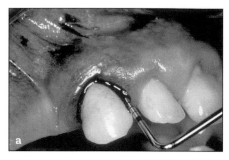
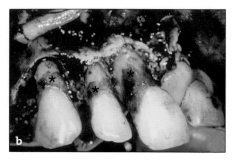
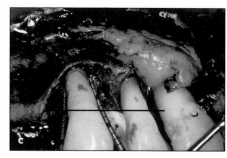

Fig 5-13a Preoperative photograph of the maxillary right canine with a 15-mm probe in place.

Fig 5-13b Intraoperative view of the maxillary incisors and canine. The base of calculus is marked (*).

Fig 5-13c Following reflection of a full-thickness flap and root debridement, 6-mm one-wall defects are visible on the mesial and distal aspects of the canine. There is a base of only 1 mm, offering complete containment for the protection of a blood clot. The *horizontal line* represents the maximum vertical level of bone.

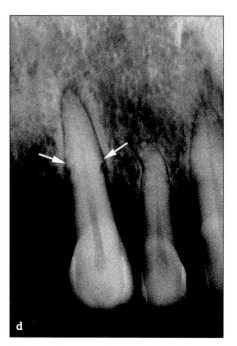
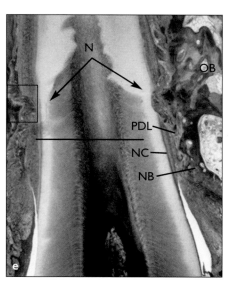
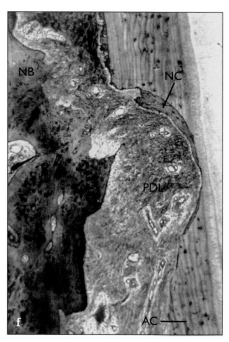

Fig 5-13d Postsurgical radiograph taken 9 months following treatment of the site with rhPDGF in the bone allograft. The notches (*arrows*) were placed at the time of surgery at the apical extent of the calculus. (Figs 5-13c and 5-13d from Nevins et al.[41] Reprinted with permission.)

Fig 5-13e Histologic section of the canine taken 9 months after treatment with rhPDGF mixed with bone allograft. Regeneration of clinically new attachment apparatus is evident. New bone (NB) is coronal to the level of old bone (OB) and the notches. The solid line demarcates the original bone from the new bone. A physiologic periodontal ligament (PDL) is clearly evident coronal to the notches (N) and adjacent new bone (toluidine blue–basic fuschin stain; original magnification ×2.5). (NC) New cementum.

Fig 5-13f Higher magnification of the boxed area in Fig 5-13e. Regeneration of attachment structures, including a thin layer of new cementum (NC), adjacent new periodontal ligament (PDL), and new bone (NB), is evident. New blood vessel formation is also apparent. The new bone is a dense construct of lamellar and woven bone and appears to be undergoing normal remodeling. The new PDL is well organized, with bundles of collagen fibers coursing perpendicularly from the new bone to the root surface (toluidine blue–basic fuschin stain; original magnification ×25). (AC) Alveolar crest.

Fig 5-14a The mandibular canine probes 8 mm at the distal surface.

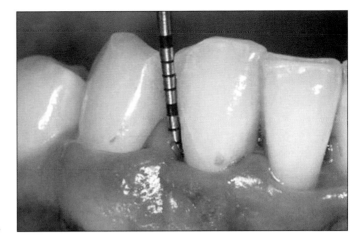

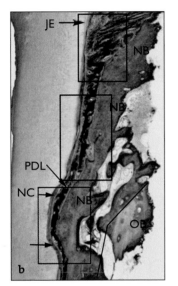

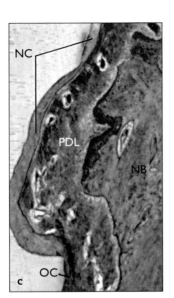

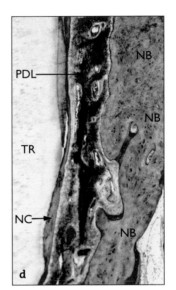

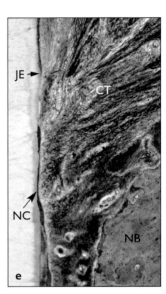

Fig 5-14b Histologic section of the infrabony defect taken at 9 months, following treatment with rhPDGF-BB. The apical extent of the calculus at the time of treatment is marked by the *arrow* at the base of the root notch. Several millimeters of dense new bone fill the original bony defect, and there is evidence of supracrestal bone apposition. The new bone (NB) is demarcated from the old bone (OB) by the *solid line*. The junctional epithelium (JE) stops just coronal to the new supracrestal bone. Thus, although no membrane was used, a long junctional epithelium did not occur. The absence of a long junctional epithelium is most likely due to growth factor stimulation (mitogenesis) and recruitment (chemotaxis) of the periodontal ligament (PDL) and bone cells, thereby allowing them to "win the race" with the epithelium (toluidine blue–basic fuschin stain; original magnification ×4). (NC) New cementum.

Fig 5-14c High-magnification view of the notch region (bottom box in Fig 5-14b). Generation of clinical new attachment apparatus is demonstrated by the presence of a thick layer of new cementum (NC), new periodontal ligament (PDL), and new bone (NB). The new bone is dense, and the PDL is vascular and well organized (toluidine blue–basic fuschin stain; original magnification ×25). (OC) Old cementum. (Figs 5-14b and 5-14c from Nevins et al.[41] Reprinted with permission.)

Fig 5-14d Higher magnification of the middle box in Fig 5-14b. Regeneration of the attachment structures, including new bone (NB), periodontal ligament (PDL), and new cementum (NC), is present. The PDL and bone are both well organized and dense. No inflammation, root resorption, or ankylosis was observed in any of the specimens (toluidine blue–basic fuschin stain; original magnification ×16). (TR) Tooth root.

Fig 5-14e Higher magnification of the top box in Fig 5-14b. Collagen fibers (Sharpey fibers) have a physiologic orientation perpendicular and inserting into the root surface. Dense bone is observed all the way to the crest. The new cementum (NC) ends adjacent to the crest of the new bone (NB). The junctional epithelium (JE) ends coronal to the new cementum and new bone (toluidine blue–basic fuschin stain; original magnification ×25). (CT) Gingival connective tissue.

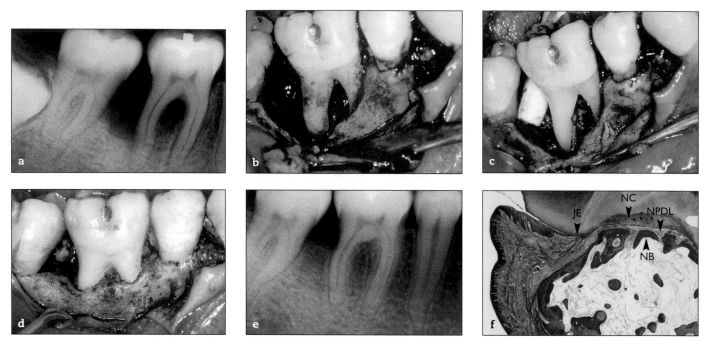

Fig 5-15a A significant class II furcation defect has compromised this mandibular molar.

Fig 5-15b Full-thickness flaps with sulcular and vertical releasing incisions are designed to achieve primary closure over the membrane and bone graft.

Fig 5-15c Meticulous root preparation has been performed, and the root has been treated with tetracycline paste for 4 minutes. All granulomatous tissue is removed and decortications are used to achieve bleeding from the bony defect. Autogenous bone harvested from the tuberosity was grafted into the class II furcation and osseous defect. A titanium-reinforced membrane was placed to cover the interproximal area and furcation.

Fig 5-15d The area is reopened after 1 year to evaluate the result. The defect shows evidence of clinical regeneration but requires minor osteoplasty to refine the interproximal bone between these molars.

Fig 5-15e Radiograph of the defect after treatment.

Fig 5-15f A surgical block section reveals new cementum (NC), new bone (NB), and a functional new periodontal ligament (NPDL). There is no evidence of root resorption or ankylosis, and the junctional epithelium (JE) ends before encroaching on the furcation (toluidine blue–basic fuschin stain).

To date, successful class I furcation treatment has not required regenerative efforts and has an endpoint goal of preventing progression to a class II furcation. The regenerative treatment of class III, or through and through, furcation invasion has remained unpredictable and evasive. Therefore the class II furcation defect was selected for experimentation, with the goal of demonstrating a successful treatment regimen that would result in defect fill, providing optimal support for the tooth and a site that is more easily maintained by the patient and clinician.

A previous observation of a successful treatment regimen included 28 consecutively treated class II furcations.[76] The clinical protocol included mechanical root planing followed by tetracycline decontamination; the harvest of autogenous bone to fill the defect; the artful placement of a nonresorbable membrane; meticulous suturing with advancement of the flaps; and lengthy surgical interventions. Clinical and radiographic suggestion of regeneration was apparent at the 1-year surgical reentry procedure, which was confirmed histologically (Fig 5-15). The definition of periodontal regeneration was satisfied with new cementum, new bone, and a new periodontal ligament with the junctional epithelium ending occlusal to the furcation entrance (see Fig 5-15f).

While interesting proof of the academic principle of cell occlusion to enhance regeneration, this treatment regimen is not user friendly, requires significant surgical time, and adds significant cost to the patient and clinician. Therefore, a more clinically viable alternative regimen was sought, and the use of rhPDGF-BB was evaluated in a similar study.[40] Following thorough debridement of the tooth and the defect, the osseous defects were filled with

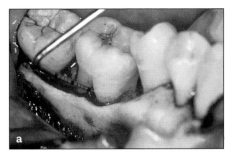

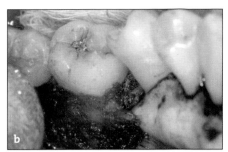

Fig 5-16a A probe reveals a 5-mm, primarily horizontal class II furcation invasion on the lingual aspect of a mandibular molar. Root conditioning for decontamination was accomplished with tetracycline paste, which was applied for 4 minutes and rinsed with saline.

Fig 5-16b rhPDGF has been applied to the root surface. The allograft was hydrated with the rhPDGF and packed into the defect.

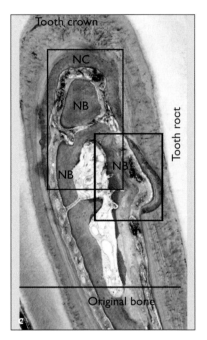

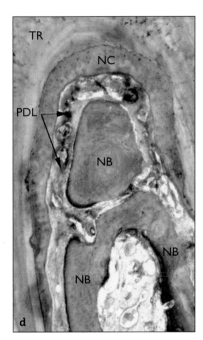

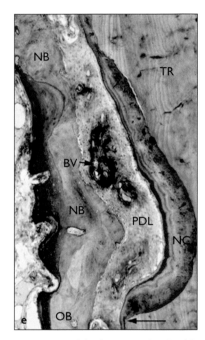

Fig 5-16c Histologic section of the molar in Fig 5-16a, obtained 9 months after treatment with rhPDGF mixed with allograft, shows complete periodontal regeneration within furcation. New bone (NB) formed in continuity with original bone, and new periodontal ligament is indistinguishable from original periodontal ligament apical to the original defect. Periodontal ligament fibers are perpendicular, traversing between new cementum (NC) and bone (toluidine blue–basic fuschin stain; original magnification ×6.3).

Fig 5-16d Higher magnification of boxed coronal area in Fig 5-16c. Complete fill of the original defect area, with new bone (NB), periodontal ligament (PDL), and new cementum (NC), is present. The new bone is equal in density to the original alveolar bone. There is no epithelial downgrowth into the furcation (long junctional epithelium), although no membrane was used (toluidine blue–basic fuschin stain, original magnification ×6). (TR) Tooth root.

Fig 5-16e Higher magnification of the boxed root notch area in Fig 5-16c, showing the tooth root (TR), newly regenerated bone (NB), new periodontal ligament (PDL), and new cementum (NC). The PDL is well organized, and its fibers are perpendicular and tangential between the NC and new bone. The new PDL is the same width as the original PDL and contains abundant blood vessels (BV) (toluidine blue–basic fuschin stain, original magnification ×25). (OB) Old bone; (arrow) base of calculus notch. (Figs 5-16c to 5-16e from Camelo et al.[40] Reprinted with permission.)

allograft that had been hydrated with rhPDGF-BB. The flaps were sutured in place, obtaining primary closure to protect the grafted site (Figs 5-16a and 5-16b).

The clinical and radiographic results were very encouraging, and the histologic evidence was compelling. The histologic definition of periodontal regeneration was fulfilled not only at the level of the notch but throughout the fundus area. The entire tooth surface was covered with cellular cementum, new bone had filled the defect, and a functional, vascular, mature PDL with Sharpey fiber attachment was evident everywhere. The bone graft scaffold was replaced, and there was no evidence of root resorption or ankylosis (Figs 5-16c to 5-16e).

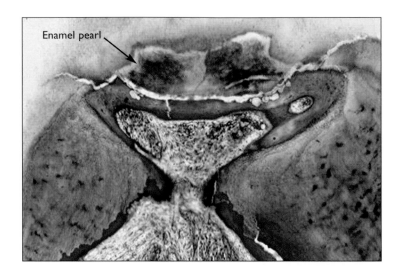

Fig 5-17 New collagen fibers insert into the cementum-like material. Separation of new cementum-like material from enamel is likely an artifact. Mild inflammation is present. The morphology of the calcified tissue in the upper right corner gives the appearance of a second osteon or new cementum bridging the narrow gap between new cementum on the root surface and that covering the enamel pearl (toluidine blue–basic fuchsin stain; original magnification ×25).

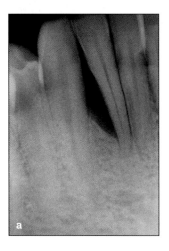

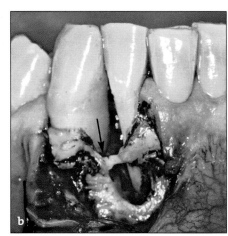

Fig 5-18a Radiograph of a mandibular lateral incisor that has been deemed hopeless and referred for extraction and implant site development.

Fig 5-18b Clinical appearance of the lateral incisor. A wide interdental crater (*arrow*) is present on the mesial surface of the canine.

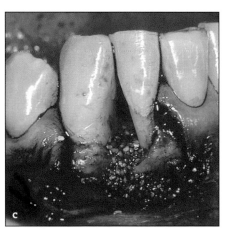

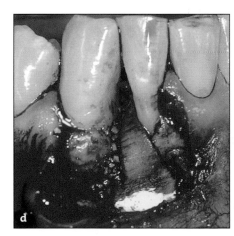

Fig 5-18c The defect has received an allograft, which has been hydrated and mixed with rhPDGF-BB. (Figs 5-18a to 5-18c from Nevins et al.[77] Reprinted with permission.)

Fig 5-18d A collagen membrane has been placed for empirical reasons.

One unique histologic observation occurred with a specimen of a class II furcation regeneration where an enamel pearl was overlooked. A bridge of cementum developed over the pearl, an indication of the powerful regenerative capacity of rhPDGF-BB[40] (Fig 5-17). Continued use of the signaling device (rhPDGF) has resulted in the treatment of severely compromised teeth with robust results.[43]

Fig 5-18e The pretreatment probing depth measures 13 mm.

Fig 5-18f Measurement after the surgical and regenerative procedure reveals a probing depth of 3 mm.

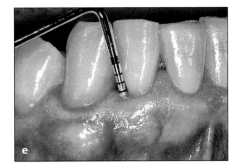
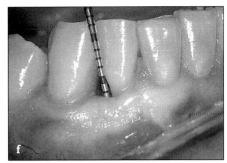

Fig 5-18g Resolution of the defect after 11 months.

Fig 5-18h The radiographic appearance at 11 months postsurgery. (Figs 5-18g and 5-18h from Nevins et al.[77] Reprinted with permission.)

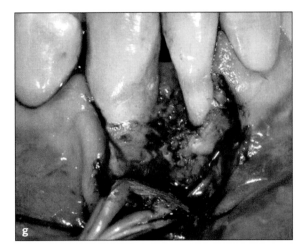
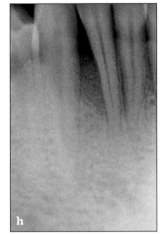

Fig 5-19a Another case treated with the protocol described in Fig 5-18. The infrabony defect threatens the prognosis of both the canine and lateral incisor.

Fig 5-19b Result of periodontal regeneration with rhPDGF-BB in combination with bone allograft. (Figs 5-19a and 5-19b from Nevins et al.[77] Reprinted with permission.)

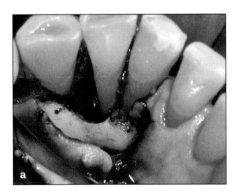
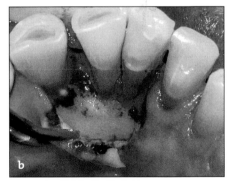

The interdental crater has not always responded to regeneration and frequently is treated with resection. However, in a case in which a mandibular incisor was referred for extraction, local bone development, and a potential implant, the patient agreed to allow treatment with rhPDGF-BB and an allograft substrate.[77] This site also received a Bio-Gide membrane for empirical reasons. The probing depth was reduced from 13 to 3 mm and reopened after 11 months (Fig 5-18). Significant regeneration was apparent not only for the lateral incisor but also for the mesial interdental crater on the canine; this was substantiated radiographically (see Fig 5-18h).

A similar case treated with the same protocol[77] involved severe bone loss associated with a mandibular lateral incisor and canine. The postsurgical result demonstrated excellent bone fill, evidence of a remarkable response to the combined treatment using rhPDGF-BB and allograft (Fig 5-19).

It is not reasonable to demand continuous histologic evidence of each case that is treated successfully. Once the proof of principle has been established, clinical and radiographic evidence is sufficient. The aforementioned regimens have significantly improved the prognosis of the treated teeth and accomplished the goal of allowing the

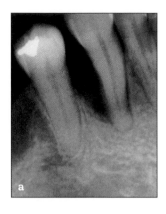
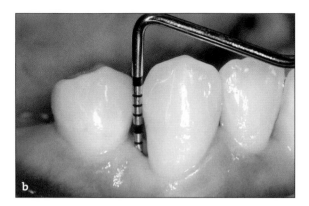

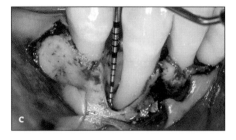
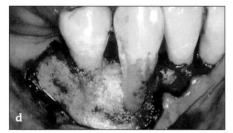

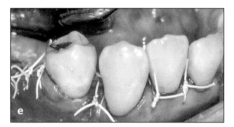
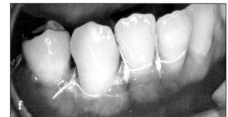

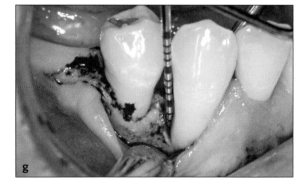
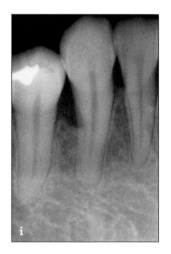

Fig 5-20a Initial pretreatment radiograph.

Fig 5-20b The distal surface of the mandibular right canine has probing depths of 8 to 9 mm.

Fig 5-20c The baseline osseous defect on the mandibular canine indicates a significant loss of periodontal attachment, and the prognosis is questionable. The osseous lesion is deep and for the most part uncontained. Meticulous debridement and root instrumentation have been completed. (Courtesy of Dr Marc L. Nevins.)

Fig 5-20d The defect has been filled with a scaffold of β-tricalcium phosphate mixed with rhPDGF.

Fig 5-20e The flaps are coapted to cover the surgical site.

Fig 5-20f Healing at 3 days.

Fig 5-20g Appearance of the defect on reopening to correct a small residual osseous discrepancy, 1-year postsurgery.

Fig 5-20h Radiographic appearance at 1 year.

Fig 5-20i Three-year postsurgical radiograph.

patient and the dental hygienist to control inflammation. The lost periodontium has been regenerated for susceptible patients with advanced defects.

The next phase of research was to test rhPDGF-BB in a large, multicenter, randomized controlled pivotal trial.[78] The regulatory process determined that β-tricalcium phosphate would be the scaffold, and 180 patients were enrolled. Only two patients were lost to the study, so 178 (97%) finished the study. No histologic blocks were necessary, because this was accomplished in earlier phases of the trial, but some areas were reopened for clinical observation.

Radiographic and clinical results were outstanding. The baseline evidence for a mandibular canine demonstrated significant loss of periodontium for a strategic tooth with an uncontained defect. The soft tissue healing at 3 days was remarkable, and the reopening and radiographic observation at 1 year provided a major upgrade of prognosis that continued at 3 years (Fig 5-20).

Freeze-dried bone allograft, a commonly used osteoconductive matrix for regenerative procedures, has been successfully used in combination with rhPDGF-BB (0.3 and 1.0 mg/mL) in treatment of severe infrabony defects. The ability of this signaling device to behave as a chemotactic and mitogenic agent when combined with such a matrix is dependent on effective absorption and release in its biologically active form. Binding and release studies of bone allograft demonstrate release with retention of potent biologic activity for the rhPDGF-BB (unpublished data, 2006). The results of patient treatments as described in this chapter demonstrate significant clinical and radiographic osteogenesis after 11 months of observation.

Conclusion

Great strides have been made toward predictable periodontal regeneration with the introduction and availability of recombinant growth factors. The observation that healing and regeneration proceed predictably without the use of barrier membranes is encouraging but does not preclude the value of membranes, as noted with some very advanced defects. Astute diagnosis, adherence to appropriate surgical protocol, and meticulous surgical technique will be dictating principles for success.

References

1. Papapanou PN, Wennstrom JL. The angular bony defect as an indicator of further alveolar bone loss. J Clin Periodontol 1991;18:317–322.
2. Goldman HM, Cohen DW. The infrabony pocket: Classification and treatment. J Periodontol 1958;29:272–291.
3. Prichard JF. The infrabony technique as a predictable procedure. J Periodontol 1957;28:202–217.
4. Prichard JF. The etiology, diagnosis, and treatment of the intrabony defect. J Periodontol 1967;38:455–465.
5. Becker W, Becker B, Berg L. Repair of intrabony defects as a result of open debridement procedures: Report of 36 treated cases. Int J Periodontics Restorative Dent 1986;6(2):8–21.
6. Becker W, Becker B, Berg L, Samsam C. Clinical and volumetric analysis of three-wall intrabony defects following open flap debridement. J Periodontol 1986;57:277–285.
7. Becker W, Becker BE, Berg L, Pritchard J, Caffesse R, Rosenberg E. New attachment after treatment with root isolation procedures: Report for treated class III and class II furcations and vertical osseous defects. J Periodontol 1988;3:9–24.
8. Becker W, Becker B. Treatment of mandibular three-wall intrabony defects by flap debridement and expanded polytetrafluoroethylene barrier membranes. Long-term evaluation of 32 treated patients. J Periodontol 1993;64:1138–1144.
9. Kim CK, Choi SH, Cho KS, Moon IS, Wikesjö UME, Kim CK. Periodontal repair in surgically created intrabony defects in dogs: Influence of the number of bone walls on healing response. J Periodontol 2004;75:31:229–235.
10. Nevins MN, Becker W, Kornman K (eds). Proceedings of the World Workshop in Clinical Periodontics, 23–27 July 1989. Chicago: American Academy of Periodontics, 1989.
11. Lynch SE. Methods for the evaluation of regenerative procedures. J Periodontol 1992;63:1085–1092.
12. Caton J, Zander H. Osseous repair of an infrabony pocket without new attachment of connective tissue. J Clin Periodontol 1976;3:54–58.
13. Ross SE, Cohen DW. The fate of a free osseous tissue autograft. A clinical and histologic case report. Periodontics 1968;6:145–151.
14. Schallhorn RG, Hiatt W, Boyce W. Iliac transplants in periodontal therapy. J Periodontol 1970;41:614–625.
15. Schallhorn RG, Hiatt W. Human allografts of iliac cancellous bone and marrow in periodontal osseous defects. 2. Clinical observations. J Periodontol 1972;43:67–81.
16. Dragoo MR, Sullivan HC. A clinical and histologic evaluation of autogenous iliac bone grafts in humans. 1. Wound healing 2 to 8 months. J Periodontol 1973;44:599–613.
17. Hiatt WH, Schallhorn RG. Intraoral transplants of cancellous bone and marrow in periodontal lesions. J Periodontol 1973;44:194–208.
18. Dragoo MR, Sullivan HC. A clinical and histological evaluation of autogenous iliac bone grafts in humans. II. External root resorption. J Periodontol 1973;44:614–625.
19. Hiatt WH, Schallhorn RG, Aaronian A. The induction of new bone and cementum formation. 4. Microscopic examination of the periodontium following human bone and marrow autograft, allograft, and non graft procedures. J Periodontol 1978;49:495–512.
20. Evans R. A clinical and histologic observation of an intra bony lesion. Int J Periodontics Restorative Dent 1981;1(1):21–26.
21. Dragoo MR, Kadahl WB. Clinical and histological evaluation of alloplasts and allografts in regenerative periodontal surgery in humans. 2. Int J Periodontics Restorative Dent 1983;3(2):9–29.
22. Bowers GM, Chadroff B, Carnevale R, et al. Histologic evaluation of new attachment formation in humans. 1. J Periodontol 1989;60:664–674.
23. Bowers GM, Chadroff B, Carnevale R, et al. Histologic evaluation of new attachment formation in humans. 2. J Periodontol 1989;60:675–682.
24. Bowers GM, Chadroff B, Carnevale R, et al. Histologic evaluation of new attachment apparatus in humans. 3. J Periodontol 1989;60:683–693.
25. Middleton CT, Bowers GM. Histologic evaluation of cementogenesis on periodontitis-affected roots. Int J Periodontics Restorative Dent 1990;10:429–436.
26. Schallhorn R, McClain P. Combined osseous composite grafting, root conditioning and guided tissue regeneration. Int J Periodontics Restorative Dent 1988;8(4):9–31.
27. McClain P, Schallhorn R. Long-term observation of combined osseous composite grafting, root conditioning and guided tissue regeneration. Int J Periodontics Restorative Dent 1993;13:9–27.
28. Schallhorn R, McClain P. Clinical and radiographic healing pattern observations with combined regenerative techniques. Int J Periodontics Restorative Dent 1994;14:391–404.
29. Cortellini P, Bowers GM. Periodontal regeneration of intrabony defects. Int J Periodontics Restorative Dent 1995;15:128–145.
30. Becker W, Becker BE, Mellonig J, et al. A prospective multi-center study evaluating periodontal regeneration for class II furcation invasions and intrabony defects after treatment with bioabsorbable barrier membranes: 1 year results. J Periodontol 1996;67:641–649.
31. Bowers GM, Schallhorn R, Mc Clain P: Factors influencing the outcome of regenerative therapy in mandibular class II furcations. I. Int J Periodontics Restorative Dent 2003;74:1255–1268.
32. Levy RM, Giannobile WV, Feres M, Haffajee A, Smith C, Socransky S. The short term effect of apically repositioned flap surgery on the composition of the subgingival microbiota. Int J Periodontics Restorative Dent 1999;19:555–567.

33. Levy RM, Giannobile WV, Feres M, Haffajee A, Smith C, Socransky S. The effect of apically repositioned flap surgery on clinical parameters and the composition of subgingival microbiota: 12-month data. Int J Periodontics Restorative Dent 2002;22:209–219.

34. Dragoo MR, Grant DA, Gutverg D, Stambaugh R. Experimental periodontal treatment in humans. I. Subgingival root planing with and without chlorhexidine gluconate rinses. Int J Periodontics Restorative Dent 1984;4(3):9–31.

35. Low SB, King CJ, Krieger J An evaluation of bioactive ceramic in the treatment of periodontal osseous defects. Int J Periodontics Restorative Dent 1997;17: 359–367.

36. Nevins ML, Camelo M, Nevins M, et al. Human histologic evaluation of bioactive ceramics in the treatment of periodontal osseous defects. Int J Periodontics Restorative Dent 2000;20:459–467.

37. Camelo M, Nevins ML, Schenk RK, et al. Clinical, radiographic, and histologic evaluation of human periodontal defects treated with Bio-Oss and Bio-Guide. Int J Periodontics Restorative Dent 1998;18:321–331.

38. Camelo M, Nevins ML, Lynch SE, Schenk R, Simion M, Nevins M. Periodontal regeneration with an autogenous bone–Bio-Oss composite graft and a Bio-Gide membrane. Int J Periodontics Restorative Dent 2001;21:109–119.

39. Nevins ML, Camelo M, Lynch SE, Schenk RK, Nevins M. Evaluation of periodontal regeneration following grafting intrabony defects with Bio-Oss collagen. A human histologic report. Int J Periodontics Restorative Dent 2003;23:9–17.

40. Camelo M, Nevins ML, Schenk RK, Lynch S, Nevins M. Periodontal regeneration in human Class II furcations using purified recombinant human platelet-derived growth factor-BB (rhPDGF-BB) with bone allograft. Int J Periodontics Restorative Dent 2003;23:213–225.

41. Nevins M, Camelo M, Nevins ML, Schenk RK, Lynch SE. Periodontal regeneration in humans using recombinant human platelet derived growth factor–BB (rhPDGF-BB) and allogeneic bone. J Periodontol 2003;74:1282–1292.

42. McGuire M, Kao R, Nevins M, Lynch SE. rhPDGF-BB promotes healing of periodontal defects: 24-Month clinical and radiographic observations. Int J Periodontics Restorative Dent 2006;26:223–231.

43. Lynch SE, Williams RC, Polson AM, et al. A combination of platelet derived growth factor and insulin-like growth factor enhances periodontal regeneration. J Clin Periodontol 1989;16:545–554.

44. Graves DT, Valentin-Opran A, Delgado R, Valente AJ, Mundy G, Piche J. The potential of platelet derived growth factor as an autocrine or paracrine factor for human bone cells. Connect Tissue Res 1989;23:209–218.

45. Lynch SE, de Castilla GR, Williams RC, et al. The effects of short–term application of a combination of platelet derived and insulin like growth factors on periodontal wound healing. J Periodontol 1991;62:458–467.

46. Oates TW, Rouse CA, Cochran DL. Mitogenic effects of growth factors on human periodontal ligament cells in vitro. J Periodontol 1993;64:142–148.

47. Graves DT, Kang YM, Kose KN. Growth factors in periodontal regeneration. Compend Suppl 1994;18:S672–S677.

48. Dennison D, Vallone D, Pinero G. Differential effect of TGF-beta 1 and PDGF on proliferation of periodontal ligaments cells and gingival fibroblasts. J Periodontol 1994;65:641–648.

49. Lynch SE, Genco R, Marx R. The role of growth factors in repair and regeneration. In: Polson AM (ed). Periodontal Regeneration: Current Status and Directions. Chicago: Quintessence, 1994:179–198.

50. Cho MI, Lin WL, Genco RJ. Platelet derived growth factor-modulated guided tissue regeneration therapy. J Periodontol 1995;66:522–530.

51. Giannobile WV. Periodontal tissue engineering by growth factors. Bone 1996;19:23S–37S.

52. Giannobile WV, Hernandez RA, Finkelman RD, et al. Comparative effects of platelet-derived growth factor, insulin-like growth factor individually and in combination on periodontal regeneration in Macaca fasicularis. J Periodontal Res 1996;31:301–304.

53. Cochrane DL, Wozney JM. Biologic mediators for periodontal regeneration. Periodontol 2000 1999;19:40–58.

54. Piche JE, Graves DT. Study of growth factor requirements of human bone–derived cells. A comparison with human fibroblasts. Bone 1989;10:131–138.

55. Rutherford RB, Niekrash CE, Kennedy JE, Charette MF. Platelet-derived and insulin like-growth factors stimulate regeneration of periodontal attachment in monkeys. J Periodontal Res 1992;27:285–290.

56. Rutherford RE, Ryan ME, Kennedy JE, Tucker MM, Charette MF. Platelet derived growth factor and dexamethasone combined with a collagen matrix induce regeneration of the periodontium in monkeys J Clin Periodontol 1993;20: 537–544.

57. Howell TH, Fiorellini JP, Paquette D, Offenbacher S, Giannobile WV, Lynch SE. A phase I/II clinical trial to evaluate a combination of recombinant human platelet derived growth factor-BB and recombinant human insulin-like growth factor-I in subjects with periodontal disease. J Periodontol 1997;68:1186–1193.

58. Pontoriero R, Lindhe J, Nyman S, Rosenberg E, Sanavi F. Guided tissue regeneration in degree 2 furcation-involved mandibular molars. J Clin Periodontol 1988;15:247–254.

59. Kalkwarf K, Kadahl, Patel KD. Evaluation of furcation region response to periodontal therapy. J Periodontol 1988;59:794–804.

60. Pontoriero R, Lindhe J, Nyman S, Karring T, Rosenberg E, Sanavi F. Guided tissue regeneration of furcation defects in mandibular molars. J Clin Periodontol 1989;16:170–174.

61. Lekovic V, Kenney EB, Kovacevic K, Caranzza FA Jr. Evaluation of guided tissue regeneration in class II furcation defects. A clinical re-entry study. J Periodontol 1989;60:694–698.

62. Pontoriero R, Lindhe J, Nyman S, Karring T, Rosenberg E, Sanavi F. Guided tissue regeneration in the treatment of furcation defects in mandibular molars. A clinical study of degree III involvements. J Clin Periodontol 1989;16:170–178.

63. Anderegg CR, Martin SJ, Gray JL Mellonig J, Gher M. Clinical evaluation of the use of decalcified freeze dried bone allograft with guided tissue regeneration in the treatment of molar furcation invasions J Periodontol 1991;62:264–268.

64. Gantes B, Synowski B, Garrett S, Egelberg J. Treatment of periodontal furcation defects. Mandibular class III defects. J Periodontol 1991;62:361–364.

65. Meltzer DG, Seamons BC, Mellonig JT, Gher M, Gray JL. Clinical evaluation of guided tissue regeneration in treatment of maxillary class II furcation invasions. J Periodontol 1991;62:353–360.

66. Black BS, Gher ME, Sandifer JB, Fucini S, Richardson AC. Comparative study of collagen and expanded polytetrafluoroethylene membranes in the treatment of human class II furcation defects. J Periodontol 1994;65:598–604.

67. Rosen PS, Marks MH, Bowers GM. Regenerative therapy in the treatment of maxillary molar class II furcations: Case reports. Int J Periodontics Restorative Dent 1997;17:517–527.

68. Haney JM, Leknes K, Wikesjö U. Recurrence of mandibular molar furcation defects following citric acid root treatment and advanced flap procedures. Int J Periodontics Restorative Dent 1997;17:529–535.

69. Sanz M, Zabalegui I, Villa A, Sicilia A. Guided tissue regeneration in human class II furcations and interproximal infrabony defects after using a bioabsorbable membrane barrier. Int. J Periodontics Restorative Dent 1997;17:563–573.

70. Garrett S, Polson AM, Stoller NH, et al. Comparison of a bioabsorbable GTR barrier to a non-absorbable barrier in treating human Class II furcation defects. A multi-center parallel design randomized single-blind trial. J Periodontol 1997; 68:667–675.

71. Giannobile WV, Ryan S, Shih MS, Su DL, Kaplan PL, Chan TCK. Recombinant human osteogenic protein-1 (OP-1) stimulates periodontal wound healing in class III furcation defects. J Periodontol 1998;69:129–137.

72. Leonardis D, Garg AK, Pedrazzoli V, Pecora GE. Clinical evaluation of the treatment of Class II furcation involvements with bioabsorbable barriers alone or associated with demineralized bone allografts. J Periodontol 1999;70:8–12.

73. Choi SH, Kim CK, Cho KS, et al. Effect of recombinant human bone morphogenetic protein-2/absorbable collagen sponge (rhBMP-2ACS) on healing of 3 wall intrabony defects in dogs. J Periodontol 2002;73:63–72.

74. Murphy KG, Gunsolley JC. Guided tissue regeneration for the treatment of periodontal intrabony and furcation defects. A systematic review. Ann Periodontol 2003;8:266–302.

75. Park JB, Cho M. Periodontal regeneration in class 3 furcation defects in beagle dogs with guided tissue regenerative therapy with periodontal growth factors. J Periodontol 1995;66:462–477.

76. Camelo M, Nevins ML, Nevins M. Treatment of class II furcations with autogenous bone grafts and ePTFE membranes. Int J Periodontics Restorative Dent 2000;20:233–243.

77. Nevins M, Hanratty J, Lynch SE. Clinical results using recombinant human platelet-derived growth factor and mineralized freeze-dried bone allograft in periodontal defects., Int J Periodontics Restorative Dent 2007;27:421–427.

78. Nevins M, Giannobile WV, McGuire MK, et al. Platelet derived growth factor stimulates bone and rate of attachment level gain: Results of a large multi-center randomized control trial. J Periodontol 2005;76:2205–2215.

Use of rhPDGF to Improve Bone and Periodontal Regeneration

Samuel E. Lynch, DMD, DMSc
Leslie A. Wisner-Lynch, DDS, DMSc
Myron Nevins, DDS

Clinicians are frequently faced with the challenge of treating patients with significant bone loss resulting from periodontal disease, congenital abnormalities, tumors, traumatic injury, or resorption secondary to tooth loss. Conventional procedures often result in inadequate bone regeneration, leaving both the clinician and the patient dissatisfied with the outcome. Growth factors have long been believed to have the potential to accelerate the healing process and augment tissue formation in challenging regenerative procedures.

One of the most extensively studied growth factors is platelet-derived growth factor (PDGF). This growth factor has well-characterized, broad wound-healing activities in both hard tissue (bone) and soft tissue (skin, gingivae). Recently, purified recombinant human PDGF (rhPDGF) has been combined with allograft tissues or synthetic ceramic matrices such as β-tricalcium phosphate (β-TCP). The efficacy of these growth factor–enhanced matrices (GEMs) has been rigorously examined in a variety of animal models and long-term human clinical studies. The results of these studies are discussed in this chapter, along with the potential for GEMs to become off-the-shelf products that can predictably and reproducibly promote bone regeneration.

Bone Regeneration

Bone grafting

A variety of biologic and synthetic materials are currently used by clinical practitioners to augment existing bone and enhance bone regeneration. Autogenous bone grafting, the gold standard for treating bone defects or deficiencies, is usually harvested from intraoral sites such as the symphysis of the chin or the ascending ramus or, as an alternative, from extraoral sites such as the iliac crest or the proximal tibia. The good clinical success rate for autogenous bone grafts is primarily due to (1) the presence of osteoblasts and osteoprogenitor cells within the graft; (2) naturally occurring growth factors and other biochemical mediators; and (3) the osteoconductive nature of the bone graft material itself.

When autogenous bone is not readily available or is of poor quality, alternative bone sources can be utilized. Tissue matrices, including allogeneic, xenogeneic, and synthetic graft materials are available for use in a variety of oral surgical and orthopedic procedures and function

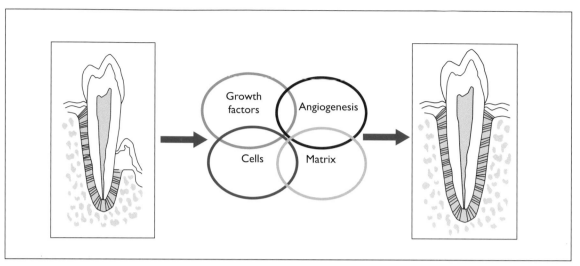

Fig 6-1 Four basic elements are required for periodontal repair and regeneration: a source of bone- and ligament-forming cells; a supporting scaffold; growth factors to regulate cellular migration, proliferation, and synthesis; and angiogenesis for revascularization of the site.

primarily by passively guiding or "conducting" cellular migration through the matrix, eventually leading to repair of the defect. These materials may be used alone, in combination with autogenous graft, or in combination with titanium cages, barrier membranes (guided tissue and guided bone regeneration), or other passive materials designed to act as a physical guide, or barrier, for cells involved in the repair and regeneration process.

Although these options are useful for maintaining space and a framework for tissue deposition, results obtained with passive therapeutic matrices have been variable, depending on their inherent physical and chemical properties as well as the patient's individual healing response.

Tissue engineering approaches

More recently, new tissue engineering techniques have been developed to regenerate bone in challenging defect sites where spontaneous repair is impossible. On a fundamental level, bone tissue engineering involves supplying the three basic elements required for bone formation to the defect site: bone-forming cells, scaffolds or matrices, and signaling molecules such as growth factors and other bone-specific proteins, including bone morphogenetic proteins (BMPs) (Fig 6-1). Osteoblasts or bone precursor cells may be provided by direct scaffold seeding (in vitro tissue engineering), or they may be induced by biochemical mediators to migrate into the scaffold from the host bone at the margins of the defect (in vivo tissue engineering).

Scaffolds provide a means to support cells in the defect site, supplying an osteoconductive foundation for newly synthesized bone and ensuring that bone-forming cells remain in place long enough to effect the desired repair. Scaffolds also prevent soft tissue collapse and facilitate blood clot stabilization. Scaffolding materials used in bone grafting include autogenous or allograft bone, synthetic porous calcium phosphate ceramics, collagen, and resorbable synthetic polymers.

Growth factors serve to stimulate migration of native cells into the defect site and increase proliferation of these cells to populate the scaffold through specific chemotactic and mitogenic effects. By increasing the number of cells in the treatment site, growth factors enhance matrix formation and increase the potential to drive the healing process toward regeneration. BMPs act primarily through osteoinduction, stimulating differentiation of pluripotent stem cells into bone-forming cells.

Periodontal and Peri-implant Regeneration

Growth factors and BMPs have been the focus of considerable attention in recent years by dental and orthopedic researchers. These biologic molecules offer the potential for off-the-shelf biomaterials that are readily available to the clinician for regenerating bone in a controlled, predictable manner. Although a considerable number of bone growth factors and morphogens have been identified, the most well-characterized growth factor being developed for clinical applications is PDGF.

In the late 1980s, Lynch and coworkers[1] first discovered that PDGF promotes regeneration of periodontal tissues, including bone, cementum, and periodontal ligament. Since then, numerous studies have been published that provide evidence for the mechanism of action of this essential growth factor.

PDGF is a naturally occurring protein that is found abundantly in bone matrix in at least three different forms: PDGF-AA, PDGF-AB, and PDGF-BB.[2–4] It is released locally during clotting by blood platelets at the site of soft or hard tissue injury, stimulating a cascade of events that leads to the wound-healing response.[5] Once it is released from the platelets, PDGF binds to well-characterized cell surface receptors, promoting rapid cellular migration (chemotaxis) and proliferation (mitogenesis) in the area of injury. In vitro studies demonstrate that PDGF is a potent chemotactic and mitogenic factor for periodontal ligament fibroblasts, cementoblasts, and osteoblasts.[1,5–9]

Although growth factor proteins have been shown to be potent stimulators of wound repair, the use of concentrated forms of these proteins contained within blood platelets, including PDGF, was not widely adopted for routine oral surgical treatment until 1998 when Marx and coworkers[10] introduced the technique of platelet concentration to dental surgeons. This early, and somewhat crude, example of tissue engineering in vivo is accomplished by first concentrating the platelets and subsequently activating them to release their growth factor contents, including PDGF, transforming growth factor β, platelet-derived endothelial cell growth factor, insulin-like growth factor 1 (IGF-1), and platelet factor 4.[11] These factors, when applied to the treatment site, provide the signal to local mesenchymal and epithelial cells to migrate, divide, and increase collagen and matrix synthesis. The thrombin-calcium preparations also initiate clotting, including the conversion of fibrinogen to fibrin, resulting in a clinically useful platelet-rich plasma gel that can improve the handling and efficacy of particulate autografts and bone substitutes.

Today, a variety of platelet concentration procedures are available that claim to increase platelet numbers by as much as fivefold to sixfold over normal circulating levels.[12] However, studies evaluating the effect of platelet gel concentrates, used alone or in combination with osteoconductive matrices, on graft maturity, bone density, and new bone formation in a number of different clinical applications have demonstrated somewhat variable outcomes ranging from excellent results in some studies to no apparent benefit in others.[13] The differences in outcomes are thought to be a result in variability in platelet concentration as well as individual patient healing responses. The platelet gel concentrate provides excellent handling characteristics alone or in combination with a variety of matrices; the primary disadvantage of the technique is the need to obtain blood from the patient, the somewhat cumbersome nature of processing the blood to make a sterile platelet gel, and lack of a predictable response following treatment.

The need to provide growth-modulating molecules (growth factors and morphogens) in a highly concentrated form is believed to be important to increase the predictability of regenerative procedures.[14] With advances in recombinant technology, proteins may now be synthesized and subsequently concentrated and purified in large quantities, allowing for the development and commercialization of recombinant growth factor–matrix combination products throughout medicine. Combination products represent an emerging trend in regenerative therapeutics and have gained increasing attention from pharmaceutical and medical device companies as a strategy to optimize tissue regeneration. These products combine tissue-specific matrices with highly concentrated bioactive proteins to actively recruit progenitor cells to the treatment site to significantly expand cell numbers. The ability to combine highly concentrated forms of signaling proteins allows clinical researchers to develop improved regenerative products that combine the physical and chemical characteristics required for specific cellular attachment, growth, and differentiation and optimal binding with ideal release of bioactive proteins, in order to achieve the greatest regeneration. To date, only three recombinant growth factor products have been commercialized for use in tissue regeneration. Two use rhPDGF-BB and one uses rhBMP-2.

rhPDGF was the first recombinant protein to be approved by the US Food and Drug Administration (FDA) for treatment of chronic foot ulcers in diabetic patients

(Regranex, Ethicon).[15] Widespread use in this application has established the safety and effectiveness of rhPDGF for soft tissue regeneration.

In addition, rhPDGF has been rigorously tested in animal studies, which indicate that PDGF has the potential to be used to direct and control bone regeneration. For example, a tibial osteotomy study in rabbits demonstrated that rhPDGF substantially increased the rate of fracture repair compared with untreated control sites.[16] In addition, the biomechanical strength of the repair tissue in rhPDGF-treated animals was not significantly different from that of normal, intact bone. Furthermore, when rhPDGF was injected subperiosteally in long bones, it induced intramembranous bone formation.[17] In a detailed study in osteoporotic animals involving dual-energy x-ray absorptiometry bone density scans, quantitative computerized tomography (CT) scans, biomechanical testing, and histologic analyses, periodic systemic injection of rhPDGF substantially increased bone density in the long bones and in the spine.[18]

Extensive in vivo animal studies and human clinical trials have been performed using rhPDGF alone and in combination with other growth factors, such as IGF, to treat periodontal defects. Lynch and coworkers[1,19] were the first to publish evidence of the regenerative potential of rhPDGF-BB when used to treat naturally occurring periodontal defects in dogs. Increased cellular activity was observed after treatment with rhPDGF-BB, leading to increased bone, cementum, and periodontal ligament regeneration. Direct application of an rhPGDF/IGF mixture around press-fit implant sites in dogs produced a two- to three-times increase in the number of peri-implant spaces filled with bone at early time points.[19] Promising results were also seen with immediate implant placement into extraction sockets treated with expanded polytetrafluoroethylene membranes and rhPDGF/IGF. Bone density and bone-to-implant contact were increased twofold for the growth factor–treated sites compared with sites treated with the membrane alone or with a combination of membranes and bone grafts.[20]

A human clinical trial of rhPDGF/rhIGF treatment applied to osseous periodontal defects was reported by Howell and coworkers.[21] The experimental sites received direct application of the growth factors, which were contained in a methylcellulose matrix to improve retention. A statistically significant increase in alveolar bone formation was observed in the growth factor–treated sites 9 months postoperatively compared with untreated control sites. New bone height for the rhPDGF/rhIGF group was measured to be 2.08 mm, and 43.2% osseous defect

fill was achieved, while the control sites exhibited 0.75 mm of new bone height and 18.5% defect fill.

Growth Factor–Enhanced Matrices

Recently, rhPDGF has been combined with tissue-specific scaffolds to take advantage of the fundamental principles of tissue engineering. Over a period of many years, Lynch and coworkers have evaluated rhPDGF in combination with osteoconductive matrices such as autograft, allograft, xenograft, or a synthetic engineered matrix such as β-TCP for use in periodontal and peri-implant procedures. In concept, PDGF stimulates cellular migration to the bone defect from the surrounding tissue margins and upregulates cellular proliferation, helping to populate the matrix with bone- and ligament-forming cells. In addition to its role as a growth factor delivery vehicle, the matrix provides support for migrating cells and helps promote new bone and ligament formation (Fig 6-2). Furthermore, PDGF may play a significant role in stimulating revascularization as bone regenerates. It has been established that PDGF has an angiogenic effect, promoting capillary budding.[15]

Animal trial

Simion and colleagues[22] used rhPDGF-BB in combination with a xenogeneic scaffold in an established canine model to study periodontal bone regeneration in surgically created severe alveolar ridge defects. An rhPDGF-BB–infused block of deproteinized bovine cancellous bone was placed in the defect site and stabilized with two titanium dental implants. The effect of rhPDGF-BB with and without a bilayer collagen membrane placed between the periosteum and the graft block was examined and compared with untreated graft blocks implanted with the collagen membrane.

The rhPDGF-BB–infused matrix significantly enhanced bone formation and gingival healing in large, critical-sized alveolar bone defects. Radiographic and histologic analyses indicated that the greatest bone regeneration occurred with the rhPDGF-BB–infused graft block without the

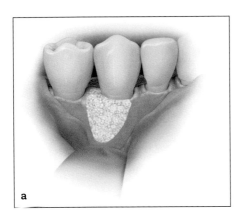
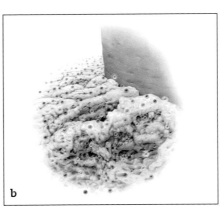
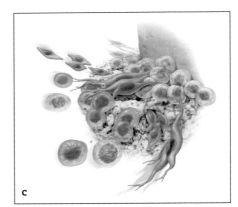
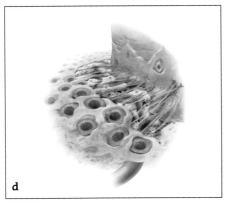
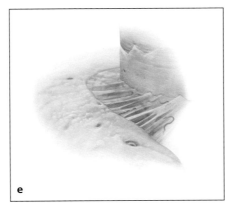
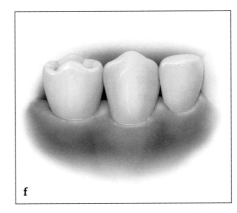

Fig 6-2 The growth factor–enhanced matrix incorporates rhPDGF in a tissue-specific scaffold material such as bone autograft, allograft, or synthetic β-TCP granules. This mixture is packed in a periodontal bone defect (*a*), and rhPDGF is released directly into the site over time (*b*). rhPDGF helps recruit and stimulate bone- and ligament-forming cells (*c*). Bone and periodontal ligament regenerate (*d*) and mature (*e*), effectively restoring normal bone structure and tooth function (*f*).

interstitial membrane (Fig 6-3). Unlike traditional guided bone regeneration procedures, the membrane appeared to block penetration of the graft by bone-forming cells. Strong evidence exists that rhPDGF-BB exerted a potent chemotactic effect when there was direct access to the periosteum and its rich supply of osteogenic cells.

Histologic analysis indicated that bone formation occurred from both the coronal and apical surfaces of the rhPDGF-BB–treated graft, demonstrating that osteoblasts and other bone-forming precursor cells were attracted into the graft from both the superior (coronal) periosteal surface and the inferior (apical) medullary spaces. Additionally, bone growth from the periosteal surface appeared more robust than the bone formation observed at the original osseous crest.

Micro-CT (SkyScan) observations confirmed the histologic findings. Regenerated bone was easily observed in the coronal region and adjacent to the native alveolar crest for the rhPDGF-BB–treated grafts, with remnants of the deproteinized bovine bone block present between the crest and the grafts. Newly formed bone filling the trabecular spaces of the intervening portions of the bone block appeared to be contiguous with the superior and inferior layers of regenerated bone. Additionally, intense bone formation activity was observed at the bone-implant interface, and a high rate of bone-to-implant contact was visible in the regenerated bone.

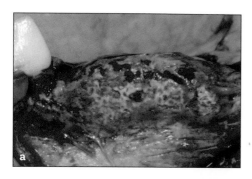

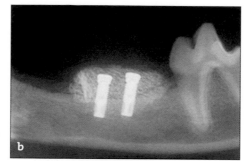

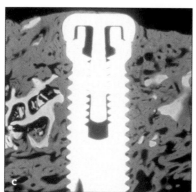

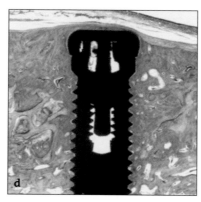

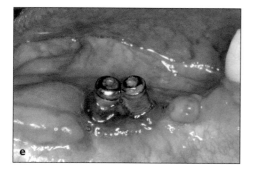

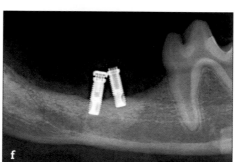

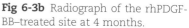

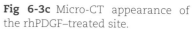

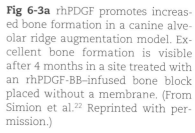

Fig 6-3a rhPDGF promotes increased bone formation in a canine alveolar ridge augmentation model. Excellent bone formation is visible after 4 months in a site treated with an rhPDGF-BB–infused bone block placed without a membrane. (From Simion et al.[22] Reprinted with permission.)

Fig 6-3b Radiograph of the rhPDGF-BB–treated site at 4 months.

Fig 6-3c Micro-CT appearance of the rhPDGF–treated site.

Fig 6-3d Histologic appearance of the rhPDGF–treated site (toludine blue/pyronine G stain; original magnification ×12.5). (From Simion et al.[22] Reprinted with permission.)

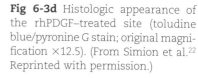

Fig 6-3e A control site is shown 4 months after treatment using guided bone regeneration with a deproteinized bovine bone block and an interstitial collagen membrane.

Fig 6-3f Radiograph of the control site at 4 months.

Clinical trials

Bone allograft

Initial human clinical studies used rhPDGF-BB combined with bone allograft. A clinical trial was completed to evaluate the effectiveness of rhPDGF-BB treatment for extensive interproximal intrabony defects and class II furcation lesions associated with advanced periodontitis.[23,24] The surgical procedure, in brief, involved reflection of full-thickness flaps and thorough debridement of the defect site. Root surfaces were scaled and root planed and then treated locally with tetracycline. Following thorough irrigation of the root surfaces, defect sites were filled with demineralized freeze-dried bone allograft that had been soaked in a solution containing rhPDGF-BB at a concentration of 0.5, 1.0, or 5.0 mg/mL (Figs 6-4a and 6-4b). Control defect sites were filled with commercially available anorganic bovine bone in collagen.

Clinical probing depths and attachment levels were assessed at periodic intervals up to 9 months postoperatively, at which time the treated teeth were removed en bloc for histologic analysis. The results indicated that substantial improvements in vertical and horizontal probing depths over baseline levels were achieved for all sites treated with rhPDGF-BB. Histologic evaluation revealed robust periodontal regeneration in the rhPDGF-BB sites, including new bone, cementum, and periodontal ligament formation (Figs 6-4c and 6-4d). Statistical analysis indicated

Fig 6-4a A class II furcation with a mesial wraparound defect is debrided.

Fig 6-4b The site is grafted with a growth factor–enhanced matrix consisting of allograft bone saturated with rhPDGF-BB. The matrix was saturated with the pure, recombinant growth factor solution prior to being packed in the defect site.

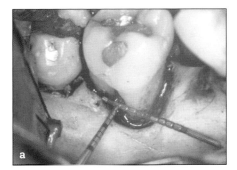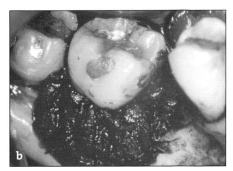

Fig 6-4c The histologic specimen reveals periodontal regeneration coronal to a reference notch placed at the base of calculus prior to treatment (toluidine blue–basic fuchsin stain; original magnification ×6.3).

Fig 6-4d Increased magnification of the boxed area in Fig 6-4c (toluidine blue–basic fuchsin stain; original magnification ×25). (Figs 6-4a to 6-4d from Camelo et al.[23] Reprinted with permission.)

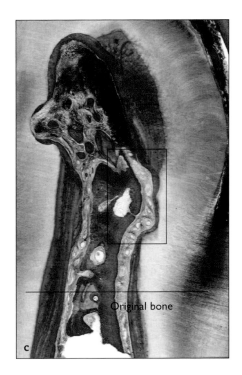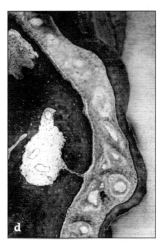

that rhPDGF-BB combined with allograft bone produced robust regeneration and improved gingival attachment in interproximal bone defects and class II furcation defects compared with baseline (Tables 6-1 and 6-2). Comparisons among doses revealed that there were no adverse reactions, even at the highest dose, indicating that rhPDGF-BB was well tolerated in oral defect sites.

The excellent results demonstrated in this study are significant, because this was the first study providing clear histologic evidence of periodontal regeneration for human class II furcation defects.[23] Previous attempts at regenerative treatments in furcation defects have met with limited and variable success because of the complicated anatomy, difficult access to the area, small size of the furcal foramen, and frequent accumulation of microbial plaque.[25]

The regenerative effects of rhPDGF in combination with mineralized freeze-dried bone allograft have been

further documented clinically in a case study reported by Nevins et al.[26] Two patients presenting with extremely severe bone loss (teeth with a guarded to hopeless prognosis) requiring surgical bone grafting were treated with mineralized freeze-dried bone allograft that was saturated with rhPDGF-BB. The GEM was packed into the defect, and a resorbable barrier membrane was placed over the defect prior to soft tissue closure. The patients were followed for 8 to 11 months, at which time a surgical reentry procedure was performed to evaluate the healing response within these previously severe defects.

Both patients exhibited excellent soft tissue healing during the entire observation period. At 8 to 11 months, probing depths for both patients measured 3 mm, and gingival recession was 0 mm and 3 mm for patient 1 and patient 2, respectively. The gains in clinical attachment level relative to baseline were 7 mm and 2 mm for patient 1

Table 6-1 Soft and hard tissue measurements for intrabony defects treated with 0.5, 1.0, or 5.0 mg/mL of rhPDGF-BB combined with allograft*

Measurement	Baseline	9 mo	Change	P†
Probing depth (mm)				
Mean	9.7	3.3	6.42	< .001
SD	1.6	1.1	1.69	
Clinical attachment level (mm)				
Mean	11.1	4.9	6.17	< .001
SD	1.7	2.3	1.94	
Radiographic bone height (mm)				
Mean	7.4	9.5	2.14	.002
SD	2.5	2.2	0.85	

*Data from Nevins et al.[24]
†P values for change from baseline from paired *t* tests.

Table 6-2 Soft tissue measurements for furcation defects treated with 0.5, 1.0, or 5.0 mg/mL of rhPDGF-BB combined with allograft*

Measurement	Baseline	9 mo	Change	P†
Probing depth (mm)				
Mean	6.2	2.8	3.40	< .001
SD	0.8	0.8	0.55	
Clinical attachment level (mm)				
Mean	6.8	2.8	4.00	.005
SD	1.3	0.8	1.58	

*Data from Nevins et al.[24]
†P values for change from baseline from paired *t* tests.

and patient 2, respectively. No adverse effects were associated with either rhPDGF-BB dose. Radiographic findings of excellent bone fill for both patients were confirmed on surgical reentry of the treated sites at 8 to 11 months. rhPDGF-BB combined with mineralized freeze-dried bone allograft proved a highly effective treatment for severe periodontal bone loss.

Synthetic GEM

An alternative to an allograft system could include the use of a completely synthetic GEM system. Recombinant human PDGF-BB has been combined with β-TCP, which is a well-established resorbable ceramic biomaterial commonly used to extend autogenous bone grafts or as a

bone graft substitute. The results of a large, multicenter, randomized controlled blinded human clinical trial evaluating the effectiveness of rhPDGF-BB with a porous β-TCP matrix (GEM 21S, BioMimetic Therapeutics) were recently reported by Nevins and coworkers.[27] The study included 180 participants with one interproximal periodontal defect of 4 mm or greater in depth after debridement. Other inclusion criteria included a baseline probing depth of 7 mm or greater, sufficient keratinized tissue to allow complete coverage of the defect, a radiographic defect base at least 3 mm coronal to the apex of the tooth, and no evidence of localized aggressive periodontitis. Class I and II furcation defects were allowable. Smokers who consumed up to one pack per day were also included in the study (Table 6-3).

Table 6-3 Characteristics of patients with intrabony periodontal defects treated by rhPDGF-BB with β-TCP*

Parameter	No. of subjects
Enrolled patients[†]	180
Completed patients[‡]	178
Smokers	43
Sex	
Male	108
Female	72
Race	
Caucasian	107
Asian	32
African American	21
Hispanic	18
Other	2

*Data from Nevins et al.[27]
[†]Mean age = 51 years.
[‡]Dropout rate of 1%.

Table 6-4 Baseline measurements and defect distribution for subjects in trial combining rhPDGF-BB with β-TCP for the treatment of intrabony periodontal defects*

Parameter	Group I (n = 60)	Group II (n = 61)	Group III (n = 59)
Clinical attachment level[†] (mm)	9.1 ± 0.2	8.8 ± 0.2	8.8 ± 0.2
Probing depth[†] (mm)	8.6 ± 0.2	8.2 ± 0.2	8.3 ± 0.2
Gingival recession[†] (mm)	0.5 ± 0.2	0.6 ± 0.2	0.5 ± 0.1
Bone defect depth[†] (mm)	6.0 ± 0.2	5.7 ± 0.2	5.7 ± 0.2
One-wall defect	20 (33.3%)	17 (27.9%)	19 (32.8%)
Two-wall defect	26 (43.3%)	32 (52.5%)	25 (43.1%)
Three-wall/circumferential defect	14 (23.3%)	12 (19.7%)	14 (24.2%)

*Data from Nevins et al.[27]
[†]Mean ± SEM.

Three treatment groups were evaluated:

1. β-TCP plus 0.3 mg/mL of rhPDGF-BB (group I)
2. β-TCP plus 1.0 mg/mL of rhPDGF-BB (group II)
3. β-TCP plus buffer alone (group III)

A summary of the baseline characteristics for subjects in each study group is provided in Table 6-4. Defects were classified as one-, two- or three-wall and circumferential, indicating the extent of involvement and severity.

At the time of surgery, β-TCP granules were saturated with the treatment solution (either buffer alone or buffer containing rhPDGF) for 10 minutes to allow rhPDGF-BB binding before the graft was placed in the defect site. The reflected gingival flap was sutured closed, producing complete soft tissue coverage. Patients were followed for a period of 6 months, with periodic clinical and radiographic evaluations to monitor the safety and effectiveness of the treatment.

Outcome measures included evaluation of soft tissue changes and assessment of bone growth. Gingival clinical attachment level and the degree of postsurgical recession were measured and compared with baseline and the β-TCP control group. Radiographic comparisons of the

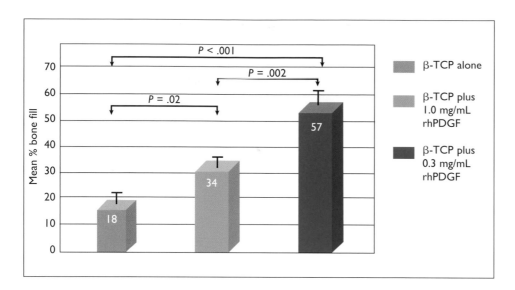

Fig 6-5 The combination of 0.3 mg/mL rhPDGF-BB and β-TCP (group I) significantly improved the percentage of bone fill of all bone defects compared with β-TCP plus buffer. (Modified from Nevins et al[27] with permission.)

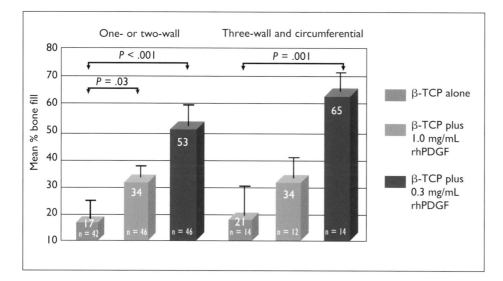

Fig 6-6 The combination of 0.3 mg/mL rhPDGF-BB and β-TCP (group I) resulted in significantly improved bone fill in one-, two-, and three-wall defects. Although there appeared to be a modest trend, there was no statistically significant difference between bone fill achieved in one- and two-wall defects and that achieved in three-wall and circumferential defects (P = .40 in group I). (Modified from Nevins et al[27] with permission.)

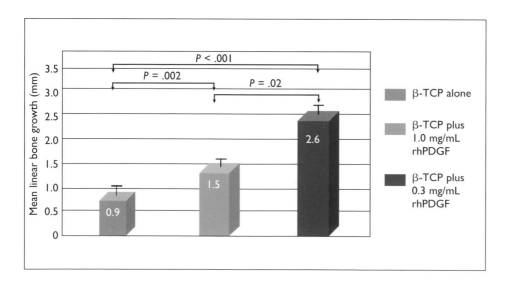

Fig 6-7 The combination of 0.3 mg/mL rhPDGF-BB and β-TCP (group I) significantly improved linear bone growth compared with β-TCP plus buffer. (Modified from Nevins et al[27] with permission.)

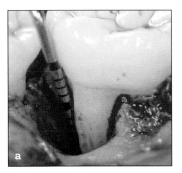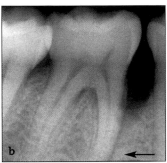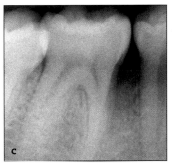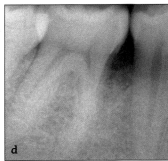

Fig 6-8a The intraoperative lingual view reveals a deep, wide intrabony defect on the mesial root surface.

Fig 6-8b The defect is easily observed on the radiograph, which shows bone loss on the mesial root surface *(arrow)* and extending to the furcation region of the mandibular right molar.

Fig 6-8c The bone level is increased 6 months after treatment with rhPDGF-BB and β-TCP.

Fig 6-8d At 18 months, the area of the furcation is completely filled, and the area of the mesial defect has increased in both height and density, providing radiographic evidence of continued bone fill and long-term maintenance of regenerated bone at an rhPDGF-BB–treated defect. (Figs 6-8a to 6-8d from McGuire et al.[28] Reprinted with permission.)

percentage of bone fill and linear bone growth between baseline and 6 months postoperatively were performed by a blinded independent radiographic center. The percentage of bone fill was calculated by dividing linear bone growth by the depth of the original bone defect. Safety was monitored throughout the trial by assessing the frequency and severity of clinical and/or radiographic adverse events.

Excellent healing was observed for all defects treated with rhPDGF-BB (see Fig 5-20). There was a significantly greater gain in clinical attachment level at 3 months for the 0.3 mg/mL rhPDGF-BB (group I) than for the β-TCP controls (group III), indicating an early benefit of rhPDGF-BB treatment. At 6 months, the clinical attachment level gain for the lower rhPDGF-BB concentration group continued to be greater than that of the control group, although statistical significance was not achieved. In addition, the rhPDGF-BB treatment group exhibited significantly less gingival recession at 3 months than did the untreated control group. This difference was no longer apparent at 6 months, however, because the control group exhibited a slight gain in gingival height over time.

The increased rhPDGF-BB concentration of 1.0 mg/mL was safe but less effective than the 0.3-mg/mL dose. Although no statistically significant differences were observed in clinical attachment level or gingival recession for the higher rhPDGF-BB concentration (group II), it did result in significant improvement in bone regeneration compared with the β-TCP controls. This observation emphasizes the need for rigorous clinical studies of new growth factor therapies that include systematic examination of dose effects.

Radiographic assessment revealed that bone fill was significantly greater at 6 months with both rhPDGF-BB concentrations than with the TCP matrix alone (Fig 6-5). A subgroup analysis further indicated that rhPDGF-BB treatment improved bone fill in smokers and for all defect types: one-, two-, and three-wall and circumferential (Fig 6-6). Similarly, linear bone growth was also significantly greater for group I than for groups II and III (Fig 6-7). No significant differences were found in the number or severity of adverse events among the three groups, indicating that both rhPDGF-BB and the β-TCP matrix were safe and well tolerated in the defect sites.

The results of this study clearly demonstrated that rhPDGF-BB in combination with a synthetic β-TCP matrix accelerates the rate of bone regeneration and improves bone fill and clinical attachment level in treated periodontal defects. These superior outcomes were maintained over time for at least 2 years after treatment (Fig 6-8). A recent case series showed that, along with continued bone fill in the defect site, there were marked changes in the radiographic appearance of the regenerated bone.[28] Radiopacity increased over time, indicating that newly formed bone continued to be deposited and mineralized as the synthetic bone matrix was replaced. In addition, a distinct trabecular pattern became more evident in the regenerated bone as it matured. Regenerated bone contained within the defect site gradually became intermingled with native bone at the margins of the original defect by 9 to 12 months postoperatively, and little difference was observed radiographically between the area of the original defect and the surrounding bone. These observations are significant because they provide clinicians with

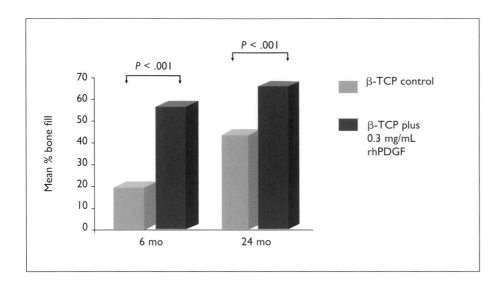

Fig 6-9 The combination of 0.3 mg/mL rhPDGF-BB and β-TCP significantly improved the percentage of bone fill compared with β-TCP plus buffer (active control) 6 months posttreatment. Both treatment groups continued to improve over the next 18 months, but the rhPDG-BB–treated group remained significantly improved over the active control.

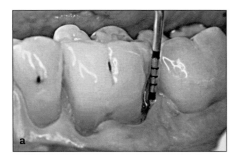

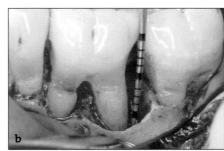

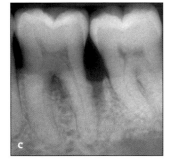

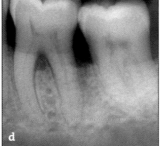

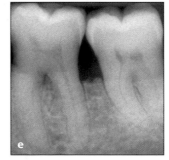

Fig 6-10a Representative case from a pivotal clinical trial of rhPDGF treatment. Periodontal defect at baseline.

Fig 6-10b The defect has been debrided.

Fig 6-10c Baseline radiograph of the defect.

Fig 6-10d Radiograph of the treated site 6 months postsurgery.

Fig 6-10e Radiograph of the treated site 18 months postsurgery. Note the progressive increase in radiopacity and trabecular bone pattern (bone fill and maturation) in the area of the original defect. (Figs 6-10b to 6-10e from McGuire et al.[28] Reprinted with permission.)

important information related to the expected time course of radiographic healing following surgical treatment with rhPDGF-enhanced matrices.

Follow-up results for patients from centers participating in a long-term (24-month) evaluation of sites treated in the pivotal clinical trial demonstrated that the significantly enhanced results in sites treated with 0.3 mg/mL of rhPDGF (GEM 21S), which were observed at the initial 6-month time point, continued to improve and remained significantly improved over results observed in the β-TCP control group (Fig 6-9). Although the β-TCP control

group did demonstrate improvement from the results observed at 6 months, the improvement remained significantly less than that which was observed in sites treated with 0.3 mg/mL of rhPDGF.

Additional clinical cases showing the long-term follow-up results in sites treated with rhPDGF are presented in Figs 6-10 to 6-14. To put these clinical results in perspective, GEM 21S compares very favorably with existing FDA-approved treatments in terms of clinical attachment level gain and bone fill (Table 6-5).

Fig 6-11a A severe intrabony defect on the distal aspect of the mandibular right first molar is evident clinically.

Fig 6-11b Baseline radiograph of the defect.

Fig 6-11c Radiograph of the treated site 6 months postsurgery.

Fig 6-11d Radiograph of the treated site 12 months postsurgery.

Fig 6-11e Radiograph of the treated site 24 months following treatment. The site appears to have increased in density (mineralization) and maturation over time, as evidenced by increased radiopacity and bony trabeculation. (Figs 6-11a to 6-11e from McGuire et al.[28] Reprinted with permission.)

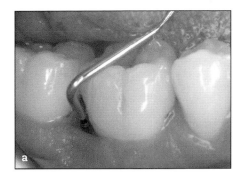

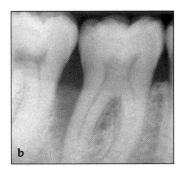
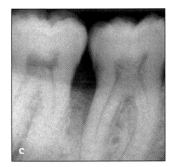
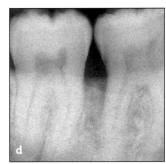
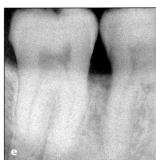

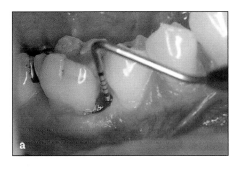
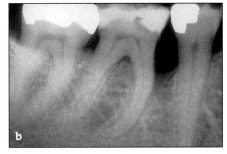
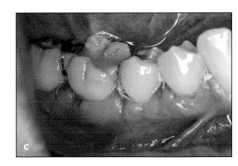

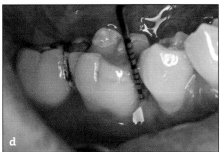
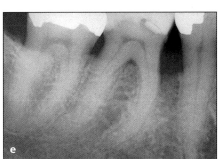
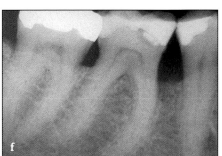

Fig 6-12a The intrabony defect will be treated with rhPDGF.

Fig 6-12b Baseline radiograph of the defect. (Figs 6-12a and 6-12b from McGuire et al.[28] Reprinted with permission.)

Fig 6-12c Early soft tissue healing is excellent, 3 to 5 days postsurgery.

Fig 6-12d Clinical healing 6 months postsurgery.

Fig 6-12e Radiograph of the treated site 6 months postsurgery.

Fig 6-12f Radiograph of the treated site 24 months postsurgery. The progressively increasing radiographic bone fill is contiguous with the surrounding bone. (Figs 6-12e and 6-12f from McGuire et al.[28] Reprinted with permission.)

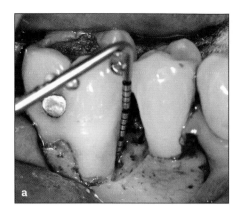

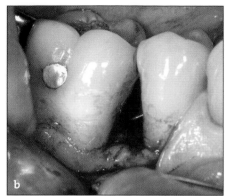

Fig 6-13a A wide, shallow defect is present at baseline.

Fig 6-13b The buccal plate has regenerated across the root prominence, and there is complete fill of the interproximal defect 24 months postsurgery.

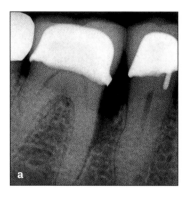

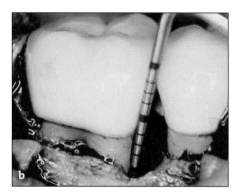

Fig 6-14a Baseline radiograph of the intrabony defect.

Fig 6-14b Clinical appearance of the defect at baseline.

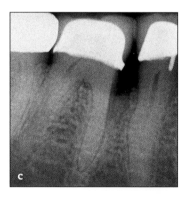

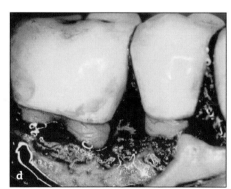

Fig 6-14c Radiograph of the treated site 6 months postsurgery.

Fig 6-14d Clinical results 6 months postsurgery.

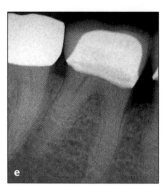

Fig 6-14e While the original defect appeared to be filled (clinically and radiographically) 6 months after treatment, there is radiographic evidence of further mineralization and maturation 24 months postsurgery.

Table 6-5 Comparison of clinical and radiographic measures of periodontal regeneration with rhPDGF-BB, FDA-cleared treatment methods, and standard surgical treatment without grafting*

Treatment modality	Gain in clinical attachment level	Radiographic linear bone gain
GEM 21S	3.7 mm	2.5 mm
Emdogain[†]	2.7 mm	1.1 mm
Pep-Gen P-15[‡]	1.1 mm	Not measured
Open flap debridement surgery	1.4 mm	0.7 mm

*Data from various sources.[27,29–32]
†Straumann.
‡Dentsply.

Conclusion

Combining rhPDGF with a tissue-specific matrix such as bone allograft or a synthetic bioresorbable ceramic such as β-TCP has the potential to fulfill the clinical need for a commercially available material that predictably stimulates bone and periodontal regeneration and improves soft tissue healing in the surgical site. The results of the large, multicenter clinical trial of rhPDGF-BB incorporated in a β-TCP matrix demonstrated that this product is safe and effective for at least 2 years following treatment. Radiographic analysis showed that rhPDGF-BB effectively and reproducibly promotes bone formation, and clinical follow-up examinations confirmed that it accelerates soft tissue attachment level gain in challenging periodontal defect sites. This treatment approach is supported by extensive and rigorous in vitro, preclinical, and clinical studies that have provided strong evidence for the mechanism of action for PDGF in periodontal and bone healing.

An off-the-shelf therapy, such as GEMs that incorporate rhPDGF, can provide substantial benefits for clinical practitioners and patients undergoing periodontal, craniomaxillofacial, or orthopedic surgery. Elimination of the pain and variable results associated with autogenous bone grafting will improve clinical outcomes and increase patient satisfaction. Extensive data, including data from level 1 randomized controlled clinical trials, indicate that rhPDGF-enhanced matrices provide clinicians with a new, highly effective treatment option for challenging bone and periodontal lesions, including class II furcation defects, which are difficult to treat through conventional methods.

The promising clinical results for rhPDGF in combination with osteoconductive matrices in a diverse array of periodontal and peri-implant sites suggest that growth factor–enhanced matrices incorporating rhPDGF have the potential to become the new standard of care.

References

1. Lynch SE, Williams RC, Polson AM, et al. A combination of platelet-derived growth factor enhances periodontal regeneration. J Clin Peridontol 1989;16:545–554.
2. Antoniades HN. Human platelet derived growth factor (PDGF): Purification of PDGF-I and PDGF-II and separation of their reduced subunits. Proc Natl Acad Sci U S A 1981;78:7314–7317.
3. Ross R, Raines EW, Bowen-Pope DF. The biology of platelet derived growth factor. Cell 1986;46:155–169.
4. Johnsson A, Heldon CH, Wasteson A, et al. The c-sis gene encodes a precursor of the B chain of platelet derived growth factor. EMBO J 1984;3:921–928.
5. Lynch SE, Genco RJ, Marx RE (eds). Tissue Engineering: Applications in Maxillofacial Surgery and Periodontics, ed 1. Chicago: Quintessence, 1999.
6. Centrella M, McCarthy TL, Kusmik WF, Canalis E. Relative binding and biochemical effects of heterodimeric and homodimeric isoforms of platelet-derived growth factor in osteoblast-enriched cultures from fetal rat bone. J Cell Physiol 1991;147:420–426.
7. Piche JE, Graves DT. Study of the growth factor requirements of human bone-derived cells: A comparison with human fibroblasts. Bone 1989;10:131–138.
8. Bowen-Pope DF, van Koppen A, Schatterman GC. Is PDGF really important? Testing the hypothesis. Trends Genet 1991;7:411–418.
9. Soriano P. Abnormal kidney development and hematological disorders in PDGF beta-receptor mutant mice. Genes Dev 1994;8:1888–1896.
10. Marx RE, Carlson ER, Eichstaedt RM, Schimmele SR, Strauss JE, Georgeff KR. Platelet rich plasma growth factor enhancement for bone grafts. Oral Surg Oral Med Oral Pathol Oral Radiol Endod 1998;85:638–646.
11. Schatteman GC, Morrison-Graham K, van Koppen A, Weston JA, Bowen-Pope DF. Regulation and role of PDGF receptor alpha-subunit expression during embryogenesis. Development 1992;115:123–131.

12. Harvest Technologies Corporation. SmartPrep 2. Available at: http://www.harvesttech.com/education/prp-brochures.html. Accessed 17 Oct 2007.

13. Sanchez AR, Sheridan PJ, Kupp LI. Is platelet-rich plasma the perfect enhancement factor? A current review. Int J Oral Maxillofac Implants 2003;18:93–103.

14. Lynch SE. Bone regeneration techniques in the orofacial region. In: Lieberman JR, Friedlaender GE (eds). Bone Regeneration and Repair: Biology and Clinical Applications. Totowa, NJ: Humana, 2005:359–390.

15. Magnusson PU, Looman C, Ahgren A, et al. Platelet-derived growth factor receptor-beta constitutive activity promotes angiogenesis in vivo and in vitro. Arterioscler Thromb Vasc Biol 2007;27:2142–2149.

16. Nash TJ, Howlett CR, Martin C, Steele J, Johnson KA, Hicklin DJ. Effect of platelet-derived growth factor on tibial osteotomies in rabbits. Bone 1994;15:203–208.

17. Joyce ME, Jingushi S, Scully SP, Bolander ME. Role of growth factors in fracture healing. Prog Clin Biol Res 1991;365:391–416.

18. Mitlak BH, Finkelman RD, Hill E, et al. The effect of systemically administered PDGF-BB on the rodent skeleton. J Bone Miner Res 1996;11:238–247.

19. Lynch SE, de Castilla GR, Williams RC, et al. The effects of short-term application of a combination of platelet-derived and insulin-like growth factors on periodontal wound healing. J Periodontol 1991;62:458–467.

20. Becker W, Lynch SE, Lekholm U, et al. A comparison of ePTFE membranes alone or in combination with platelet derived growth factor and insulin-like growth factor-I or demineralized freeze-dried bone in promoting bone formation around immediate extraction socket implants. J Periodontol 1992;63:929–940.

21. Howell TH, Fiorellini JP, Paquette DW, Offenbacher S, Giannobile WV, Lynch SE. Evaluation of a combination of recombinant human platelet-derived growth factor-BB and recombinant human insulin-like growth factor-I in patients with periodontal disease. J Periodontol 1997;68:1186–1193.

22. Simion M, Rocchietta I, Kim D, Nevins M, Fiorellini J. Vertical ridge augmentation by means of deproteinized bovine bone block and recombinant human platelet-derived growth factor-BB: A histologic study in a dog model. Int J Periodontics Restorative Dent 2006;26:415–423.

23. Camelo M, Nevins ML, Schenk RK, Lynch SE, Nevins M. Periodontal regeneration in human Class II furcations using purified recombinant human platelet-derived growth factor-BB (rhPDGF-BB) with bone allograft. Int J Periodontics Restorative Dent 2003;23:213–225.

24. Nevins M, Camelo M, Nevins ML, Schenk RK, Lynch SE. Periodontal regeneration in humans using recombinant human platelet-derived growth factor-BB (rhPDGF-BB) and allogenic bone. J Periodontol 2003;74:1282–1292.

25. Novaes AB, Palioto DB, Andrade PF, Marchesan JT. Regeneration of Class II furcation defects: Determinants of increased success. Braz Dent J 2005;16:87–97.

26. Nevins M, Hanratty J, Lynch SE. Clinical results using recombinant human platelet-derived growth factor and mineralized freeze-dried bone allograft. Int J Periodontics Restorative Dent 2007;27:421–427.

27. Nevins M, Giannobile WV, McGuire MK, et al. Platelet-derived growth factor stimulates bone fill and rate of attachment level gain: Results of a large multicenter randomized controlled trial. J Periodontol 2005;76:2205–2215.

28. McGuire MK, Kao RT, Nevins M, Lynch SE. rhPDGF-BB promotes healing of periodontal defects: 24-month clinical and radiographic observations. Int J Periodontics Restorative Dent 2006;26:223–231 [erratum 2007;27:88].

29. Straumann (applicant). Emdogain US FDA Premarket Approval [PMA no. P930021], 30 Sept 1996 (last supplement 24 April 2006). Available from: http://www.accessdata.fda.gov/scripts/cdrh/cfdocs/cfPMA/pma.cfm. Accessed October 15, 2007.

30. Zetterstrom O, Andersson C, Eriksson L, et al. Clinical safety of enamel matrix derivative (EMDOGAIN) in the treatment of periodontal defects. J Clin Periodontol 1997;24:697–704.

31. Heijl L, Heden G, Svardstrom G, Ostgren A. Enamel matrix derivative (EMDOGAIN) in the treatment of intrabony periodontal defects. J Clin Periodontol 1997;24:705–714.

32. Ceramed, Dentsply (applicants). PepGen P-15 US FDA Premarket Approval [PMA no. P990033], 25 Oct 1999 (last supplement 9 Aug 2007). Available from: http://www.accessdata.fda.gov/scripts/cdrh/cfdocs/cfPMA/pma.cfm.

Soft Tissue Engineering Applications in Dentistry

Michael K. McGuire, DDS

Current surgical techniques, effective in most ridge augmentation, free gingival graft, and root coverage procedures, require a remote surgical harvest site for donor tissue. From the patient's perspective, the donor site is often more uncomfortable postoperatively than the graft site; from the clinician's viewpoint, the donor site is more prone to postoperative problems, such as excessive bleeding. In addition to these concerns, only a finite amount of donor tissue is available to be harvested at any one time. Because the amount of donor tissue available is insufficient to meet the needs of most patients requiring multiple grafts, the patient is required to go through multiple surgical harvesting procedures. For other soft tissue defects, such as the open interproximal space, no augmentation techniques are currently available to achieve predictable correction.

The hope is that tissue engineering will provide an unlimited supply of "off the shelf" donor tissue, or other therapeutics, to allow resolution of oral defects such as the open interproximal space. The first tissue to be successfully engineered in the laboratory and applied in routine patient care was the body's largest organ, skin.[1] Tissue engineered skin products have been used in wound-healing centers for treating burns, venous stasis, pressure and diabetic ulcers, and other maladies.[2,3] It is reasonable to assume that this technology could be har-

nessed for dentistry, where the development of soft tissue engineering has followed three lines of basic research: the application of acellular allografts, the application of growth factors and extracellular matrix proteins, and the application of live, cell-based therapies. This chapter will report on researchers' latest efforts to resolve soft tissue defects by employing these novel approaches in the oral environment.

Acellular Allografts

Skin allografts can incorporate into full-thickness skin wounds, but they are eventually rejected because the cells of the epidermal and dermal graft tissue, primarily responsible for this rejection, elicit an immune response. The noncellular component of the dermis, consisting of extracellular matrix proteins and collagen, is relatively nonimmunogenic.

Transplantation of nonimmunogenic extracellular tissue matrix has been successfully demonstrated with freeze-dried demineralized bone grafts.[4] The cells in these allografts are destroyed during the freeze-drying process, but the structural organization of the extracellular matrix remains intact and does not elicit a specific immune response. The extracellular matrix, in addition, may provide an environment for osteoinduction and osteogenic cell repopulation.

Similarly, an acellular skin substitute may provide a biocompatible surface capable of producing chemical or physical signals that direct cells into desired activities, such as proliferation, migration, and differentiation. An example of a biologically based skin substitute that has been used for soft tissue applications in dentistry is acellular dermal matrix (Alloderm, Life Cell). Acellular dermal matrix is made by removing cells from cadaver skin and leaving the extracellular matrix proteins of the dermis to produce an immunologically inert allograft, which can support fibroblastic migration and revascularization. This allograft can be used as donor material for soft tissue ridge augmentation, but most studies have evaluated it as a donor material for root coverage grafts. Mean root coverage in these studies ranges from 66% to 99%, and the mean for all studies is 86%.[5–12] At the present time, controlled studies indicate stable results for up to 1 year, but further studies are needed to confirm long-term stability.[8,9,11]

Growth Factors and Extracellular Matrix Proteins

Tissue engineering strategies to regenerate or repair tissue often mimic the body's natural process (biomimetics) to grow or regenerate tissue, frequently incorporating signaling molecules or extracellular matrix molecules.

Enamel matrix derivative

One of the early examples of the use of biomimetics in dentistry is the sequence of events that occurs after enamel matrix derivative (EMD; Emdogain, Straumann) is applied to the root surface to promote selective cellular repopulation during the early stages of periodontal healing.[13] Various reports have shown that EMD enhances proliferation, differentiation, and migration of osteoblasts and periodontal ligament (PDL) cells, mimicking the natural process of tooth development.[14–17]

EMD has been evaluated for its potential both in regeneration of intrabony defects and more recently in gingival recession.[18,19] In 1997, Heijl[20] demonstrated new cementum and bone gain histologically in one experimentally created recession defect. Rasperini et al[21] added EMD to a subepithelial connective tissue graft and found histologic evidence of new cementum, bone, and connective tissue fibers. Modica et al[22] compared the results of coronally advanced flaps with and without EMD and concluded that EMD did not significantly improve the clinical outcome of gingival recession treated by a coronally advanced flap, even though the test group demonstrated slightly better results in root coverage.

Based on this information, the author compared coronally advanced flaps plus EMD to subepithelial connective tissue grafts.[19] A randomized, controlled, single-center, split-mouth design study was undertaken to compare the clinical efficacy of EMD placed under a coronally advanced flap (test group) with that of subepithelial connective tissue placed under a coronally advanced flap (control group) in patients with recession type defects. All patients were followed for 12 months.

Twenty patients with incisors or premolars presenting with a facial recession of 4 mm or more in contralateral quadrants of the same jaw were treated, and 17 patients completed the study. Clinical parameters, measured at baseline and at 6, 9, and 12 months, included the amount of recession; the width at the coronal extent of the gingival defect; the width of keratinized tissue; the probing depth; the clinical attachment level; the inflammation score; the plaque score; the plaque index; the alveolar bone level; the tissue texture and color; and the patient's perception of pain, bleeding, swelling, and sensitivity.

Results for both the test and control groups were similar for all measured clinical parameters with the exception of early healing, self-reported discomfort, and the amount of keratinized tissue obtained. The coronally advanced flap with EMD resulted in better early healing and less patient-reported discomfort than did the subepithelial connective tissue graft, whereas the sites treated with a subepithelial connective tissue graft demonstrated a greater amount of keratinized tissue during the 12-month evaluation period (Fig 7-1).

There was no statistically significant difference in the percent of root coverage obtained between the control and test groups at the end of 12 months. Of the root surfaces treated with subepithelial connective tissue grafts, 93.8% were covered, whereas 95.1% of the root surfaces treated with a coronally advanced flap plus EMD were covered. Both test and control groups demonstrated an

Figs 7-1a and 7-1b Baseline appearance of maxillary lateral incisors that have been randomized to receive test treatment (EMD) (a) or control treatment (subepithelial connective tissue graft) (b).

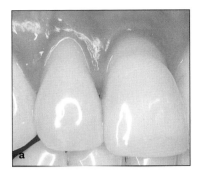
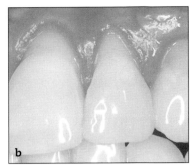

Figs 7-1c and 7-1d Results after 1 week. Teeth subjected to the test treatment (c) exhibit fewer clinical signs of inflammation than do the control teeth (d).

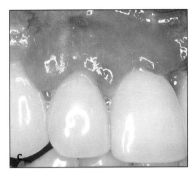
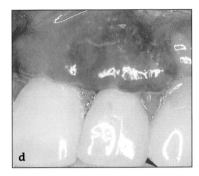

Figs 7-1e and 7-1f Test (e) and control (f) teeth at 4 weeks. The test treatment continues to exhibit superior wound healing.

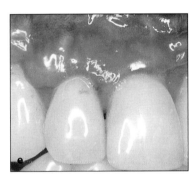
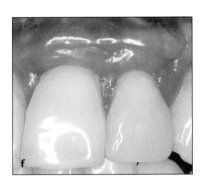

Figs 7-1g and 7-1h Results 12 months postsurgery. The re-creation of a functional and esthetic morphology of the mucogingival complex is clinically demonstrated with both test (g) and control (h) treatments. (Figs 7-1a to 7-1g from McGuire and Nunn.[19] Reprinted with permission.)

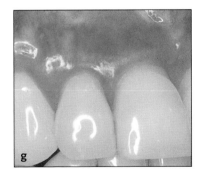
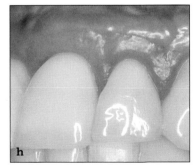

average gain in attachment of 4.5 mm (range of 4.0 to 8.0 mm). There were no statistically significant differences in clinical attachment gain, root hypersensitivity, or probing depth. Within the limitations of this study, the findings indicated that the addition of EMD to a coronally advanced flap resulted in root coverage similar to that obtained with a subepithelial connective tissue graft, without the morbidity and potential clinical difficulties associated with donor site surgery.

Trombelli[23] stated that the goal of root coverage grafts is to re-create the functional and esthetic morphology of the mucogingival complex and regenerate the lost attach-

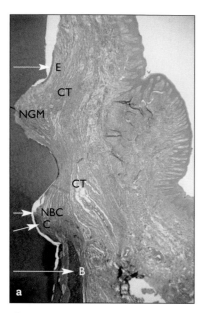
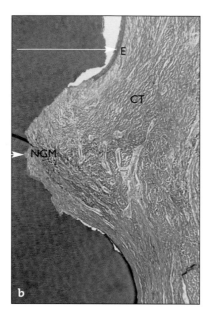
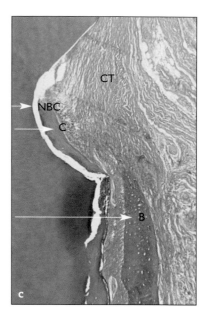

Fig 7-2a Low-power magnification of the connective tissue graft (CT). (E) Epithelium; (NGM) notch at original gingival margin; (NBC) notch at bone crest; (C) cementum; (B) bone (hematoxylin-eosin [H&E] stain; original magnification ×25).

Fig 7-2b Notch at original gingival margin (NGM). Junctional epithelium ends at the coronal aspect of the notch. (CT) Connective tissue graft; (E) epithelium. (H&E stain; original magnification ×250).

Fig 7-2c Notch at the original alveolar crest (NBC). Cementum (C) formation is seen in the notch. (CT) Connective tissue graft; (B) bone (H&E stain; original magnification ×250). (Figs 7-2a to 7-2c from McGuire and Cochran.[24] Reprinted with permission.)

ment apparatus, including the formation of new cementum with inserting connective tissue fibers and regeneration of alveolar bone. In another study, two hopeless teeth in one patient were randomly selected to receive a subepithelial connective tissue graft or a coronally advanced flap plus EMD.[24] The surgery was accomplished in accordance with the protocol previously described. The teeth and a small collar of tissue were removed at 6 months and underwent histologic analysis.

The histologic analysis of the subepithelial connective tissue graft revealed connective tissue attachment intimately opposed to the dentin, with a long junctional epithelium limited to the most coronal portion of the graft. There were large, noninflamed connective tissue bundles that made up the bulk of the new tissue, and the new tissue extended above the original gingival margin. This histologic evidence of root coverage reinforced the clinical findings. However, the analysis also revealed a long junctional epithelium against the root surface and evidence of root resorption in the notched area. There was some cementum formation (likely reparative cementum) in the notch made adjacent to the alveolar crest, most likely due to the acute trauma of making the notch, but

there was no evidence of a new attachment apparatus comprising new cementum, bone, or inserting PDL fibers. In fact, the alveolar crest level did not appear to be altered despite the open flap procedure[24] (Fig 7-2).

The histologic analysis of the coronally advanced flap plus EMD was compromised because postoperative fenestration of the flap rendered the reference notches useless. (Although unfortunate, the absence of reference notches is not unusual; approximately 50% of the human histologic evaluations of root coverage grafts reported in the literature lack reference notches.) Without reference points, the researcher was unable to prove the exact location on the root surface from which the sections were taken, but intraoperative photographs demonstrated that there was no bone on the facial or mesial side of the tooth. In addition, an apicoectomy performed many years prior to extraction left the tooth without bone at the apex. Based on these clinical observations, any bone observed histologically on these surfaces would represent new bone formation.[24]

The histologic analysis demonstrated that the cementum lining the treated root surface was primarily cellular.[24] Although EMD is purported to foster the development

Fig 7-3a Low-power magnification of the coronally advanced flap plus EMD (H&E stain; original magnification ×25).

Fig 7-3b Increased magnification of the boxed area in Fig 7-3a. Islands of condensing bone (B) have formed a uniform distance from the root (R) surface. New cementum (C) and an organizing PDL are also evident. (CT) Connective tissue (H&E stain; original magnification ×250). (Fig 7-3b from McGuire and Cochran.[24] Reprinted with permission.)

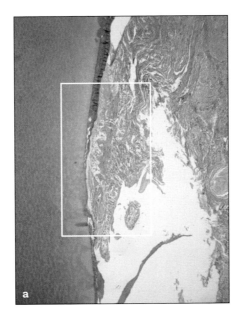
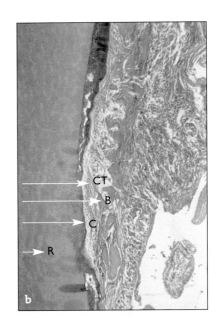

of acellular cementum, it is not uncommon to find both cellular and acellular forms deposited on both old cementum and dentin.[25,26] In addition, new cementum that occurs with bone grafts is usually cellular. Especially interesting were the islands of condensing bone observed at a uniform distance from the root surface.[24] This type of de novo bone formation in humans, to the best of the author's knowledge, has never before been reported in the literature. All other reports of bone formation in conjunction with any type of root coverage graft represent an extension of or apposition to the existing alveolar crest. The only time in nature that bone forms at a fixed distance from the root surface is during tooth development. These histologic sections strongly suggest that EMD may result in regeneration, although further studies would be required to confirm this single observation (Fig 7-3).

Connective tissue, presumably organizing PDL fibers, was observed running parallel between the cementum on the root surface and the islands of condensing bone.[24] A requirement of regeneration is functionally oriented PDL fibers, but most histologic studies evaluating root coverage procedures, whether with a coronally advanced flap, guided tissue regeneration, connective tissue, or EMD, report fiber orientation that is predominantly parallel to the tooth rather than perpendicular.[25,27–30] Perhaps a longer period of healing is necessary for the fibers to properly orient themselves, particularly in the presently described report, because the bone tissue was immature.

To summarize, histologic sections of the coronally advanced flap plus EMD demonstrated the presence of cementum, interspersed connective tissue (interpreted to be organizing PDL by its location), and islands of condensing bone found at a fixed distance from the root surface. While the absence of reference notches on the tooth treated with coronally advanced flap plus EMD precluded clear interpretation of results, the healing results suggest that EMD may possess potential for enhancing periodontal regeneration of coronally advanced flaps over denuded root.[24]

Root coverage with rhPDGF

Growth factors play a critical role in tissue engineering. Platelet-derived growth factor (PDGF) is the most thoroughly studied growth factor in periodontics. Since PDGF was first discovered to promote regeneration of bone, cementum, and periodontal ligament in the late 1980s, nearly 100 studies have been published on its effects on periodontal ligament and alveolar bone cells and its role in the regeneration of the periodontium in both animals and humans.[31] These studies have clearly demonstrated the mechanism of action of PDGF, including the presence of cell surface receptors for PDGF on PDL and alveolar

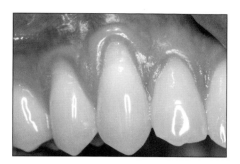

Fig 7-4a Preoperative view of a control tooth (canine).

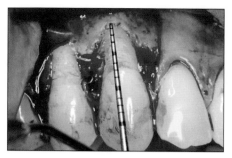

Fig 7-4b Intraoperative measurement following partial-thickness flap.

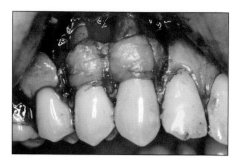

Fig 7-4c Connective tissue sutured over denuded root surfaces.

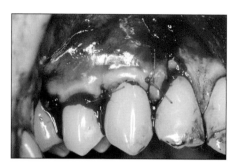

Fig 7-4d Mucogingival flap repositioned over the connective tissue.

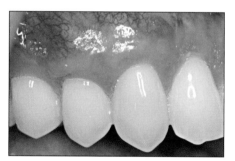

Fig 7-4e Six-month postoperative view of the connective tissue graft. (Figs 7-4a to 7-4e from McGuire and Scheyer.[43] Reprinted with permission.)

bone cells and the stimulatory effect of PDGF on the proliferation and chemotaxis of these cells.[32] Additionally, recombinant human PDGF-BB (rhPDGF-BB) has been shown in numerous animal studies and in landmark human histologic reports to promote the regeneration of periodontal tissues, including bone, cementum, and periodontal ligament.[33–41]

β-Tricalcium phosphate (β-TCP) is a purified, multicrystalline, porous form of calcium phosphate with a calcium-to-phosphate ratio similar to that of natural bone mineral. When placed under a membrane, β-TCP prevents membrane collapse against the root surface, provides a matrix or scaffold for new bone formation, and facilitates the stabilization of the blood clot. In a recent 180-patient clinical trial, the combination of β-TCP and rhPDGF-BB (GEM 21S, BioMimetic Therapeutics) was shown to accelerate clinical attachment level gain and significantly increase linear bone growth and percentage of bone fill in severe intrabony defects when compared with

β-TCP alone as well as with currently used grafting materials.[42]

Based on these findings, McGuire and Scheyer[43] published a case series evaluating rhPDGF-BB plus β-TCP and a collagen membrane with a coronally advanced flap and comparing the results with those obtained with a subepithelial connective tissue graft with a coronally advanced flap in patients with recession-type defects. Because of the limited number of cases treated in this feasibility study and the small differences in clinical results, statistical comparisons were not made between the test and control groups, as would be done in a larger, more adequately powered trial. Nevertheless, both procedures predictably achieved root coverage; at the end of 6 months of healing, all patients, test and control, had no more than 1 mm of residual recession. All tissues appeared healthy and stable, and the test grafts appeared less bulky and more esthetic (Figs 7-4 and 7-5). The case series provided proof of principle for successful treatment of peri-

Fig 7-5a Preoperative view of a test tooth (canine).

Fig 7-5b Appearance after reflection of a full-thickness flap and root preparation. (Figs 7-5a and 7-5b from McGuire and Scheyer.[43] Reprinted with permission.)

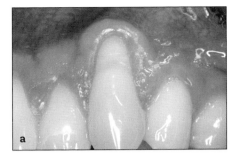
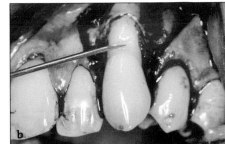

Figs 7-5c and 7-5d Mixture of rhPDGF and β-TCP placed over the root surface.

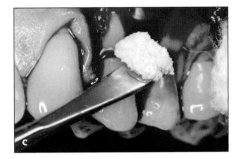
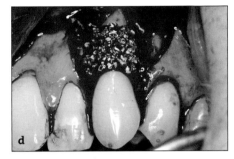

Figs 7-5e and 7-5f Collagen membrane, saturated in rhPDGF, trimmed, and sutured over the denuded root.

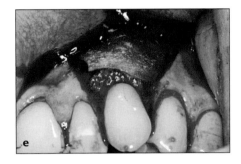
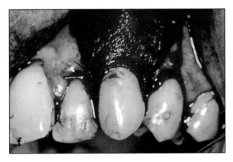

Fig 7-5g Mucogingival flap advanced over the membrane and sutured to the papilla.

Fig 7-5h Six-month postoperative view of rhPDGF plus β-TCP and collagen membrane graft. (Figs 7-5d to 7-5h from McGuire and Scheyer.[43] Reprinted with permission.)

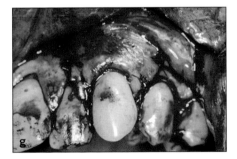
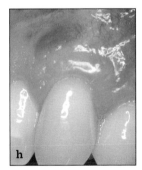

odontal recession-type defects with rhPDGF-BB plus β-TCP and a collagen membrane without the need for autogenous tissue harvested from a second surgical site. The positive results of this feasibility study support the need for a properly powered clinical study to determine the viability of this approach for root coverage.

The evidence from these two studies suggests that tissue engineering strategies that employ extracellular matrix molecules and growth factors to facilitate coverage of denuded root surfaces hold promise for achieving improved outcomes with less invasive surgical procedures.

Live, Cell-Based Therapies

The third line of research in soft tissue engineering has been the implantation of live cells. Live, cell-based skin substitutes and the in vitro construction of a transplantable, vital tissue have been major goals in tissue engineering. One of the first bioengineered skin substitutes consisted of autologous cultures grown from small biopsies.

Autologous fibroblast transplantation

To date, all attempts to rebuild the interproximal papilla have met with limited success. In a small number of case reports, only a few clinicians have been able to regenerate a deficient papillary form caused by hard or soft tissue loss, and none have been able to regenerate the papilla predictably. Most studies consist of a single case report, and few provide long-term results. These attempts have used traditional periodontal plastic surgery approaches and some nonsurgical approaches to preserve the papilla.[44] Modified flap designs or surgical manipulations have been the traditional approach,[45–48] while some researchers have attempted hard and soft tissue grafts. Poor vascularity and limited surgical access have frustrated these efforts. Still, the patient's desire to close open interproximal spaces compels clinicians to attempt papillary regeneration procedures.

Gingival fibroblasts have considerable phenotypic heterogeneity and, theoretically, could contribute to papillary regeneration. With the proper stimulation, undifferentiated mesenchymal cells could differentiate into fibroblastic, cementoblastic, and osteoblastic phenotypes.[49–54] In a healthy site, fibroblasts are responsible for the production and maintenance of the connective tissue matrix.[55]

A recent plastic surgery technique involves the injection of autologous fibroblasts expanded in vitro for soft tissue contouring[56–58] (Isolagen, Isolagen Inc). In a phase I study, this technique was found to be safe in the oral environment.[59]

In an attempt to expand interdental gingival soft tissue volumes, the author has recently completed a randomized, double blind, placebo-controlled study with a novel fibroblast injection technique.[60] To assist the cell transplantation process, a transient inflammatory response was induced in the papilla.

Twenty patients with interdental papillary recession defects were enrolled in the study. Two primary interproximal recession defects were identified in each patient and randomized for either cell transplantation or placebo treatment. The change in papillary height between baseline and 4 months was measured as the distance from the tip of the interproximal papilla to the base of the contact area. The patient's and the clinician's perceptions of change were also recorded. Measurements were made with a UNC 15 periodontal probe (Hu-Friedy), with a digital caliper on plaster casts, and on digital photographs. A visual analog scale evaluation was completed by the examiner and by the patient for each site. The subjects and examiner were blinded as to test and control sites.

Following cultivation and expansion of gingival fibroblasts obtained from a biopsy, a laboratory produced an autologous cell suspension. Five to seven days prior to the initial injection of cells or placebo solution, the papilla was surgically insulted. This papilla-priming procedure was intended to induce a transient inflammatory response to temporarily increase tissue volume and enable the injection of the cell suspension. The suspension was injected at a dose of 20 million cells per milliliter. The first treatment occurred 5 to 7 days after the papilla-priming procedure. Second and third treatments were administered at 1- to 2-week intervals following the first injection. On average, 0.4 to 0.6 mL of solution was injected into the papilla at each of the three injections. Study results were recorded at each treatment visit and 2, 3, and 4 months following the initial injection.

In a study conducted previously at the University of Medicine and Dentistry of New Jersey, 94 patients graded their perceived degree of correction of facial rhytids and dermal depressions, their satisfaction with results, and their perception of continuing improvements.[59] On a scale of 0 to 10, with 10 representing total and complete correction, the average grade for degree of correction was 7.8. In addition, 92% of the patients were satisfied with the overall results, and 78% perceived an ongoing improvement for up to 24 months.

Similarly, in the author's study,[60] both the investigator's and the patients' visual analog scores showed statistically significant improvement with the injection of autologous fibroblasts. By the second month in the study, the mean visual analog score improved in both test and placebo sites, but improvement was greater in the test sites ($P = .02$, signed rank test). In addition, the placebo sites deteriorated in months 3 and 4, while the test sites continued to improve and maintain their statistically significant differ-

Fig 7-6a Preoperative view of an open interproximal space.

Fig 7-6b Four months after three injections into the papilla with the patient's own fibroblasts. Note the improved papillary form. (Figs 7-6a and 7-6b from McGuire and Scheyer.[60] Reprinted with permission.)

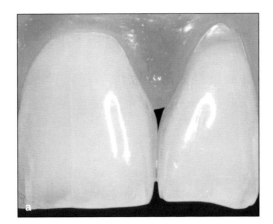 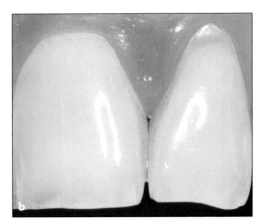

ence (P = .02 for month 3 and P = .006 for month 4) over the placebo sites (Fig 7-6). These preliminary results indicate that novel tissue engineering techniques may hold promise in resolving open interproximal spaces. Further research is underway to refine the technique and confirm the results.

Autologous cell biosynthetics

The periodontal literature contains a few reports of surgeons using tissue engineering techniques to biopsy and then grow the patient's own cells as donor tissue for grafts. Pini Prato et al[61] reported on a patient in whom a biopsy specimen of attached gingiva was taken from the side of the mouth opposite that requiring gingival augmentation. Fibroblasts were obtained from the biopsy specimen and were seeded onto a nonwoven, three-dimensional hydroxyapatite matrix (benzyl ester of hyaluronic acid). Ten days following the biopsy, the graft of cultured fibroblasts on the three-dimensional resorbable membrane was sutured to the periosteal bed.[61] The authors suggested that this technique of obtaining a large amount of donor tissue from a small biopsy specimen was a potentially significant improvement over past techniques and greatly decreased postoperative patient discomfort.

Pini Prato et al[62] also published a case report in which the same technique was used to generate keratinized tissue in six sites from five patients. In this study, small biopsy specimens of epithelium and connective tissue were taken. The keratinocytes and fibroblasts were separated, and only the fibroblasts were cultivated, seeded onto the hydroxyapatite scaffold, and ultimately used as donor material. The seeded scaffold was sutured to the periosteal bed. At the conclusion of the study (3 months), histologic examination revealed an increase in the amount of fully keratinized tissue at all treated sites.

In another study, Momose et al[63] used a similar technique to biopsy attached gingiva (epithelium and connective tissue) from the retromolar pad. The epithelial cells were seeded onto a collagen-silicone bilayer membrane, and the cultures were expanded and then used as donor tissue for soft tissue grafts. The study reported that significant amounts of vascular endothelial growth factor, transforming growth factor α, and transforming growth factor $\beta 1$ were released from the tissue-engineered human gingival epithelial sheets. The authors postulated that the grafting material might have the potential to promote wound healing and tissue regeneration.

Human fibroblast–derived dermal substitute

The first controlled, randomized study to evaluate the safety and effectiveness of a live, cell-based skin substitute in the oral environment was published by McGuire and Nunn.[64] It evaluated a living, tissue-engineered human fibroblast–derived dermal substitute (HF-DDS; Dermagraft, Advanced Tissue Sciences) and its ability to increase the amount of keratinized tissue around teeth that did not require root coverage and compared the results with those of a gingival autograft using donor tissue harvested from the patient's palate.

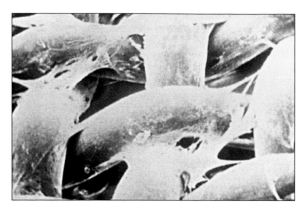

Fig 7-7 Electron microscopic view of polyglactin mesh with fibroblasts stretching across the spaces of the scaffold, 2 days after seeding (original magnification ×2,000). (From McGuire and Nunn.[64] Reprinted with permission.)

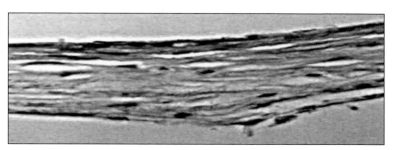

Fig 7-8 Histologic section of HF-DDS demonstrating fibroblasts lying in parallel in a collagen matrix (H&E stain; original magnification ×500).

The tissue-engineered human dermal replacement graft used in this study was manufactured through a three-dimensional cultivation of human diploid fibroblast cells on a polymer scaffold. The scaffold is a bioabsorbable polyglactin mesh (Vicryl, Ethicon), which degrades by hydrolysis and is lost after transplantation, leaving the cellular and extracellular matrix components (Fig 7-7). The human fibroblast cell strains used to produce this material come from newborn foreskins and are cultured by standard methods. The fibroblasts secrete a mixture of growth factors and matrix proteins to create a living dermal structure[65] (Fig 7-8) that, following cryopreservation, remains metabolically active after being implanted on the graft bed.

The proposed mechanism of action of the HF-DDS material involved multiple components acting in concert, including colonization of the wound bed by cells, angiogenesis, and promotion of re-epithelialization.[66] The biologic activity was designed to work simultaneously along two fronts[2]: First, the dermal tissue would fill the bed, producing a substrate that encouraged keratinocyte migration of epithelium over the graft. The collagen and fibronectin provided by the HF-DDS were required for optimal keratinocyte attachment and migration. Second, the living fibroblasts were included to produce a variety of growth factors, including angiogenic factors such as vascular endothelial growth factor, matrix-stimulating factors such as transforming growth factor β1, and keratinocyte-stimulating factors such as keratinocyte growth factor.[65,67] These factors work synergistically to promote regenera-

tion.[68] In the case of HF-DDS, the surface receptors of the fibroblasts are able to communicate with the native cells of the defect and modulate the secretion of growth factors, extracellular matrices, and glycosaminoglycans to ensure that the exact amount needed is received and that secretion is modulated on an ongoing basis.[69]

Twenty-five patients with insufficient attached gingiva associated with at least two teeth in contralateral quadrants of the same jaw were treated.[64] One tooth in each patient was randomized to receive either a gingival autograft (control) or an HF-DDS graft (test). Clinical parameters measured at baseline and 3, 5, 7, 9, and 12 months included recession, clinical attachment level, keratinized tissue height, and plaque index. Probing depth was measured at 7, 9, and 12 months. The inflammation of each site was scored, and texture and color of the grafted tissue were compared with the surrounding tissue. Resistance to muscle pull was evaluated, and a questionnaire was used to determine the preference of the patient. The surgical position of the graft and alveolar bone level were recorded at the surgical visit. Patients were evaluated weekly for the first 4 weeks, at which time the recession and level of oral hygiene were measured.

Biopsies were performed at both the test and control sites of three patients 6 months following surgery. Histologically, the biopsies of the gingival autograft and the HF-DDS appeared similar: connective tissue covered by keratinized epithelium. In addition to the soft tissue biopsies, the study also evaluated 2-mm punch biopsies of the test graft in seven female patients, from 3 to 18 months

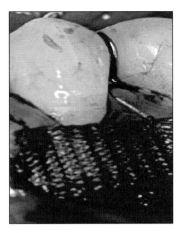

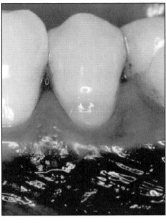

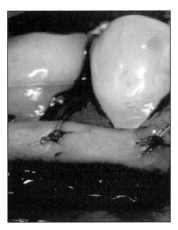

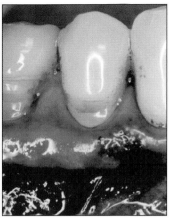

Fig 7-9a HF-DDS sutured to the interproximal papillae following preparation of the bed.

Fig 7-9b Result at 12 months. A band of keratinized tissue is evident after staining with Schiller iodine stain.

Fig 7-9c Free gingival graft sutured to the interproximal papillae following preparation of the bed

Fig 7-9d Result at 12 months. A band of keratinized tissue is evident following staining with Schiller iodine stain. (Figs 7-9a to 7-9d from McGuire and Nunn.[64] Reprinted with permission.)

after surgery, to determine if any of the fibroblasts from the graft remained in the patient. The capacity of these fibroblasts to colonize the implantation site and survive was investigated by detection of the Y-chromosome marker SRY in the biopsy sample using a nested polymerase chain reaction technique capable of detecting single molecules. Fibroblasts from the cultured implant were not detected in any patient in any biopsy. Furthermore, no adverse events were observed at any time.

Results for both test and control groups were similar for all measured clinical parameters, with the exception of the amount of keratinized tissue and the percent of shrinkage of keratinized tissue. The control group exhibited an average of 1.0 to 1.2 mm more keratinized tissue over time than did the test group ($P < .001$), and the control group had about half as much shrinkage as did the test group over time ($P < .001$). The study also demonstrated that the use of multiple layers of the material resulted in less shrinkage and more keratinized tissue. Test sites demonstrated significantly better color match over time than did control sites ($P = .01$). Similarly, tissue texture was significantly better at test sites than at control sites over time ($P = .001$). The results of this study clearly indicate that the use of a single layer of HF-DDS graft resulted in more shrinkage and less keratinized tissue than the gingival autograft.

Limited information exists in the literature regarding a tissue-engineered material's ability to create keratinized tissue around teeth. Three case reports seem to bear out the observations of the author's aforementioned study—

that keratinized tissue can be generated with these tissue-engineered materials but not in great quantities.[67,69,70] The author's study[64] represents the first attempt at using an off-the-shelf tissue-engineered material in the oral environment, and better results might have been obtained if a flap had covered the test material. Overall, the investigation showed that the tissue-engineered HF-DDS graft was safe and capable of generating keratinized tissue without the morbidity and potential clinical difficulties associated with donor site surgery. The gingival autograft generated more keratinized tissue and shrank less than the HF-DDS graft, but the test graft generated tissue that appeared more natural (Fig 7-9).

HF-DDS was also evaluated in a controlled, randomized feasibility study in which it was placed under a coronally advanced flap and compared with a subepithelial connective tissue graft.[71] The purpose of this randomized, controlled, split-mouth study was to test the feasibility of human fibroblast–derived dermal substitute placed under a coronally advanced flap as a potential substitute for a subepithelial connective tissue graft placed under a coronally advanced flap in patients with recession-type defects.

Thirteen patients were selected for this study. Each patient had Miller class I or II bilateral facial recession defects of 3 mm or more on two nonadjacent teeth. The test tooth received an HF-DDS graft, while a connective tissue graft was placed on the control site. One operator performed the 10 test surgeries, and another surgeon performed three surgeries. Eight of the HF-DDS sites received a single thickness of material; five received a

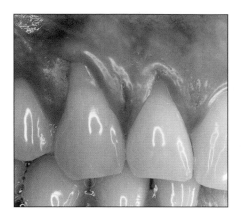

Fig 7-10a Preoperative view of a denuded root surface on a test tooth.

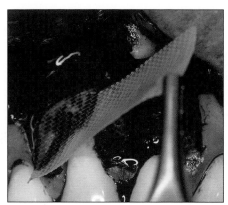

Fig 7-10b HF-DDS placed over the denuded root surface and sutured interproximally after root preparation and elevation of a partial-thickness flap.

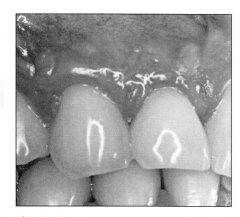

Fig 7-10c One-year postoperative view demonstrating excellent root coverage. (Figs 7-10a to 7-10c from Wilson et al.[71] Reprinted with permission.)

double thickness. Clinical measurements were taken at baseline, 1 week, and 1, 3, and 6 months following surgery. The parameters measured were plaque index, recession depth, clinical attachment levels, recession width, probing depth, and width of keratinized tissue. All clinical readings were taken by a masked, calibrated examiner.

No statistically significant differences were found between the test and control groups. The amount of root coverage was slightly greater for the control group than for the test group, but statistically the difference was insignificant. The width of the recession defect, measured at the cementoenamel junction, was slightly smaller in the test group at the conclusion of the study. The amount of keratinized tissue was the same in both groups at 6 months. The probing depth was slightly greater in the control group, as was the gain in clinical attachment, but neither difference was statistically significant. The greater amount of root coverage obtained when two layers of HF-DDS were used rather than one layer approached statistical significance, but the small sample size may have been responsible for the difference.

The clinical handling characteristics of the HF-DDS were better than those of a connective tissue graft. The membrane was easy to trim and place on the bed. Because it was very thin, the HF-DDS permitted easier advancement of the coronal flap than did the connective tissue graft. Figure 7-10 demonstrates the use of HF-DDS to cover a denuded root.

Within the limits of this study, the human fibroblast–derived dermal substitute may present an acceptable substitute for connective tissue grafts for covering recession defects.[71] The coronally advanced flap with HF-DDS represents a simpler technique for the clinician and a less invasive surgery for the patient. A larger, multicenter trial is necessary to validate the results of this feasibility study.

Living, bilayered skin substitute (bilayered cell therapy)

A study is currently underway (McGuire MK, Scheyer ET, unpublished data, 2007) to evaluate the safety and efficacy of a bilayered cell therapy (BCT; Apligraf, Organogenesis). The test device is being compared with gingival autografts for the ability to generate attached gingiva around teeth that do not require root coverage.

Bilayered cell therapy was the first biomedical device containing viable human cells to be approved by the US Food and Drug Administration. It is a living, bilayered, tissue-engineered skin substitute composed of a dermal layer of human fibroblasts and an overlying cornified epidermal layer of living human keratinocytes on a bovine type I collagen lattice (Fig 7-11). The keratinocytes and fibroblasts used in BCT are derived from neonatal foreskin. It is currently approved for the treatment of venous stasis ulcers and diabetic foot ulcers and has been used more recently to treat a variety of acute wounds.[72] The effects of BCT on these wounds are believed to be related to its structural similarities to human skin. It is delivered "live" as evidenced by the fact that if it is injured in its package, it "heals itself" on the shelf. It is shipped in a

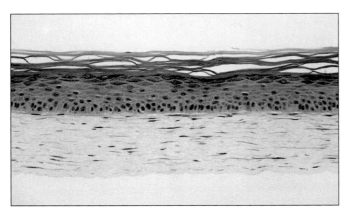

Fig 7-11 Histologic cross section of bilayered cell therapy demonstrating a distinct dermis and epidermis. Compare with the HF-DDS graft, which is composed of dermis only, in Fig 7-8.

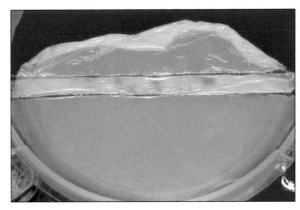

Fig 7-12 Bilayered cell therapy material. The material is folded into three layers and then cut to the appropriate length in the bioreactor.

special container that allows a 10-day shelf life without the need for refrigeration (Fig 7-12).

The epidermis is primarily composed of differentiating keratinocytes, which produce growth factors and cytokines that act as signals between cells and help to regulate skin function.[3] Fibroblasts, the major cell type of the dermis, are responsible for producing and maintaining most of the extracellular matrix. Dermal cells produce and use cytokine and growth factors as signals to regulate processes critical to skin function. Bilayered cell therapy is a tissue-engineered, gingiva-like product that exhibits a synergistic interaction between the epidermal and dermal layers (eg, the product produces cytokine and growth factors not produced by either of the component cells alone).

The efficacy of BCT appears to be related less to the structural functionality of oriented epidermis over dermis and more to the cross talk between the cells of each layer. As such, it appears to produce results regardless of its orientation in the wound bed. Bilayered cell therapy enhances cell and tissue differentiation through cell-matrix, cell-cell, and cell-environment interactions. Although the layers closely resemble human skin, there are some inherent differences in cellular composition. Bilayered cell therapy does not contain blood vessels, sweat glands, or hair follicles. Although BCT does not contain cells such as Langerhans cells, melanocytes, macrophages, or lymphocytes, which may explain its low immunogenic profile, it possesses a cytokine profile similar to that of human skin. The living cells in the graft produce cytokines and growth factors involved in normal wound healing. Research has also revealed that the product is dynamic, with a cytokine profile that changes in response to injury.

To date, preliminary periodontal results appear encouraging (Fig 7-13). If these positive results are confirmed, larger multicenter trials involving a variety of applications are anticipated.

Conclusion

Tissue engineering, more than anything else on the horizon, holds the promise of rewriting the rules of regeneration. The surgical limits of what clinicians can and cannot do are primarily based on available blood supply, but in the future it is likely that surgeons will have materials capable of enhancing blood supply to the defect so that the limits of repair and regeneration will be redefined.

The implantation of live cells in the defect adds an entirely new dimension to treatment, although near-term ability to gain regulatory approval for products of this type may be challenging. The advantage of cell-based therapies is that cells communicate with each other and with the native cells of the defect, ensuring the delivery of metabolically active molecules exactly where needed and in the exact amounts required. Recombinant protein therapeutics, especially rhPDGF-BB, with its well-established effects on hard and soft tissue cells, have the advantage of providing tissue engineering in vivo, utilizing cells within the treatment site as the population to expand (through proliferative effects), thereby removing the need to expand cells in culture prior to treatment.

In the past, regeneration was promoted by excluding a single factor such as epithelial cells (guided tissue regen-

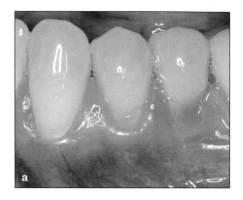

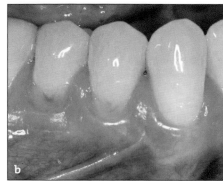

Figs 7-13a and 7-13b Baseline appearance of mandibular first premolars and canine that have been randomized to receive test treatment (bilayered cell therapy) (a) or control treatment (gingival autograft) (b).

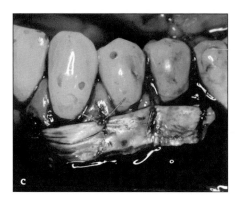

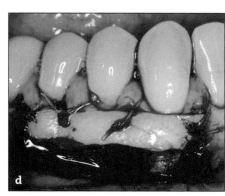

Figs 7-13c and 7-13d Test graft (c) and free gingival graft (d) sutured interproximally following bed preparation.

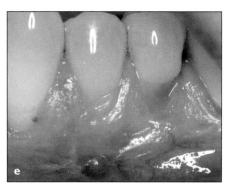

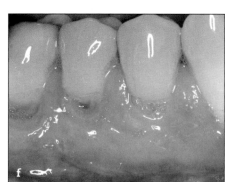

Figs 7-13e and 7-13f One-month postoperative view of test (e) and control (f) grafts.

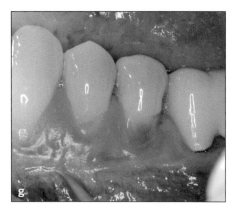

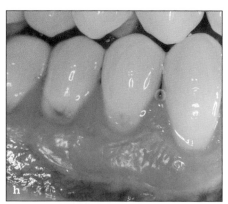

Figs 7-13g and 7-13h Six-month postoperative view of test (g) and control (h) grafts.

Figs 7-13i and 7-13j Six-month postoperative view of test *(i)* and control *(j)* grafts after staining with Schiller iodine stain. An increase in keratinized tissue has been obtained with each graft.

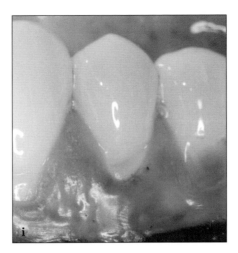
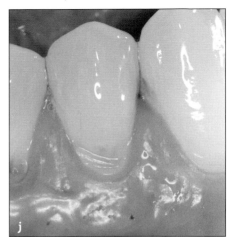

eration) or by including a single growth factor such as bone morphogenetic protein. It was naive to think that the exclusion or inclusion of a single factor could trigger an entire regenerative cascade, but that was the best the profession could do. That will not be the case in the future.

The field of soft tissue engineering is advancing rapidly. Commercial products based on directive matrices, metabolically active molecules, and live cells are reaching the market. These new devices will improve the ability to regenerate soft tissue by providing templates, migration pathways, adhesive substrates, and growth factors. This new dimension in treatment should broaden the scope of practice and, more importantly, provide patients with predictable regenerative solutions.

References

1. Rhenwald JG. Methods for clinical growth and dermal cultivation of normal human epidermal keratinocytes and mesothelial cells. In: Baserga R (ed). Cell Growth and Division: A Practical Approach. New York: Oxford University Press, 1989:156–164.

2. Gentzkow G, Jensen J, Pollak R, et al. Improved healing of diabetic foot ulcers after grafting with a living human dermal replacement. Wounds 1999;11:77–84.

3. Tenner J, Hardin-Young J, Parenteau NL. Tissue engineered skin. In: Patrick CW Jr, Midos AG, McIntire LV (eds). Frontiers in Tissue Engineering. New York: Elsevier Science, 1998:664–677.

4. Quattlebaum JB, Mellonig JT, Hensel NF. Antigenicity of freeze-dried cortical bone allograft in human periodontal osseous defects. J Periodontol 1998;59:394–397.

5. Harris RJ. A comparative study of root coverage obtained with an acellular dermal matrix versus a connective tissue graft: Results of 107 recession defects in 50 consecutively treated patients. Int J Periodontics Restorative Dent 2000;20:51–59.

6. Aichelmann-Reidy ME, Yukna RA, Evans GH, Nasr HF, Mayer ET. Clinical evaluation of acellular allograft dermis for the treatment of human gingival recession. J Periodontol 2001;72:998–1005.

7. Novaes AB, Grisi DC, Molina GO, Souza SL, Taba M, Grisi MF. Comparative 6-month clinical study of a subepithelial connective tissue graft and acellular dermal matrix graft for the treatment of gingival recession. J Periodontol 2001;72:1477–1484.

8. Paolantonio M, Dolci M, Esposito P, et al. Subpedicle acellular dermal matrix graft and autogenous connective tissue graft in the treatment of gingival recessions: A comparative 1-year clinical study. J Periodontol 2002;73:1299–1307.

9. Tal H, Moses O, Zohar R, Meir H, Nemcovsky C. Root coverage of advanced gingival recession: A comparative study between acellular dermal matrix allograft and subepithelial connective tissue grafts. J Periodontol 2002;73:1405–1411.

10. Woodyard JG, Greenwell H, Hill M, Drisko C, Iasella JM, Scheetz J. The clinical effect of acellular dermal matrix on gingival thickness and root coverage compared to coronally positioned flap alone. J Periodontol 2004;75:44–56.

11. Henderson RD, Greenwell H, Drisko C, et al. Predictable multiple site root coverage using an acellular dermal matrix allograft. J Periodontol 2001;72:571–582.

12. Harris RJ. Acellular dermal matrix used for root coverage. 18-month follow-up observation. Int J Periodontics Restorative Dent 2002;22:156–163.

13. Van der Pauw MT, Van der Bos T, Everts V, Beersten W. Enamel matrix-derived protein stimulates attachment of periodontal ligament fibroblasts and enhances alkaline phosphate activity and transforming growth factor β1 release of periodontal ligament and gingival fibroblasts. J Periodontol 2000;71:31–43.

14. Lyngstadaas SP, Andersson C, Lundberg E, Ekdahl H. Interleukin expression in cultured human PDL cells growing on Emdogain [abstract 2986]. J Dent Res 2000;79(special issue):517.

15. Hoang AM, Oates TW, Cochran DL. In vitro wound healing responses to enamel matrix derivative. J Periodontol 2000;71:1270–1277.

16. Yoneda S, Kasugai S, Itoh D, et al. Effect of enamel matrix derivative (Emdogain) on osteoblastic cells [abstract 2641]. J Dent Res 2000;79(special issue):474.

17. Schwartz Z, Carnes DL Jr, Pulliam R, et al. Porcine fetal enamel matrix derivative stimulates proliferation but not differentiation of pre-osteoblastic 2T9 cells, inhibits proliferation and stimulates differentiation of osteoblast-like MG63 cells and increases proliferation and differentiation of normal human osteoblast NHOst cells. J Periodontol 2000;71:1287–1296.

18. Heijl L, Heden G, Svärdström G, Östrgren A. Periodontal plastic surgery for treatment of localized gingival recessions: A systematic review. J Clin Periodontol 2002;29(suppl 3):178–194.

19. McGuire MK, Nunn M. Evaluation of human recession defects treated with coronally advanced flaps and either enamel matrix derivative or connective tissue. I. Comparison of clinical parameters. J Periodontol 2003;74:1110–1125.

20. Heijl L. Periodontal regeneration with enamel matrix derivative in one human experimental defect. A case report. J Clin Periodontol 1977;24(pt 2):693–696.

21. Rasperini G, Silvestri M, Schenk RK, Nevins ML, Nevins M. Histological evaluation of human gingival recession treated with subepithelial connective tissue graft plus enamel matrix derivative. A case report. Int J Periodontics Restorative Dent 2000;20:3–9.

22. Modica F, Del Pizzo M, Rocuzzo M, Romagnoli R. Coronally advanced flap for treatment of buccal gingival recession with and without enamel matrix derivative. A split mouth study. J Periodontol 2000;71:1693–1698.

23. Trombelli L. Periodontal regeneration in gingival recession defects. Periodontol 2000 1999;19:138–150.

24. McGuire MK, Cochran DL. Evaluation of human recession defects treated with coronally advanced flaps and either enamel matrix derivative or connective tissue. Part 2: Histological evaluation. J Periodontol 2003;74:1126–1135.

25. Rasperini G, Silvestri M, Schenk RK, Nevins ML. Clinical and histological evaluation of human gingival recession treated with a subepithelial connective tissue graft and enamel matrix protein derivative (Emdogain): A case report. Int J Periodontics Restorative Dent 2000;20:269–275.

26. Bowers GM, Chadroff B, Carnevale R, et al. Histologic evaluation of new attachment apparatus formation in humans. 2. J Periodontol 1988;60:675–672.

27. Bruno JF, Bowers GM. Histology of a human biopsy section following the placement of a subepithelial connective tissue graft. Int J Periodontics Restorative Dent 2000;20:225–231.

28. Pasquinelli KL. The histology of a new attachment utilizing a thick autogenous soft tissue graft in an area of deep recession: A case report. Int J Periodontics Restorative Dent 1995;15:248–257.

29. Cortellini P, Clauser C, Pini Prato G. Histologic assessment of new attachment following the treatment of human buccal recession by means of a guided tissue regeneration procedure. J Periodontol 1993;64:387–391.

30. Harris RJ. Histologic evaluation of root coverage obtained with GTR in humans: A case report. Int J Periodontics Restorative Dent 2001;21:240–251.

31. Lynch SE, Williams RC, Polson AM, et al. A combination of platelet-derived growth factor and insulin-like growth factor enhances periodontal regeneration. J Clin Periodontol 1989;16:545–554.

32. Matsuda N, Lin WL, Kumar MI, Cho MI, Genco RJ. Mitogenic, chemotactic and synthetic responses of rat periodontal ligament fibroblastic cells to polypeptide growth factors in vitro. J Periodontol 1992;63:515–525.

33. Lynch SE, Castill GR, Williams RC, et al. The effect of short term application of a combination of platelet-derived and insulin-like growth factors on periodontal wound healing. J Periodontol 1991;62:458–467.

34. Lynch SE. The role of growth factors in periodontal repair and regeneration. In: Polson A (ed). Periodontal Regeneration: Current Status and Directions. Chicago: Quintessence, 1994:179–198.

35. Lynch SE. Introduction. In: Lynch SE, Genco RJ, Marx RE (eds). Tissue Engineering: Applications in Maxillofacial Surgery and Periodontics. Chicago: Quintessence, 1999:xi–xviii.

36. Giannobile W. Periodontal tissue regeneration by polypeptide growth factors and gene transfer. In: Lynch SE, Genco RJ, Marx RE (eds). Tissue Engineering: Applications in Maxillofacial Surgery and Periodontics. Chicago: Quintessence, 1999:231–243.

37. Park JB, Matshuhra M, Hank Y, et al. Periodontal regeneration in Class III furcation defects of beagle dogs using guided tissue regeneration therapy with platelet-derived growth factor. J Periodontol 1995;66:462–477.

38. Cho MI, Lin WL, Genco RJ. Platelet-derived growth factor–modulated guided tissue regeneration therapy. J Periodontol 1995;66:522–530.

39. Rutherford RB, Nickrash CE, Kennedy JE, Charette MF. Platelet-derived and insulin-like growth factors stimulate regeneration of periodontal attachment in monkeys. J Periodontol 1992;27:285–290.

40. Nevins M, Camelo M, Nevins ML, Schenk RK, Lynch SE. Periodontal regeneration in humans using recombinant human platelet-derived growth factor-BB (rhPDGF-BB) and allogeneic bone. J Periodontol 2003;74:1282–1292.

41. Camelo M, Nevins ML, Schenk RK, Lynch SE, Nevins M. Periodontal regeneration in human Class II furcations using purified recombinant human platelet-derived growth factor-BB (rhPDGF-BB) with bone allograft. Int J Periodontics Restorative Dent 2003;23:213–225.

42. Nevins M, Giannobile WV, McGuire MK, et al. Platelet-derived growth factor stimulates bone fill and rate of attachment level gain: Results of a large multicenter randomized controlled trial. J Periodontol 2005;76:2205–2215.

43. McGuire MK, Scheyer ET. Comparison of rhPDGF-BB plus beta tricalcium phosphate and a collagen membrane to subepithelial connective tissue grafting for the treatment of recession defects: A case series. Int J Periodontics Restorative Dent 2006;26:127–133.

44. Shapiro A. Regeneration of interdental papilla using periodic curettage. Int J Periodontics Restorative Dent 1985;5(5):27–33.

45. Takei HH, Han TJ, Carranza FA Jr, Kenny EB, Lekovic V. Flap technique for periodontal bone implants. Papilla preservation technique. J Periodontol 1985;56:204–210.

46. Cortellini P, Pini Prato G, Tonetti MS. The modified papilla preservation technique. A new surgical approach for interproximal regeneration procedures. J Periodontol 1995;66:261–266.

47. Cortellini P, Tonetti MS. Microsurgical approach to periodontal regeneration. Initial evaluation in a case cohort. J Periodontol 2001;72:559–569.

48. Cortellini P, Pini Prato G, Tonetti MS. The simplified papilla preservation flap. A novel surgical approach for the management of soft tissues in regenerative procedures. Int J Periodontics Restorative Dent 1999;19:589–599.

49. McCullouch CAG, Knowles G. Role of fibroblasts in subpopulations in periodontal physiology and pathology. J Periodontal Res 1991;76:144–154.

50. Otsuka K. Pitaru S, Overall CR, et al. Biochemical comparison of fibroblast populations from different tissues: Characterization of matrix protein and collagenolytic enzyme synthesis. Biochem Cell Biol 1988;66:167–176.

51. Irwin CR, Picardo M, Ellis I, et al. Inter- and intra-site heterogeneity in the expression of fetal-like phenotypic characteristics by gingival fibroblasts: Potential significance for wound healing. J Cell Sci 1994;107:1333–1346.

52. Tipton DA, Stricklin GP, Dabbous MK. Fibroblast heterogeneity in collagenolytic response to cyclosporine. J Cell Biochem 1991;46:152–165.

53. Pender HN. Migration and proliferation of progenitor cells in the connective tissue of rat gingival papilla. J Periodontal Res 1995;30:312–318.

54. Carnes DL, Maeder CL, Graves DT. Cells with osteoblastic phenotypes can be expanded from human gingival and periodontal ligament. J Periodontol 1997;68:701–707.

55. Biagini G, Checci L, Pelliccioni GA, Solmi R. In vitro growth of periodontal fibroblasts on treated cementum. Quintessence Int 1992;23:335–340.

56. Boss WK, Marko D. Isolagen. In: Klein AW (ed). Tissue Augmentation in Clinical Practice. New York: Dekker, 1998:335–347.

57. Boss WK, Usal H, Fodor PB, Chernoff G. Autologous cultured fibroblasts as cellular therapy in plastic surgery. Clin Plast Surg 2000;27:613–626.

58. Boss WK, Usal H, Fodor PB, Chernoff G. Autologous cultured fibroblasts. A protein repair system. Ann Plast Surg 2000;44:536–542.

59. Bowsma O, D'Sousa R, Meyerat BS. Treatment of deep periodontal pockets with autologous fibroblasts or placebo [abstract 1180]. J Dent Res 2005;84(special issue A).

60. McGuire MK, Scheyer ET. A randomized, double-blind, placebo-controlled study to determine the safety and efficacy of cultured and expanded autologous fibroblast injections for the treatment of interdental papillary insufficiency associated with the papilla priming procedure. J Periodontol 2007;78:4–17.

61. Pini Prato GP, Rotundo R, Magnani C, Soranzo C. Tissue engineering technology for gingival augmentation procedures: A case report. Int J Periodontics Restorative Dent 2000;20:553–559.

62. Pini Prato GP, Rotundo R, Magnani C, Soranzo C, Muzzi L, Cairo F. An autologous cell hyaluronic acid graft technique for gingival augmentation: A case series. J Periodontol 2003;74:262–267.

63. Momose M, Murata M, Kato Y, et al. Vascular endothelial growth factors and transforming growth factor-α and β_1 are released from human cultured gingival epithelial sheets. J Periodontol 2002;73:749–775.

64. McGuire MK, Nunn ME. Evaluation of the safety and efficacy of periodontal applications of a living tissue–engineered, human fibroblast–derived dermal substitute. 1. Comparison to the gingival autograft: A randomized controlled pilot study. J Periodontol 2005;76:867–880.

65. Mansbridge J, Lim K, Patch R, Symons K, Pinney E. Three-dimensional fibroblast culture implant for the treatment of diabetic foot ulcers: Metabolic activity and therapeutic range. Tissue Eng 1998;4:403–413.

66. Naughton G, Mansbridge J, Gentzkow G. A metabolically active human dermal replacement for treatment of diabetic foot ulcers. Artif Organs 1997;21:1203–1210.

67. Naughton G, Bartel R, Mansbridge J. In: Atala A, Mooney D (eds). Synthetic Biodegradable Polymer Scaffolds. Boston: Birkhauser, 1997:121–147.

68. Mansbridge JN, Liu K, Pinney RE, Patch R, Ratcliffe A, Naughton GK. Growth factors secreted by fibroblasts: Role in healing diabetic foot ulcers. Diabetes Obes Metab 1999;1:265–279.

69. Hansborough J. Current status of skin replacements for coverage of extensive burn wounds. J Trauma 1990;30:155–162.

70. Oliver RC, Löe H, Karring T. Microscopic evaluation of the healing and revascularization of free gingival grafts. J Periodontal Res 1968;3:84–95.

71. Wilson TG, McGuire MK, Nunn ME. Evaluation of the safety and efficacy of periodontal applications of a living tissue–engineered human fibroblast–derived dermal substitute. 2. Comparison to the subepithelial connective tissue graft: A randomized controlled feasibility study. J Periodontol 2005;76:881–889.

72. Sabolinski ML, Alvarez O, Auletta M, et al. Cultured skin as a smart material for healing wounds: Experience in venous ulcers. Biomaterials 1996;17:311–320.

Site Development for Implant Placement: Regenerative and Esthetic Techniques in Oral Plastic Surgery

Marc L. Nevins, DMD, MMSc

James T. Mellonig, DDS, MS

The replacement of teeth with dental implants has evolved from treatment of complete edentulism with hybrid prostheses to the replacement of single teeth with implant-supported crown restorations. Accordingly, esthetic demands have evolved to require inconspicuous implant restorations that adapt to the natural contours of the marginal soft tissues. The treatment demands increase when multiple teeth are replaced in the esthetic zone.[1,2] Therefore, diagnostic procedures and techniques should be utilized to determine the course of treatment that will optimize the results of implant therapy.

Guided bone regeneration (GBR) procedures to augment deficient alveolar ridges and ridge preservation techniques to maintain adequate ridge volume at tooth extraction sites are well-established means of enhancing the esthetics and function of dental implant restorations. More recently, clinicians have begun to apply principles of tissue engineering, particularly treatment with growth factors, to improve the outcome of implant site preparation. This chapter will discuss currently applied techniques for implant site development and present the results of clinical application of recombinant human platelet-derived growth factor BB (rhPDGF-BB) for tissue regeneration.

Guided Bone Regeneration

GBR using autografts and membranes is a predictable procedure for regenerating horizontal ridge defects.[3] Vertical bony defects present a greater challenge for regeneration and can be treated with GBR in staged or simultaneous procedures.[4–6] Newer techniques such as distraction osteogenesis have been reported to successfully treat advanced vertical defects; however, their predictability may be limited for sites requiring three-dimensional regeneration.[7,8]

Guidelines for successful GBR treatments have been published previously.[9–11] Large contained defects can be predictably treated with autografts and nonresorbable membranes (Fig 8-1). Large noncontained defects may benefit from the use of block grafts to support additional particulate graft material—either autogenous or allogeneic bone replacement grafts.[3,12,13] These procedures can be successful with either nonresorbable or resorbable membranes. Figure 8-2 depicts advanced vertical and lateral ridge resorption in the maxillary central incisor region. The site was treated successfully with autogenous corticocancellous block bone grafts and particulate

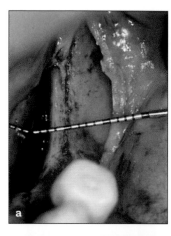 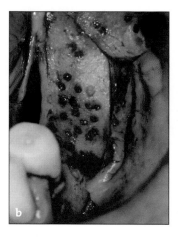 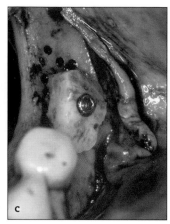 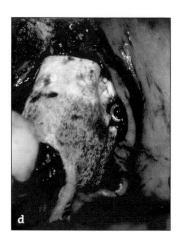

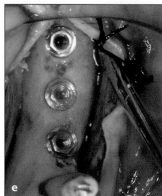

Fig 8-1a The mandibular ridge is too narrow to allow implant placement.

Fig 8-1b The ridge is perforated to open the marrow spaces.

Fig 8-1c An autogenous block graft is placed and affixed with a miniscrew.

Fig 8-1d The block graft and autogenous bone chips are covered with a nonresorbable membrane.

Fig 8-1e The site is reopened at second-stage surgery to reveal adequate bony width for implant placement.

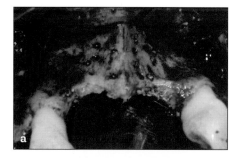 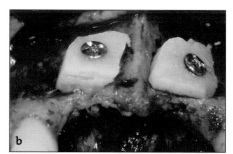

Fig 8-2a The knife-edged anterior maxillary site is unsuitable for implant placement.

Fig 8-2b Autogenous block grafts are fixed with miniscrews.

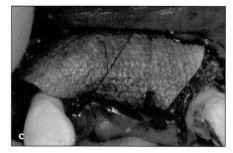 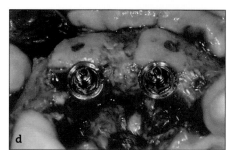

Fig 8-2c The block grafts are contoured with autogenous bone chips and covered with a resorbable membrane.

Fig 8-2d The reentry surgery for implant placement 6 months after grafting reveals sufficient reconstruction of the alveolar process to proceed with implant placement.

autogenous bone chips combined with freeze-dried bone allograft (FDBA) and protected by a resorbable membrane. There was sufficient restoration of the alveolar process to proceed with implant placement.

Significant morbidity can be associated with the donor site for block bone grafting. This includes bruising, paresthesia, hypoesthesia, muscle prolapse, or altered facial contours.[14] In most cases, alternative techniques that

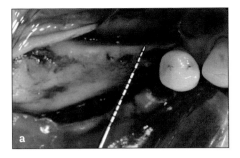
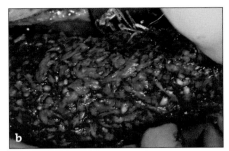
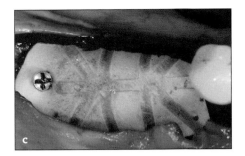

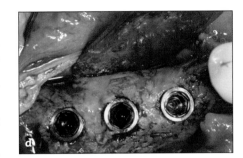
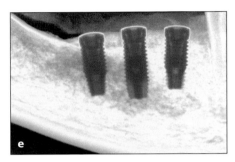

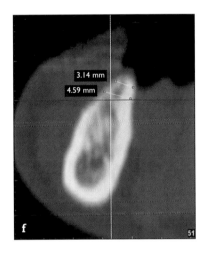
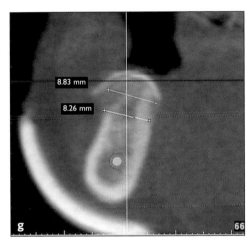

Fig 8-3a A modified split-crest technique is performed on a noncontained, lateral ridge defect. The surface of the bony ridge is incised to a depth of 5 to 7 mm, and the bone crest is moved approximately 45 degrees buccally to open the marrow space on the coronal aspect of the ridge.

Fig 8-3b An autogenous particulate graft is placed laterally and crestally.

Fig 8-3c The graft is protected with a non-resorbable, titanium-reinforced expanded polytetrafluoroethylene membrane.

Fig 8-3d Implants are placed 6 months after grafting.

Fig 8-3e Colorized digital radiograph of the ridge reveals adequate lateral and crestal bony volume.

Fig 8-3f The initial CT indicates the lack of bone volume.

Fig 8-3g The CT taken 5 months post-grafting reveals the increase in bone volume.

involve particulate grafts and GBR techniques can be used. For noncontained defects, treatment options include split-crest techniques with simultaneous implant placement or vertical ridge augmentation with simultaneous implant placement.[15–18] It is important to consider management of complications when combining implant placement and bone grafting. A wound dehiscence or partial healing of the bone graft may result in an integrated fixture that is an esthetic or biologic failure. Such complications can be difficult to resolve.

The modified split-crest technique is a conservative, staged approach for treating noncontained lateral ridge defects. The technique can result in both lateral and vertical ridge augmentation. The surface of the bony ridge is incised to a depth of 5 to 7 mm, and the bone crest is moved approximately 45 degrees buccally to open the marrow space on the coronal aspect of the ridge. Apical to the ridge split on the buccal surface, intramarrow penetration is performed with a No. 1/2 round bur or a 1.0-mm twist drill. Either autogenous or other bone replacement particulate grafts are placed laterally and crestally on the prepared ridge. The graft is then covered with a nonresorbable or resorbable membrane. This modified approach allows for significant ridge enhancement with particulate grafting in a staged approach (Fig 8-3).

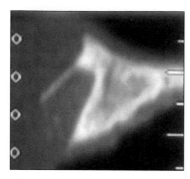

Fig 8-4a The buccal wall of the extraction socket is intact at baseline.

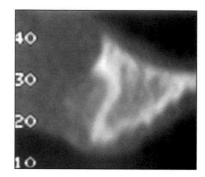

Fig 8-4b The buccal wall has been resorbed and the crestal height is clearly reduced after 37 days. (Figs 8-4a and 8-4b from Nevins et al.[21] Reprinted with permission.)

Ridge Preservation Techniques

Most treatment protocols for lateral and vertical ridge augmentation have been developed to manage an edentulous site that is deficient in bone volume.[3–6] However, the clinician has the opportunity to intercept the alveolar resorption that will result in a ridge defect subsequent to tooth extraction. The goal at the time of tooth extraction should be to use techniques and procedures that preserve the ridge volume, facilitate implant treatment, and optimize function and esthetics.

The process of ridge resorption can occur just weeks after tooth extraction.[19–22] When a tooth with a thin buccal plate is extracted, ridge resorption is inevitable (Fig 8-4). Soft tissues that have lost their bony support will collapse into the bone defect, resulting in a volumetric deficiency for both hard and soft tissue. The resultant scar tissue complicates the surgical procedure, especially wound closure. Soft tissue manipulation has been such a prevalent problem that specialized tissue-expanding devices have been developed and advocated.[23]

Thus, the goal of extraction socket management should include bone and soft tissue preservation, which may require grafting to prevent ridge defects of hard and soft tissues. Clinical findings, such as the presence or absence and thickness of the buccal and lingual plates and the presence or absence and extent of apical pathosis, dictate the appropriate management of extraction sites. An extraction site with intact bony walls can "self-heal" with bone fill.[24,25] Immediately after extraction of a tooth, a blood clot or coagulum develops within the extraction site. This coagulum is then replaced with provisional connective tissue. Woven bone forms and remodels to become mature bone within the alveolus.[24,25]

Preferences vary as to the ideal time for implant placement following extraction. Options include immediate placement at the time of extraction, delayed placement after soft tissue healing, or placement after bone fill or maturation.[3,26–28] When teeth are being extracted because of dental caries and the alveolar process and soft tissues are healthy, either delayed or immediate implant placement can provide ridge preservation.

If a pathologic condition is present and/or there is a thin bony buccal plate at risk for resorption, the course of treatment may be significantly simplified if ridge preservation procedures are performed at the time of extraction. These procedures will result in increased bone and/or soft tissue volume for future implant support and emergence profile esthetics.

Where bone loss necessitates soft tissue healing prior to bone augmentation, site preservation can be achieved with connective tissue grafting (Fig 8-5). Once the area has healed, there will be adequate soft tissue to protect a bone graft utilized for future implant placement. Even in severely compromised sites, this approach can provide enhanced esthetics.

In rare instances in which surgical access is not needed for debridement or the identification of anatomic obstacles, a nonsurgical approach can be used in the extraction socket. Figure 8-6 demonstrates the use of a nonsurgical treatment with immediate implant placement and bone grafting to replace a tooth with a root fracture defect. The postoperative radiograph reveals trabeculation consistent

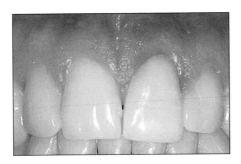

Fig 8-5a The maxillary left central incisor is to be extracted.

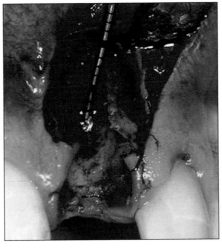

Fig 8-5b Bone loss requires soft tissue healing prior to bone augmentation. The site will be preserved with connective tissue grafting.

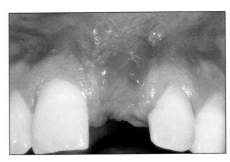

Fig 8-5c The grafted area is healed.

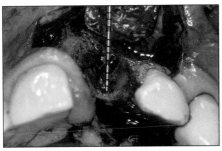

Fig 8-5d There is adequate soft tissue to protect a bone graft.

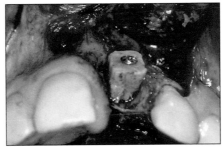

Fig 8-5e A block bone graft is secured with a miniscrew.

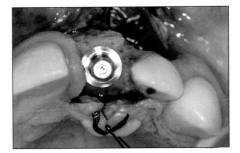

Fig 8-5f An implant is placed.

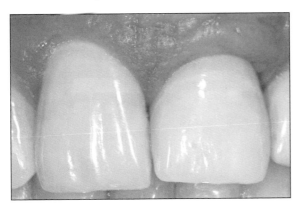

Fig 8-5g Four years postoperatively, the cosmetic result is excellent.

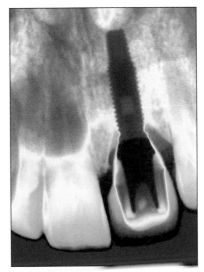

Fig 8-5h On the colorized digital radiograph taken 4 years postoperatively, function appears satisfactory.

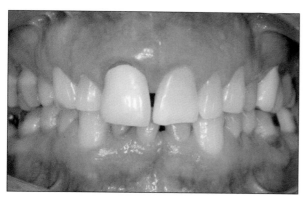

Fig 8-6a A nonsurgical approach to site preservation, with immediate implant placement and bone grafting, is planned for the maxillary right central incisor.

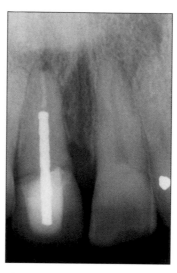

Fig 8-6b The tooth is to be extracted because of a root fracture defect.

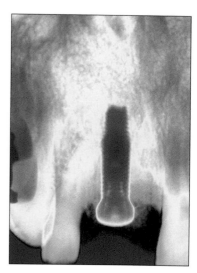

Fig 8-6c An implant is inserted in the extraction socket.

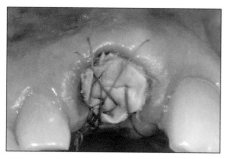

Fig 8-6d The site is filled with freeze-dried bone allograft and covered with a gingival graft.

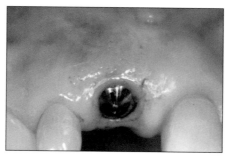

Fig 8-6e After the second stage of surgery, there is a need for soft tissue conditioning.

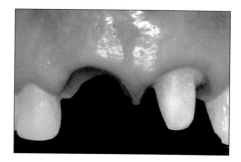

Fig 8-6f The site is shown following papilla formation 3 months after provisionalization.

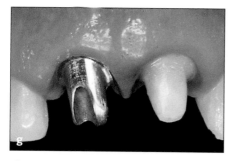

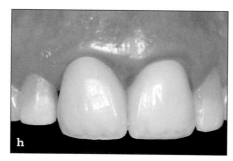

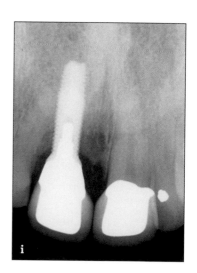

Fig 8-6g A custom abutment is made for the single-stage implant.

Fig 8-6h The esthetic implant-supported crown is in place. (Restoration by Dr Jenny Chang, Natick, Massachusetts.)

Fig 8-6i The postoperative radiograph reveals trabeculation consistent with bone fill in the region of the defect.

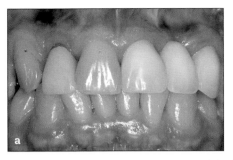
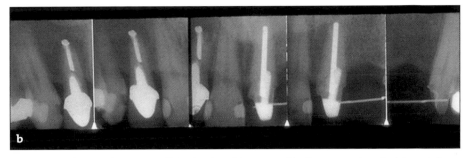

Fig 8-7a In a staged approach, successful ridge augmentation can be accomplished using GBR around lesions associated with root fractures or endodontic failures.

Fig 8-7b The radiographs reveal the extensive periapical pathoses.

Figs 8-7c and 8-7d Sites are thoroughly debrided following extraction.

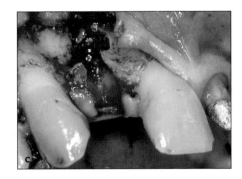
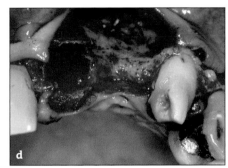

Figs 8-7e and 8-7f Following ridge augmentation, barrier membranes are placed (e) and remain in place until re-entry at 9 months (f).

(Fig 8-7 continued on next page.)

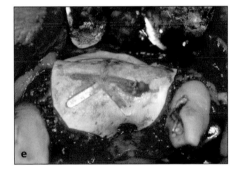
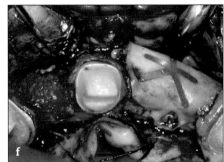

with bone fill in the region of the defect. Provisional restorations helped to develop the tissue prior to fabrication and delivery of the final abutment and crown.

For sites with extensive periapical pathosis, a staged approach is favored over immediate implant placement. Thorough and complete degranulation and debridement of infected lesions associated with root fractures or endodontic failures will facilitate successful ridge augmentation procedures. The buccal flap is advanced coronally to provide complete wound closure. Periosteal releasing incisions may be necessary to accomplish this goal.[9]

Figure 8-7 demonstrates successful implant placement 6 months after extraction and GBR. Previously deficient sites now have sufficient hard and soft tissue to receive implants. In this case, where there was initially significant alloy tattooing, the soft tissue is augmented with a free gingival graft to enhance the zone of keratinized tissue and improve the esthetics prior to prosthetic treatment. The final result reveals the benefit of well-planned, evidence-based GBR therapy. The implants are clinically and radiographically successful.

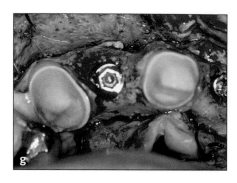

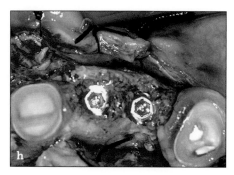

Figs 8-7g and 8-7h Implants are placed 6 months after GBR.

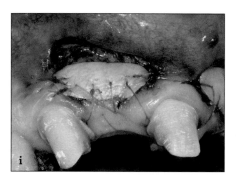

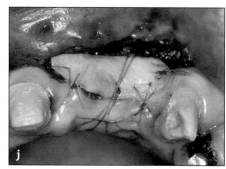

Figs 8-7i and 8-7j The soft tissue is augmented with a free gingival graft to enhance the zone of keratinized tissue and improve the esthetics prior to prosthetic treatment.

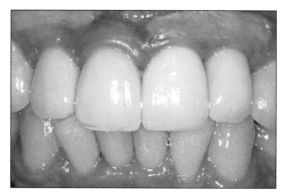

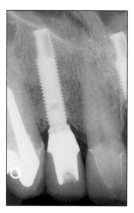

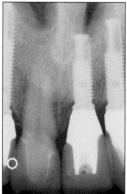

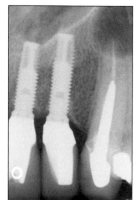

Fig 8-7k The final result reveals the benefit of well-planned, evidence-based GBR therapy.

Fig 8-7l Radiographs show the success of implant treatment.

Recombinant Protein Therapies

With the current understanding of the biologic basis of oral wound healing, regeneration of bone and soft tissues can be enhanced to enable successful, long-term implant treatments. Newer techniques and technologies that take advantage of well-understood cellular and molecular mediators of tissue regeneration continue to increase the effectiveness and predictability of implant site preparation. Combination therapies, described elsewhere in this book, now provide dental surgeons with access to pure recombinant tissue growth factors. These developments have allowed a progression from previously passive therapies

Fig 8-8a An augmentation procedure is to be performed in the area of the mandibular left first and second molars to restore vertical and horizontal bone height in advance of implant placement. The first molar requires extraction due to a hopeless prognosis.

Fig 8-8b The site is shown 3 months after tooth extraction and placement of rhPDGF-BB–enhanced particulate FDBA.

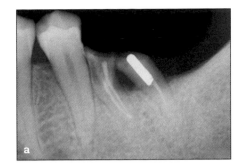

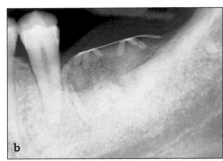

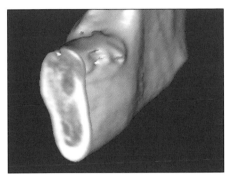

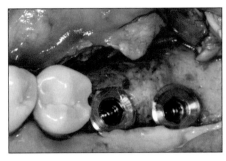

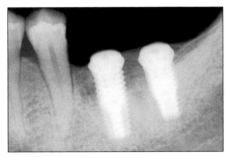

Fig 8-8c The three-dimensional CT of the site reveals evidence of excellent bone fill 6 months postsurgery.

Fig 8-8d Bone fill is confirmed on surgical reentry at the time of implant placement.

Fig 8-8e Radiograph taken 6 months postsurgery.

to new active treatments, thereby enhancing the opportunity for bone and tissue regeneration and providing faster and more predictable outcomes for patients.

The following three clinical cases demonstrate the use of rhPDGF-BB in combination with appropriate tissue matrices, providing examples of the outcomes that may be achieved with recombinant protein therapeutics.

Case 1

The first patient, a 27-year-old healthy, nonsmoking woman, presented with radiographic and clinical evidence of a class III furcation lesion on the mandibular left first molar and a vertically and horizontally atrophied ridge in the area of the second molar, which had been extracted previously (Fig 8-8a).

The tooth roots of the first molar were extracted, and the alveolar ridge in the area of the second molar was expanded with a modified split-crest technique. The defects and deficient ridges were augmented with particulate FDBA that had been fully saturated with 0.3 mg/mL of rhPDGF-BB. The graft was then protected with a nonresorbable titanium-reinforced expanded polytetrafluoroethylene (e-PTFE) membrane that remained in place for a period of 6 months.

Figure 8-8b demonstrates the healing 3 months postsurgery. The site healed without complication. The 6-month postsurgical periapical radiograph and computerized tomograph (CT) revealed excellent bone fill, which was confirmed on surgical reentry at the time of implant placement (Figs 8-8c to 8-8e).

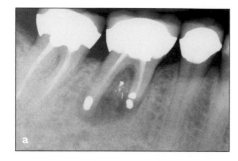

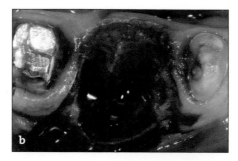

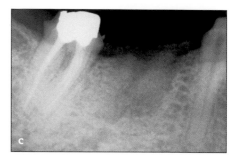

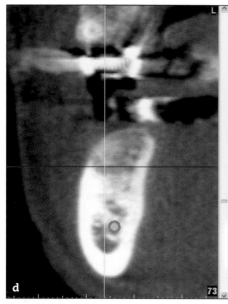

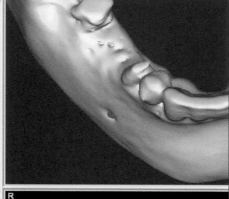

Fig 8-9a An augmentation procedure is to be performed in the area of the mandibular right first molar following extraction due to unsuccessful endodontic treatment.

Fig 8-9b The tooth has been extracted. On surgical exposure a large dehiscence defect was revealed on the buccal surface of the tooth.

Fig 8-9c The 2-month postsurgical radiograph reveals excellent healing.

Fig 8-9d The 6-month postsurgical CT evaluation reveals evidence of excellent bone fill.

Fig 8-9e The bone fill is confirmed on surgical reentry 6 months postsurgery, and the endosseous implants are easily placed.

Figs 8-9f and 8-9g Postoperative views of the implant *(f)* and crown restoration *(g)*.

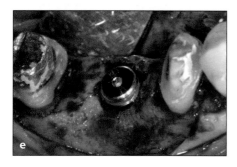

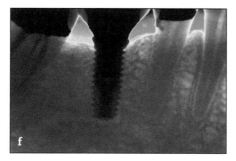

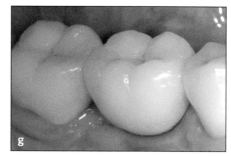

Case 2

A 49-year-old healthy, nonsmoking woman presented with radiographic evidence of periapical pathosis associated with the mandibular right first molar. There was an 8-mm clinical vertical probing measurement on the buccal surface of the tooth and a class II buccal furcation involvement (Fig 8-9a).

Surgical exposure revealed complete loss of the buccal plate (measuring 9 mm vertically). After the tooth was extracted (Fig 8-9b), the site was treated with FDBA that

had been fully saturated with 0.3 mg/mL of rhPDGF-BB. Space maintenance was provided for the grafted site with a titanium-reinforced e-PTFE membrane. Two weeks postsurgery, the e-PTFE membrane became exposed and had to be removed.

A periapical radiograph obtained 8 weeks postsurgery revealed excellent healing and no evidence of pathosis (Fig 8-9c). Six months postsurgery, the CT scan, reentry surgery, and radiography revealed excellent bone fill in the area of the large dehiscence defect, resulting in an edentulous ridge that exhibited sufficient bone height and width for implant placement (Figs 8-9d to 8-9g).

Fig 8-10a An augmentation procedure is necessary in the area of the mandibular left lateral incisor following extraction. The tooth has a hopeless prognosis following unsuccessful root canal therapy performed 3 years earlier.

Fig 8-10b The radiograph provides evidence of extensive bone loss associated with the lateral incisor (*arrow*).

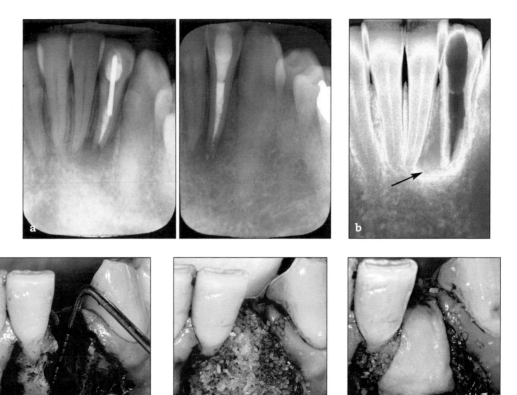

Fig 8-10c On surgical exposure and tooth extraction, a large dehiscence defect is revealed on the buccal surface of the tooth. The extraction defect is approximately 15 mm deep. The facial dehiscence measures approximately 10 mm vertically and 5 mm horizontally.

Fig 8-10d The defect is augmented with rhPDGF-BB–enhanced particulate FDBA.

Fig 8-10e The graft is protected by a resorbable collagen membrane that has been saturated with 0.3 mg/mL of rhPDGF-BB.

Fig 8-10f The flaps are replaced and sutured.

(*Fig 8-10 continued on next page.*)

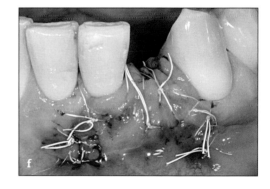

Case 3

A 51-year-old healthy, nonsmoking man had undergone a repeat root canal therapy on the mandibular left lateral incisor 3 years previously (Fig 8-10a). A radiograph revealed extensive bone loss associated with the lateral incisor (Fig 8-10b), which was confirmed on surgical exposure of the defect.

The large dehiscence defect and associated periapical lesion resulted in a hopeless prognosis for the tooth, which was extracted. The resultant defect was approximately 15 mm in depth and had a facial dehiscence defect measuring 10 mm vertically and 5 mm horizontally at the coronal extent of the defect (Fig 8-10c). The defect was treated with 0.3 mg/mL of rhPDGF-BB–enhanced FDBA (Fig 8-10d). The augmented site was then covered with a resorbable collagen membrane that had been saturated with 0.3 mg/mL of rhPDGF-BB solution (Fig 8-10e), and the flaps were replaced (Fig 8-10f).

Healing proceeded uneventfully, and 2 months postsurgery the site appeared very healthy; the gingival tissues

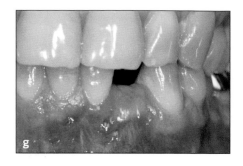

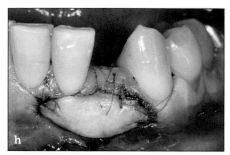

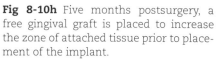

Fig 8-10g Healing has proceeded without complication, and 2 months postsurgery the site appears very healthy. The gingival tissues appear pink and firm, and the edentulous ridge has sufficient width and height to accommodate placement of an endosteal implant.

Fig 8-10h Five months postsurgery, a free gingival graft is placed to increase the zone of attached tissue prior to placement of the implant.

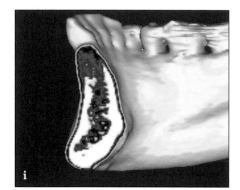

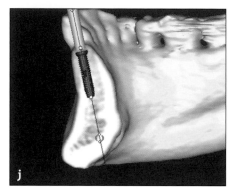

Fig 8-10i Three-dimensional CT evaluation 6 months postoperatively demonstrates the reconstruction of the alveolar bone.

Fig 8-10j Demonstration of implant placement in the newly reconstructed alveolar bone 6 months postoperatively.

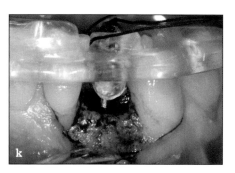

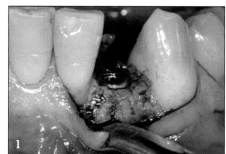

Fig 8-10k Re-entry surgery after 6 months of healing revealed adequate bone volume for ideal implant placement using a surgical guide.

Fig 8-10l There was almost complete reconstruction of the damaged alveolar process.

were pink and firm, and the edentulous ridge had sufficient width and height to accommodate placement of an endosteal implant (Fig 8-10g). Five months postsurgery, a free gingival graft procedure was performed to increase the zone of attached tissue prior to placing the implant (Fig 8-10h). The 6-month postoperative CTs demonstrated successful reconstruction of the alveolar bone (Figs 8-10i and 8-10j), which allowed for ideal implant placement (Figs 8-10k and 8-10l). The new bone appeared to have undergone significant remodeling; no particulate graft material was evident at the 6-month re-entry.

Conclusion

Over the years, traditional guided bone regeneration techniques and ridge preservation strategies have helped to enhance the functional and esthetic outcomes of dental implant therapy. The availability of recombinant therapeutics represents a major evolution in regenerative therapies from previously passive therapies to new, active treatments. Regenerative therapeutics for use in craniomaxillofacial and orthopedic indications will develop further as the physical and biologic requirements for regenerative cells in specific tissue locations are further elucidated. These advances will enhance the opportunity for bone and tissue regeneration and provide faster and more predictable outcomes for patients.

References

1. Tarnow DP, Cho SC, Wallace SS. The effect of inter-implant distance on the height of inter-implant bone crest. J Periodontol 2000;71:546–549.
2. Grunder U, Gracis S, Capelli M. Influence of the 3-D bone-to-implant relationship on esthetics. Int J Periodontics Restorative Dent 2005;25:113–119.
3. Buser D, Dula K, Hirt HP, Schenk RK. Lateral ridge augmentation using autografts and barrier membranes: a clinical study with 40 partially edentulous patients. J Oral Maxillofac Surg 1996;54:420–432.
4. Simion M, Trisi C, Piatelli M. Vertical ridge augmentation using a membrane technique associated with osseointegrated implants. Int J Periodontics Restorative Dent 1994;14:497–512.
5. Jovanovic SA, Nevins M. Bone formation utilizing titanium-reinforced barrier membranes. Int J Periodontics Restorative Dent 1995;15:57–69.
6. Tinti C, Parma-Benfenati S, Polizzi G. Vertical ridge augmentation: surgical protocol and retrospective evaluation of 48 consecutively inserted implants. Int J Periodontics Restorative 1998;18:435–443.
7. Jensen OT, Cockrell R, Kuhlke L, Reed C. Anterior maxillary alveolar distraction osteogenesis: A prospective 5-year clinical study. Int J Oral Maxillofac Implants 2002;17:52–68.
8. McAllister BS. Histologic and radiographic evidence of vertical ridge augmentation utilizing distraction osteogenesis: 10 consecutively placed distractors. J Periodontol 2001;72:1767–1779.
9. Buser D, Dula K, Belser UC, Hirt HP, Berthold H. Localized ridge augmentation using guided bone regeneration. 1. Surgical procedure in the maxilla. Int J Periodontics Restorative Dent 1993;13:29–45.
10. Buser D, Dula K, Belser UC, Hirt HP, Berthold H. Localized ridge augmentation using guided bone regeneration. 2. Surgical procedure in the mandible. Int J Periodontics Restorative Dent 1995;15:11–29.
11. Nevins M, Mellonig JT. Enhancement of the damaged edentulous ridge to receive dental implants: A combination of allograft and the Gore-Tex membrane. Int J Periodontics Restorative Dent 1992;12:97–111.
12. Lyford R, Mills M, Knapp C, Scheyer E, Mellonig J. Clinical evaluation of freeze-dried block allografts for alveolar ridge augmentation: A case series. Int J Periodontics Restorative Dent 2003;23:417–425.
13. Keith JD, Petrungaro P, Leonetti JA, et al. Clinical and histologic evaluation of a mineralized block allograft: Results from the developmental period (2001–2004). Int J Periodontics Restorative Dent 2006;26:321–327.
14. Hunt D, Jovanovic S. Autogenous bone harvesting: A chin graft technique for particulate and monocortical bone blocks. Int J Periodontics Restorative Dent 1999;19:165–173.
15. Simion M, Baldoni M, Zaffe D. Jawbone enlargement using immediate implant placement associated with a split-crest technique and guided tissue regeneration. Int J Periodontics Restorative Dent 1992;12:463–473.
16. Simion M, Trisi C, Piatelli M. Vertical ridge augmentation using a membrane technique associated with osseointegrated implants. Int J Periodontics Restorative Dent 1994;14:497–512.
17. Scipioni A, Bruschi GB, Calesini G. The edentulous ridge expansion technique: A five-year study. Int J Periodontics Restorative Dent 1994;14:451–459.
18. Scipioni A, Bruschi GB, Calesini G, Bruschi E, De Martino C. Bone regeneration in the edentulous ridge expansion technique: Histologic and ultrastructural study of 20 clinical cases. Int J Periodontics Restorative Dent 1999;19:269–277.
19. Carlsson H, Thilander H, Hedegard B. Histologic changes in the upper alveolar process after extractions with or without insertion of an immediate full denture. Acta Odontol Scand 1967;25:21–43.
20. Amler MH, Johnson PL, Salsman I. Histologic and histochemical investigation of human alveolar socket healing in undisturbed extraction wounds. J Am Dent Assoc 1960;61:46–48.
21. Nevins M, Camelo M, De Paoli S, et al. A study of the fate of the buccal wall of extraction sockets of teeth with prominent roots. Int J Periodontics Restorative Dent 2006;26:19–29.
22. Fiorellini JP, Howell TH, Cochran D, et al. Randomized study evaluating recombinant human bone morphogenetic protein-2 for extraction socket augmentation. J Periodontol 2005;76:605–613.
23. Bahat O, Handelsman M. Controlled tissue expansion in reconstructive surgery. Int J Periodontics and Restorative Dent 1991;11:32–47.
24. Evian CI, Rosenberg ES, Coslet JG, Corn H. The osteogenic activity of bone removed from healing extraction sockets in humans. J Periodontol 1982;53:81–85.
25. Cardaropoli G, Araujo M, Lindhe J. Dynamics of bone tissue formation in tooth extraction sites. An experimental study in dogs. J Clin Periodontol 2003;30:809–818.
26. Lazzara RJ. Immediate implant placement into extraction sites: Surgical and restorative advantages. Int J Periodontics Restorative Dent 1989;9:332–343.
27. Gelb D. Immediate implant surgery: 3-year retrospective evaluation of 50 consecutive cases. Int J Oral Maxillofac Implants 1993;3:389–399.
28. Wagenberg B, Froum SJ. A retrospective study of 1925 consecutively placed immediate implants from 1988 to 2004. Int J Oral Maxillofac Implants 2006;21:71–80.

9

Use of PRP in Oral and Maxillofacial Surgery and Periodontology

Robert E. Marx, DDS

Platelet-rich plasma (PRP) represents the first autologous growth factor source available to dental and medical clinicians.[1] First introduced in 1998, it has since proven to be an effective osteopromoter in several standard bone regeneration techniques[1–3] and in osseointegration[4,5] as well as a wound-healing enhancer in numerous soft tissue applications.[6–9] PRP also has a wider application across more specialties of medicine and dentistry than any other source of growth factors, with reports of efficacy not only in oral and maxillofacial surgery and periodontology but also in plastic surgery, ophthalmology, orthopedic surgery, cardiovascular surgery, and dermatology, among others.

The widespread application and acceptance of PRP are the result of its efficacy, safety, and cost effectiveness. The advantage of PRP over other growth factor sources and recombinant human growth factors is that it contains seven native growth factors in their natural ratios in a concentrated form. In addition, PRP contains concentrated vitronectin and native levels of fibronectin and fibrin, which are the essential cell adhesion molecules for cell migration, capillary ingrowth, and bone deposition. It is safe because it is derived from the patient's own blood and now has been applied an estimated 2 million times without serious adverse reactions. This chapter will explain the biology of PRP as well as its clinical application for the enhancement of a variety of healing processes.

Biology of PRP

Development

PRP is developed from an autologous blood draw of 20 mL, which will yield 3 mL of PRP; 60 mL, which will yield 7 to 10 mL of PRP; or 120 mL, which will yield 14 to 20 mL of PRP. The blood should be drawn with an 18-gauge or larger needle to avoid hemolysis or platelet activation, and a large vein should be chosen. The syringe should contain anticoagulant citrate dextrose-A in amounts recommended by the manufacturer of the PRP device. Other anticoagulants, such as citrate phosphate dextrose or ethylenediaminetetraacetic acid (EDTA), should not be used, because they do not support platelet viability.

The anticoagulated autologous blood is placed in the PRP processing device, which will separate and concentrate the platelets. Because PRP processing first requires separation of the platelets from the red blood cells and then concentration of the separated platelets in the plasma, the device must be a dual-spin differential centrifuge. Several reports of poor or inadequate results with PRP can be traced to the use of the wrong anticoagulant or a centrifuge that is not a dual-cycle device or does not meet rigid specifications of centrifugal time and rate.[10–13]

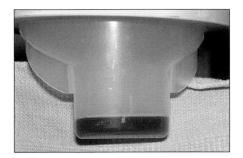

Fig 9-1 PRP is initially a platelet concentrate where the differential centrifugation concentrates the platelets in the upper level of the red blood cell column and in the "buffy coat," or white line, of the concentrated white blood cells.

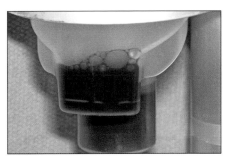

Fig 9-2 The concentrated platelets are resuspended in a small volume of plasma, creating PRP. (From Marx and Garg.[5] Reprinted with permission.)

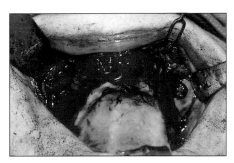

Fig 9-3 PRP must be applied in the clotted state for growth factor release. (From Marx and Garg.[5] Reprinted with permission.)

The resultant platelet concentrate appears as a small red blood cell button and white line representing a small amount of residual red blood cells, white blood cells, and the compacted platelets below an amber-colored plasma (Fig 9-1). The amber plasma represents platelet-poor plasma (PPP). A volume of PPP is then aspirated from levels above this concentrate and placed in a sterile container. The residual plasma is then mixed into the platelet concentrate to resuspend the compacted platelets, thus producing PRP (Fig 9-2). The PRP and PPP therefore are both anticoagulated and can remain on the sterile field for up to 8 hours without loss of activity.[14]

For clinical application, it is necessary to use clotted PRP, which activates the platelets so that they secrete their growth factors. This is accomplished by the addition of 2 to 4 drops of a solution obtained by placing 5 mL of 10% calcium chloride into 5,000 units of topical bovine thrombin or by the use of a suspension of type I collagen and 0.25 mL of a 10% calcium chloride solution. The calcium reverses the anticoagulant effect of citrate dextrose-A, and the thrombin or the collagen initiates the cascade of coagulation that results in clotting. Because the platelets in PRP can only secrete their growth factors after clotting, it becomes imperative that PRP be applied in the clotted state (Fig 9-3). Failure to clot the PRP will result in a graft or wound that does not demonstrate enhanced healing; this has been the reason for some reports that PRP has no benefit.[5,14,15]

Components

All of the growth factors and cell adhesion molecules in PRP are proteins. The platelets synthesize and secrete seven growth factors—the three isomers of platelet-derived growth factor (PDGF-AA, PDGF-AB, and PDGF-BB), two growth factors of the transforming growth factor β family (TGF-β1 and TGF-β2), vascular endothelial growth factor (VEGF), and epidermal growth factor (EGF)—as well as one cell adhesion molecule, vitronectin. PRP also contains the cell adhesion molecules fibrin and fibronectin, which are soluble proteins in the plasma component of PRP. Therefore, PRP represents a complete package for wound-healing acceleration; this explains its application for so many different indications.

PDGFs

The three isomers of PDGF act differently and at different times in bone regeneration and soft tissue healing. Their actions overlap and are somewhat dependent on the cells in the wound. Therefore, it is impossible to separate the actions of these three proteins. However, their most important common actions are mitogenesis and chemotaxis.[16] That is, they recruit cells from the local wound space (tooth socket, sinus walls, bony pockets

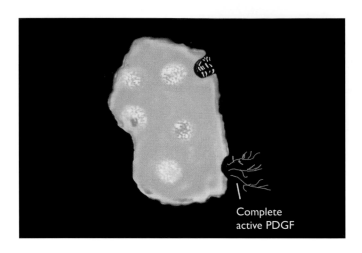

Complete
active PDGF

Fig 9-4 During blood clotting, the alpha granules in platelets migrate and fuse to the cell membranes, where histones and carbohydrate side chains are added to the incomplete growth factors to make them complete and biologically active. (From Marx and Garg.[5] Reprinted with permission.)

around teeth, etc) and induce cell division. They essentially induce cell division only in cells that possess cell membrane receptors specific to them. Therefore, the PDGF will enhance all wound healing by increasing the stem cell population, bone regeneration by increasing the osteoblastic population, capillary ingrowth by stimulating endothelial cell proliferation, and connective tissue regeneration and collagen synthesis by replicating and stimulating fibroblasts.

TGF-βs

TGF-β1 and TGF-β2 are the least specific of the TGF-β family, which also includes the 46 recognized bone morphogenetic proteins (BMPs). These two growth factors are mitogenic and angiogenic, but they also stimulate matrix production and guide differentiation toward bone and/or cartilage formation.[17] Therefore, these TGF-βs are also morphogens.

VEGF

VEGF is a more specific angiogenic growth factor. Its actions are limited to endothelial cells, almost all of which have membrane receptors for VEGF. The result is proliferation of endothelial cells and synthesis of basal lamina, resulting in capillary budding and ingrowth into the wound.

EGF

EGF is also a specific growth factor limited to the basal cells of skin and mucous membrane. It induces replication and migration of epithelial cells over a matrix of cell adhesion molecules. It further stimulates these cells to secrete the complex structures of the basement membrane and to proliferate in a sheet over the basement membrane to resurface a wound.

Vitronectin

Vitronectin is synthesized and secreted by platelets; with fibronectin and fibrin, which are synthesized in the liver and part of the plasma fraction, vitronectin makes up the cell adhesion molecular triad of the clot matrix. This matrix serves as the biologic scaffold for bone regeneration in all grafts and in osseointegration. It also serves as the matrix for epithelial migration in mucosal grafts and skin grafts and as the support for new blood vessels to grow into an area. This cell adhesion molecule, as well as fibrin and fibronectin, are the matrix molecules that distinguish PRP from recombinant human PDGF-BB (rhPDGF-BB) and recombinant human BMP-2 on an absorbable collagen sponge (rhBMP-2/ACS), both of which require carriers as a matrix, which limits their applications and outcomes.

Secretion and release of growth factors

When PRP is clinically applied in the clotted state, the clotting process causes migration of the alpha granules in the platelets to the cell membrane where fusion with the platelet cell membrane occurs. These preformed and incomplete growth factors are then completed by the cell membrane by the addition of histone and carbohydrate side chains into a biologically active molecule (Fig 9-4). It is known that this growth factor release begins within 10 minutes and that 90% of the growth factors are secreted in the first hour. Afterward, new growth factors are synthesized and released for the remaining life span of the platelet, which is about 7 days.

Mechanism of growth factors

The mechanism of action of all growth factors is well known and is almost identical. That is, the growth factors in PRP as well as all of the commercially prepared animal growth factors and recombinant human growth factors, such as rhPDGF-BB (Gem 21S, BioMimetic Therapeutics) and rhBMP-2/ACS (InFuse, Medtronic Sofamor Danek), act on specific transmembrane receptors with dual or adjacent active sites. These growth factors are dimers that bind to these two active sites on the external surface of the cell membrane. This binding activates the transmembrane receptors and induces a high-energy phosphate bond to dormant signaling molecules within the cytoplasm of the cells (see Fig 4-2b). These now activated signaling molecules are released and float to the nucleus, where they act to express a specific normal gene function, such as controlled cell replication, capillary budding, osteoid production, or collagen synthesis (see Fig 4-2c). Therefore, growth factors control and regulate all biosynthesis, and platelets regulate all wound healing. PRP is merely a means to upregulate the amount of active growth factors to accelerate the rate and degree of healing.

Applications and Effects of PRP

Bone regeneration procedures

PRP has shown efficacy when added to a variety of nonviable graft materials such as demineralized allogeneic bone, mineralized allogeneic bone, hydroxyapatite preparations, and xenogenic bone preparations as well as viable autogenous bone grafts in human clinical applications.[2,3,6,10] Over the past 8 years, the Division of Oral and Maxillofacial Surgery and the Tissue Bank at the University of Miami Miller School of Medicine have conducted extensive randomized controlled studies measuring the degree of clinical outcomes enhanced by PRP with both viable autogenous and nonviable graft materials.

Enhancement of nonviable graft materials

Most of the literature supporting or refuting PRP-induced enhancement of bone regeneration involves either short case studies or uncontrolled clinical data. Therefore, the author and colleagues completed a 5-year randomized prospective controlled clinical study comparing five nonviable graft materials with and without PRP to viable autogenous grafts with and without PRP in the classic human sinus augmentation model (unpublished data, 2006). The outcome revealed the relative value of each graft material alone and the degree of enhancement of each when PRP was added.

The materials tested were particle-sized nondemineralized freeze-dried bone allograft (FDBA); heated-treated anorganic xenogencic bovine bone (Bio-Oss, Osteohealth); heat-treated anorganic xenogeneic bovine bone with a 15–amino acid sequence of collagen on its surface (Pep-Gen P-15, Dentsply); porous sea algae–produced hydroxyapatite (C-graft, ScionX); resorbable bioactive glass (Biogran, 3i/BIOMET); and viable autogenous bone harvested from the left proximal tibia. Thirty sinus augmentations were accomplished with each tested material. For each graft material, 15 sinus augmentations were accomplished without the addition of PRP, and 15 included 7 mL of PRP containing at least 1 million platelets/μL. At 6 months, dental implants were placed in the grafted areas and core bone biopsies taken for histomorphometry.

The results clearly revealed the superiority of 100% autogenous bone over all of the nonviable graft materials (Table 9-1). Without the addition of PRP, autogenous bone resulted in a mean viable new trabecular bone area (TBA) of 52%, more than double the TBA achieved by any of the other materials. This result is not surprising and reinforces the "gold standard" reputation attributed to autogenous grafts.

These results further showed that bone regeneration with nonviable graft materials is limited to 24% TBA at best and defined the upper limit of osteoconduction in the closed system of the sinus augmentation procedure.

Table 9-1 New TBA after sinus augmentations with or without PRP

Graft material (n = 30)	New TBA		
	Without PRP (n = 15)	With PRP (n = 15)	P
Autograft	52%	78%	.005
FDBA	21%	36%	.01
Bio-Oss	24%	39%	.01
Pep-Gen P-15	18%	23%	.02
Biogran	15%	21%	.02
C-graft	22%	41%	.01

These results also identified a relative underperformance from Pep-Gen P-15 and Biogran.

The results also revealed that PRP enhanced bone regeneration in all six graft materials. PRP enhanced the bone regeneration of autogenous bone TBA by 26% (a gain of 50% more bone), which is consistent with the 19% enhancement reported[1] for grafts in continuity defects of the mandible to which PRP was added. However, PRP also significantly increased the regenerated TBA of FDBA (Fig 9-5), Bio-Oss (Fig 9-6), Pep-Gen P-15 (Fig 9-7), Biogran, and C-graft (see Table 9-1).

The qualitative PRP enhancement effect that was observed in all six graft materials tested included not only more bone but also an increased thickness of the bony trabeculae and a greater resorption of the nonviable graft particles. These results are consistent with the known mechanism of action of growth factors and cell adhesion molecules. The wide-ranging enhancement of bone re-generation when nonviable graft materials are used is the result of two separate actions of PRP. First, the growth factors in PRP upregulate the marrow stem cells and endosteal osteoblasts from the exposed bony walls of the sinus after the membrane is elevated. These cells are the source cells of bone formation in sinus augmentation when any nonviable graft material is used. The mitogene-sis, angiogenesis, and differentiation properties of the growth factors in PRP increase their number and the amount of osteoid they produce, resulting in the increase in bone regeneration observed in this study.

Second, the cell adhesion molecules—vitronectin, fibro-nectin, and fibrin—adhere to the surface of the nonviable graft particles and to the bony sinus walls (see Fig 4-9a). The endosteal osteoblasts and marrow stem cells prolif-erate along these strands, which act as a scaffold connect-ing the sinus bony walls to the graft particles and one particle to another (see Figs 4-9b and 4-9c). This is usual-ly achieved to some degree by the normal blood clot when PRP is not used. When PRP is used, there is a much denser network of these scaffolding molecules and a more complete coating of the graft particles for viable osteoid deposition.

The second mechanism explains the relative under-performance of Pep-Gen P-15 and of Biogran with and without PRP. That is, each of these materials binds cell adhesion molecules to itself less completely and less tight-ly. The higher heat treatment of Pep-Gen P-15 and the 15–amino acid sequence on the surface of the particle renders its surface smoother than most other materials. Therefore, cell adhesion molecules are less able to adhere to the particle.

In addition, the 15–amino acid sequence added to the surface of Pep-Gen P-15 is theorized to add osteoblast-binding sites to the surface. However, osteoblasts do not directly bond to a nonviable substance. Instead, osteo-blasts first bind to cell adhesion molecules. They then deposit osteoid on these same molecules rather than on the surface of any graft particle (see Fig 4-7). The adher-ence of cell adhesion molecules is crucial to every depo-sition of osteoid and relates to titanium implant surfaces. This is why every implant manufacturer has advanced to a textured surface that binds cell adhesion molecules bet-ter than the original machined surfaces.

Biogran's underperformance can be explained by a similar mechanism. That is, bioactive glasses undergo a surface change within the first 36 to 48 hours after place-ment. Their surface actually becomes more liquid in a phase change. This inherent property interferes with the surface adherence of cell adhesion molecules, resulting in reduced osteoconduction and less osteoid deposition.

The results of the study underscore the main advan-tages of PRP, which are an increase of seven growth fac-tors and an upregulation of osteoconduction by three cell adhesion molecules. However, although radiographic bone density and TBAs are good indicators of bone regenera-tion, the clinician is more interested in the usefulness of the regenerated bone measured by implant survival. Therefore, these patients were followed for 3 years after implant placement in the augmented sinuses, and func-tionally loaded implant survival was recorded.

Once again, the results allowed a comparison of the performance of the five nonviable graft materials and autogenous grafts with regard to their ability to osseoin-tegrate dental implants and to maintain the osseointegra-

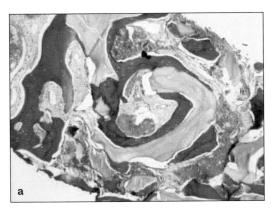
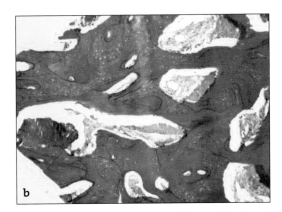

Fig 9-5 Core biopsy specimens 6 months after a sinus augmentation graft using FDBA without PRP (*a*) and with PRP (*b*). (*a*) A small amount of viable new bone is represented by thin trabeculae. Many residual nonviable bone particles are present (hematoxylin-eosin [H&E] stain; original magnification ×4). (*b*) A greater amount of viable new bone is visible as well as thicker bone trabeculae and a nearly complete resorption of the nonviable bone particles (H&E stain; original magnification ×4).

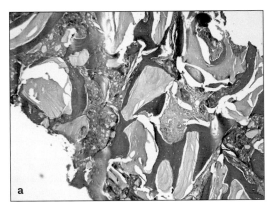
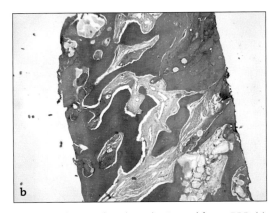

Fig 9-6 Core biopsy specimen 6 months after a sinus augmentation graft using Bio-Oss without PRP (*a*) and with PRP (*b*). (*a*) A small amount of viable new bone is represented by thin trabeculae. Many residual nonviable bone particles are evident (H&E stain; original magnification ×10). (From Marx.[19] Reprinted with permission.) (*b*) A greater amount of new viable bone is present, represented by thicker bony trabeculae. There is also a greater resorption of the nonviable Bio-Oss particles (H&E stain; original magnification ×10). (From Marx.[18] Reprinted with permission.)

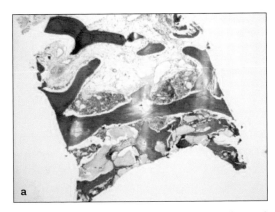
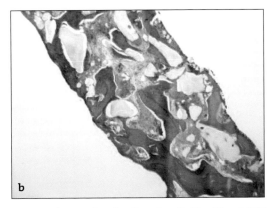

Fig 9-7 Core biopsy specimen 6 months after a sinus augmentation graft using Pep-Gen P 15 without PRP (*a*) and with PRP (*b*). (*a*) Less formation of new viable bone, very thin bony trabeculae, and many residual nonviable graft particles are evident. (*b*) As with the other graft materials, there is an enhancement of viable new bone, including thicker bony trabeculae and a greater resorption of the nonviable graft particles.

Table 9-2 Survival rates at 3 years of functional loading for implants placed after sinus augmentation with or without PRP

Graft material (n = 30)	Survival rate		
	Without PRP (n = 15)	With PRP (n = 15)	P
Autograft	83%	94%	.01
FDBA	77%	89%	.01
Bio-Oss	77%	90%	.01
Pep-Gen P-15	62%	70%	.01
Biogran	58%	65%	.01
C-graft	77%	90%	.01

tion over 3 years (Table 9-2). Implant survival under functional loading directly correlated to the amount of new bone regeneration induced by each graft material. That is, Pep-Gen P-15 and Biogran, which regenerated the least new bone, also had the lowest implant survival rates. Although the implant survival rates of FDBA, Bio-Oss, and C-graft were slightly lower than those of implants placed in an autogenous graft, the rates were comparable (77% to 83%). This suggests that implant survival does not increase proportionately in trabecular bone once a TBA greater than 35% is achieved.

Comparison of the 3-year implant survival rates of each graft material with and without the use of PRP also indicated an increase in implant survival across the board (see Table 9-2). Once again, the PRP-induced enhancement of Pep-Gen P-15 and Biogran was significantly less than the effect for FDBA, Bio-Oss, and C-graft. In addition, the implant survival of implants placed in FDBA, Bio-Oss, and C-graft graft materials with PRP approached the implant survival rate in autogenous bone (89% or 90% to 94%). This outcome supports the conclusion that only 35% to 50% of viable TBA is required for osseointegration. Results demonstrated that PRP upregulation places many nonviable graft materials in this range, so that in some cases the addition of PRP can even avoid the need for autogenous bone. The findings also indicate that the increase in implant survival observed when implants are placed in grafts enhanced by PRP is due as much to the more rapid development of mature bone and increase in bone density, and therefore primary stability, as it is to the absolute increased amount of regenerated bone.

Enhancement of viable autogenous grafts

Because autogenous grafts are the gold standard and recognized to predictably regenerate the most bone, studies demonstrating the presence or absence of an enhancement effect from PRP are difficult. The study that identified the enhanced bone regeneration from PRP in autogenous grafts was conducted on 88 randomized cancer patients with mandibular continuity defects that were more than 6 cm in length.[1] This defect is recognized to be the most challenging type in which to regenerate useful bone. In this study, bone regeneration occurred 1.62 times faster and produced 19% more bone (74% TBA versus 55% TBA, an increase of 35%) and denser bone after placement of PRP-enhanced autogenous grafts than after placement of autogenous grafts without PRP. This study launched the era of PRP and PDGFs but did not relate to the more common implant-related grafting performed by most of the dental profession.

Therefore, a second 5-year study was conducted by the Division of Oral and Maxillofacial Surgery at the University of Miami, Miller School of Medicine. This study used the most challenging population of patients requiring a sinus augmentation procedure—women with documented osteoporosis. The study population included 76 women aged 60 years or older who had been diagnosed as having osteoporosis with dual-energy x-ray absorptiometry scan values of −2.5 or less.

The patients, scheduled to receive autogenous grafts for sinus augmentation, were randomized to receive a viable autogenous graft alone or a graft with the addition of 7 mL of PRP containing at least 1 million platelets/µL. At 6 months, the gain in bone height was measured with computerized tomography. At that time, implants were placed and bone core biopsy specimens were taken for histomorphometry. After dental implants were placed, implant survival was recorded at 1 year and 3 years.

The radiographic and histomorphometric data showed a clear enhancement of outcome when PRP was added to the autogenous graft (Table 9-3). Grafts without PRP showed a mean gain in bone height of 8 mm while grafts

Table 9-3 Outcomes after autogenous graft sinus augmentations with or without PRP in women with osteoporosis*

Graft	Mean gain in bone height	Mean new TBA
Without PRP (n = 38)	8 mm	52%
With PRP (n = 38)	12 mm	78%
P	.01	.005

*Women aged 60 years or older with dual-energy x-ray absorptiometry scan values of −2.5 or less.

Table 9-4 Survival rates of implants placed after sinus augmentation with or without PRP in women with osteoporosis*

Graft	Survival at 1 y	Survival at 3 y
Without PRP (n = 38)	79%	64%
With PRP (n = 38)	91%	89%
P	.02	.01

*Women aged 60 years or older with dual-energy x-ray absorptiometry scan values of −2.5 or less.

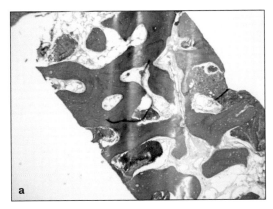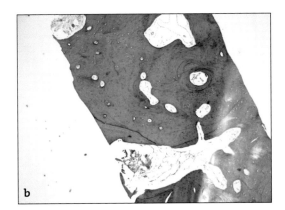

Fig 9-8 Core biopsy specimen 6 months after an autogenous bone graft without PRP (*a*) and with PRP (*b*) in a woman with osteoporosis. (*a*) Mature bone of about 50% TBA is visible. (*b*) Mature bone of about 75% TBA is visible (H&E stain; original magnification ×4).

with PRP gained 12 mm, an increase of 50%. In addition, the mean TBA of grafts with PRP (78%) was also 50% higher than that of grafts without PRP (52%) (Fig 9-8).

The 1-year survival rate of functionally loaded implants in this patient population was 79% when PRP was not added to the autogenous graft but 91% in PRP-enhanced grafts (Table 9-4). By 3 years, the implant survival rate deteriorated to 64% in the grafts where PRP was not used but was nearly maintained in grafts enhanced by PRP (89%).

These data are consistent with those of previous studies of autogenous grafts using PRP[1] and indicate a clinical benefit of enhanced implant survival corresponding to a greater trabecular bone density when PRP is used in the most challenging patient population.

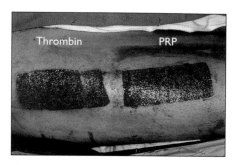

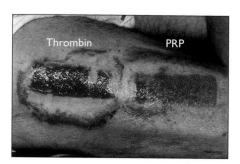

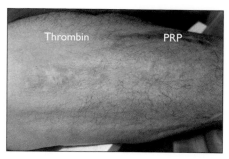

Fig 9-9a One of these adjacent split-thickness skin graft donor sites has been treated with only topical thrombin for hemostasis and the other with PRP activated with topical thrombin.

Fig 9-9b At 6 days, the site treated with PRP evidences enhanced healing, represented by an absence of the peripheral inflammation apparent in the adjacent site. In addition, the PRP-treated site exhibits the sheen of a thin epithelial cover, in contrast to the residual granulation tissue cover at the adjacent site.

Fig 9-9c At 6 months, the donor site treated with PRP shows far less scarring and less pigment change than does the adjacent site. (Figs 9-9a to 9-9c from Marx and Garg.[5] Reprinted with permission.)

Enhancement of soft tissue healing

It would be wrong for the student of tissue engineering and regeneration to separate soft tissue regeneration from bone regeneration, yet this is commonly done (even in this chapter) for the sake of clarity and convenience. In clinical situations in the oral cavity, the soft tissue cover promoting vascular ingrowth and preventing saliva and the oral flora from gaining access to a bone graft is crucial. PRP has numerous applications for soft tissue healing enhancement in oral and maxillofacial and periodontal procedures that address the cover over grafts and promote more rapid soft tissue healing. This is particularly well illustrated by skin graft healing, root coverage procedures, and dermal fat grafts.

Split-thickness skin grafts are the human clinical model for soft tissue healing and epithelial regeneration and closely parallel mucosal healing as represented by palatal graft harvests. In a study similar to those involving bone regeneration discussed earlier in this chapter, a comparison study of split-thickness skin graft donor site healing compared native healing rates and the degree to which healing was enhanced with the addition of PRP. In this study, 20 skin graft donor sites in cancer patients were dressed with PRP and compared with adjacent donor sites dressed without PRP. Clinical observations and photography at 1 week, 45 days, 3 months, and 6 months were supplemented with volunteered human biopsy specimens at 1 week.

The outcome showed a remarkable elimination of inflammation and a much more rapid epithelialization in the PRP-enhanced sites (Fig 9-9). Even at 1 week, the PRP-treated skin graft donor sites exhibited a thin but complete surface re-epithelialization not observed in the no-PRP control sites. This was confirmed by the human biopsy specimens, which revealed residual granulation tissue and no epithelial budding in the 1-week, no-PRP control sites and epithelial budding migrating over a more mature collagen connective tissue in the PRP-treated sties (Figs 9-10 and 9-11). This was clinically evident as a thin epithelial covering in the PRP-treated site that contrasted with the red exuberant granulation tissue covering the donor site of the no-PRP controls (see Fig 9-9b).

At 1 month, the maturity and thickness of the epithelial covering in the PRP-treated sites were indicated by the absence of hypervascular granulation tissue visible though a thin skin covering, which was evident in the no-PRP control sites (Fig 9-12). At 6 months, both sites were healed and mature. However, the control sites without PRP exhibited greater scarring and significantly more pigment changes than did the PRP-treated group (see Fig 9-9c). This faster rate of healing was clinically correlated to less pain: The patients reported a mean pain score of 7 (on a scale of 0 to 10) for the no-PRP control site versus 2 for the PRP-treated site.

These results underscore the basic clinical value of PRP in generating faster and more complete tissue regeneration. In this clinical trial, the addition of PRP translated into less wound care, less pain, and less scar tissue formation.

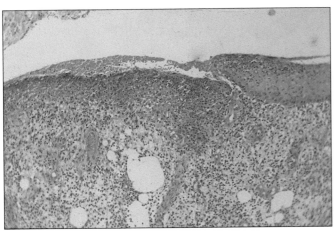

Fig 9-10a Biopsy specimen of a split-thickness skin graft donor site that was not treated with PRP. At 6 days, there is no evidence of epithelial budding or migration, and the base consists of immature fibroblasts and macrophages (H&E stain; original magnification ×4).

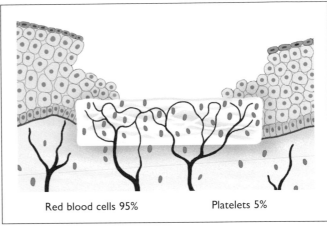

Red blood cells 95%   Platelets 5%

Fig 9-10b Representation of the incomplete epithelialization and connective tissue immaturity of a controlled skin wound where PRP was not used. (Figs 9-10a and 9-10b from Marx and Garg.[5] Reprinted with permission.)

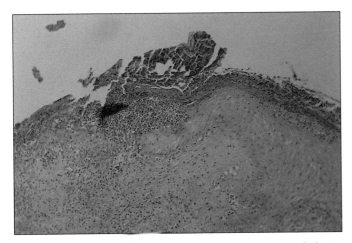

Fig 9-11a Biopsy specimen of a split-thickness skin graft donor site treated with PRP. At 6 days, obvious epithelial budding and migration are present. The subepithelial connective tissue also shows mature fibroblasts with collagen production (H&E stain; original magnification ×4).

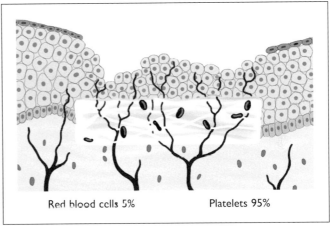

Red blood cells 5%   Platelets 95%

Fig 9-11b Representation of the more complete epithelialization and connective tissue maturity of a controlled skin wound where PRP was used. (Figs 9-11a and 9-11b from Marx and Garg.[5] Reprinted with permission.)

Although not studied in a controlled fashion, this acceleration of soft tissue healing has been applied to root coverage procedures with lyophilized human dermis (Alloderm, Life Cell) and palatal connective tissue grafts. Anecdotal reports of more predictable clinical outcomes imply that the same enhancement of healing as was proven for skin grafts applies to mucosal grafts and mucosal healing (Fig 9-13). The growth factors in PRP promote rapid revascularization and epithelialization of the wound; these qualities provide resistance to infection in the short term and reduce scarring in the long term.

The same cell adhesion molecules that provided the scaffold for osteoconduction in bone regeneration also provide the biologic scaffold for connective tissue ingrowth and epithelial migration in soft tissue healing.

Another example of the soft tissue benefits of PRP is in dermal fat grafts. Dermal fat grafts are grafts of subcutaneous fat rather than visceral fat, as exists near internal organs. It is a desirable graft for soft tissue defects because it replaces what is mostly missing—subcutaneous fat—and it has the proper texture and contour. However, until PRP came into use, these grafts fell out of favor because of

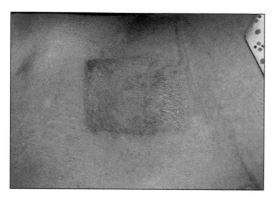

Fig 9-12a Even at 45 days, a split-thickness skin graft that was not enhanced with PRP shows evidence of slow re-epithelialization and wound immaturity, evidenced by the hypervascularity showing through the thin epithelial cover.

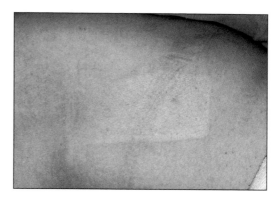

Fig 9-12b At 45 days, a split-thickness skin graft that was enhanced with PRP shows a thicker epithelial cover and a more mature wound, as evidenced by an absence of hypervascularity and greater normalization of color. (Figs 9-12a and 9-12b from Marx and Garg.[5] Reprinted with permission.)

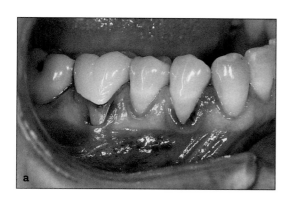

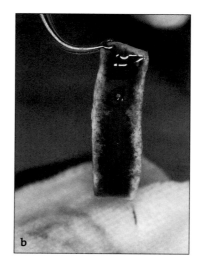

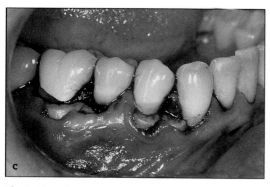

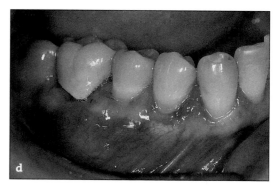

Fig 9-13a These exposed roots are candidates for a root coverage procedure.

Fig 9-13b Allogeneic dermis (Alloderm) is coated with PRP for use in the root coverage procedure.

Fig 9-13c The allogeneic dermis, coated with PRP, is placed in areas of root exposure.

Fig 9-13d Successful, rapid, and mature root coverage has been obtained using allogeneic dermis enhanced with PRP. (Figs 9-13a to 9-13d from Marx and Garg.[5] Reprinted with permission.)

Fig 9-14a This patient has hemifacial atrophy as a result of Parry-Romberg syndrome.

Fig 9-14b A rhytidectomy-type dissection develops a pocket between the dermis and the superficial musculoaponeurosis system as a recipient bed for a dermal fat graft.

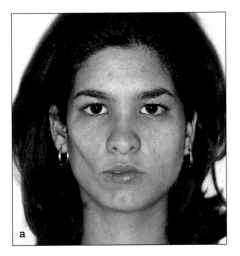

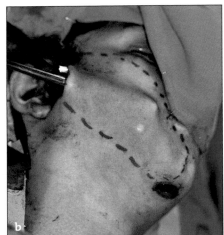

Fig 9-14c The dermal fat graft and PRP are inserted.

Fig 9-14d The dermal fat graft enhanced with PRP has restored normal facial contours and texture without overcontouring or undercontouring. (Figs 9-14a to 9-14d from Marx and Garg.[5] Reprinted with permission.)

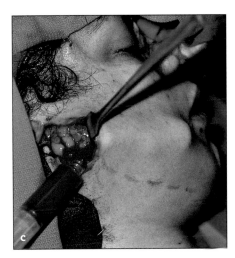

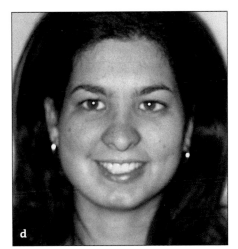

unpredictable outcomes and shrinkage and were replaced by the higher-morbidity and complication-prone free microvascular grafts.

The biologic problem with dermal fat grafts that has been overcome by the addition of PRP is delayed revascularization. That is, a dermal fat graft of a clinically useful size (4 × 4 cm or larger) is not penetrated quickly enough by new perfusing capillaries, resulting in central fat necrosis. This causes shrinkage of the graft or even a sterile abscess after the graft is placed. To compensate, clinicians have oversized dermal fat grafts by as much as 30%. The usual outcome is either overcontour or undercontour, requiring a second surgery.

Some clinicians have resorted to using particulated fat or liposuctioned fat to encourage early revascularization. However, this strategy has actually been counterproductive, resulting in rapid necrosis of the fat and a rapid loss of the contour and texture gained. This occurs because particulated fat and, even more so, liposuctioned fat break up the cell membranes of the fat cells. The released triglycerides provoke an intense inflammation, which leads to necrosis of the fat cells, resulting in loss of nearly the entire graft.

Therefore, clinicians are restricted to single-unit dermal fat grafts that must be rapidly penetrated by new capillaries to survive the transplantation. The larger the graft, the more rapid the revascularization required. PRP added to dermal fat grafts of even large sizes promotes early and complete revascularization so that fat necrosis is avoided. This has brought back the use of simple dermal fat grafts with a predictable outcome, so that free microvascular tissue transfers and their attendant morbidity can be avoided in many cases. The contour gained at the time of placement is the final contour realized by the patient; overcontouring and second surgeries are rarely needed (Fig 9-14).

Conclusion

PRP is a source of at least seven native growth factors and three cell adhesion molecules. The development of PRP from autologous blood by simple, sterile, office-based and Food and Drug Administration—cleared devices produces a concentration of platelets that must be activated with a clotted plasma fraction to be biologically effective. PRP works through transmembrane receptors and intracytoplasmic signaling pathways, as do all other growth factor preparations. Because PRP and all growth factor preparations work through normal regulated genes and are not mutagens, they have no risk of promoting neoplasias and are safe promoters of biologic healing.

The enhancement of bone regeneration has been shown to apply to all nonviable graft materials as well as viable autogenous grafts by prospective randomized human clinical trials of large numbers of patients. This enhancement translates to improved short-term and long-term implant survivals.

The enhancement of soft tissue healing parallels that of bone in mechanism and in degree. The clinical applications are limited only by the limitations and needs of the patient. PRP will enhance the rate and degree of soft tissue healing in soft tissue wounds as well as in bone regeneration. Therefore, it is more universally applicable than recombinant proteins, which are limited in their clinical applications and require synthetic carriers, allogeneic carriers, or animal product carriers. Applications in skin graft healing, mucosal healing, and dermal fat grafts are examples of the benefits of PRP in soft tissue healing, as are upregulation and improved outcomes of autogenous, xenogeneic, and synthetic bone graft materials.

References

1. Marx RE, Carlson ER, Eichstaedt RM, Schimmele SR, Strauss JE, Georgeff KR. Platelet-rich plasma: Growth factor enhancement for bone grafts. Oral Surg Oral Med Oral Pathol Oral Radiol Endod 1998;85;638–646.
2. Kassolis JD, Rosen PS, Reynolds MA. Alveolar ridge and sinus augmentation utilizing platelet-rich plasma in combination with freeze-dried bone allografts. Case series. J Periodontol 2000;71:1654–1661.
3. Camargo PM, Lekovic V, Weinlaender M, Vasilic N, Madzarevic M, Kenney EB. Platelet-rich plasma and bovine porous bone mineral combined with guided tissue regeneration in the treatment of intrabony defects in humans. J Periodontal Res 2002;37:300–306.
4. Rodriguez A, Anastassov Ge, Lee H, Buchbinder D, William H. Maxillary sinus augmentation with deproteinated bovine bone and platelet rich plasma with simultaneous insertion of endosseous implants. J Oral Maxillofac Surg 2003; 61:157–163.
5. Marx RE, Garg AD. Dental and Craniofacial Applications of Platelet-Rich Plasma. Chicago: Quintessence, 2005.
6. Jackson RF. Using platelet rich plasma to promote healing and prevent seroma formation in abdominoplasty procedures. Am J Cosmet Surg 2003;20:187–192.
7. Yazawa M, Ogata H, Nakajima T, Mori T, Watanabe N, Handa M. Basic studies on the clinical applications of platelet-rich plasma. Cell Transplant 2003;12:509–518.
8. Anitua E, Andea I, Ardanza B, Nurden P, Nurden AT. Autologous platelets as a source of proteins for healing and tissue regeneration. Thromb Haemost 2004;91:4–15.
9. Trowbridge CC, Stammers AH, Woods E, Yen BR, Klayman M, Gilbert C. Use of platelet gel and its effects of infections in cardiac surgery. J Extra Corp Technol 2005;37:381–386.
10. Sanchez AR, Eckert SE, Sheridan PJ, Weaver AL. Influence of platelet-rich plasma added to xenogeneic bone grafts on bone mineral density associated with dental implants. Int J Oral Maxillofac Implants 2005;20:526–532.
11. Jensen SS, Broggini N, Weibrich G, Hjørting-Hansen E, Schenk R, Buser D. Bone regeneration in standardized bone defects with autografts or bone substitutes in combination with platelet concentrate: A histologic and histomorphometric study in the mandibles of minipigs. Int J Oral Maxillofac Implants 2005;20: 703–712.
12. Aghaloo TL, Moy PK, Freymiller EG. Investigations of platelet-rich plasma in rabbit cranial defects. A pilot study. J Oral Maxillofac Surg 2002;60:1176–1181.
13. Froum SJ, Wallace SS, Tarnow DP, et al. Effect of platelet-rich plasma on bone growth and osseointegration in human maxillary sinus grafts: Three bilateral case reports. Int J Periodontics Restorative Dent 2002;22:45–51.
14. Marx RE. Platelet-rich plasma: Evidence to support its use. J Oral Maxillofac Surg 2004;62:489–496.
15. Kevy S, Jacobson M. Preparation of growth-factor-enriched autologous platelet gel. Presented at the Society for Biomaterials 27th Annual Meeting, Minneapolis, April 2001.
16. Lui Y, Kalen A, Resto O, Wahlstrom O. Fibroblast proliferation due to exposures to a platelet concentrate in vitro is pH dependent. Wound Repair Regen 2002;10:336–340.
17. Celeste AJ, Iannazzi JA, Taylor RC, et al. Identification of transforming growth factor β family members present in bone inductive protein purified from bovine bone. Proc Natl Acad Sci U S A 1990;87:9843–9847.
18. Marx RE. Tibia bone grafting for sinus augmentation. In: Jensen OT (ed). The Sinus Bone Graft, ed 2. Chicago: Quintessence, 2006:147–156.
19. Marx RE. PRP and BMP: A comparison of their use and efficacy in sinus grafting. In: Jensen OT (ed). The Sinus Bone Graft, ed 2. Chicago: Quintessence, 2006: 289–304.

Minimally Invasive Strategies for Vertical Ridge Augmentation

Massimo Simion, MD, DDS

Isabella Rocchietta, DDS

The use of osseointegrated dental implants anchored in the jawbone with direct bone-to-implant contact became an increasingly important treatment modality for the replacement of missing teeth in completely and partially edentulous patients in the 1980s. The prime prerequisite for long-term success of osseointegrated implants is a sufficient volume of healthy bone at the recipient sites. However, patients frequently lack a sufficient amount of bone volume as a result of trauma or infectious diseases such as advanced periodontitis. A number of different techniques have been developed to reconstruct deficient alveolar ridges to allow dental implant placement in either a simultaneous or staged approach.

Guided Bone Regeneration

Basic principles

Guided bone regeneration (GBR), a regenerative procedure derived from guided tissue regeneration around natural teeth, is used for ridge augmentation. The biologic principles of guided tissue regeneration were applied by Nyman et al[1] in the early 1980s. The surgical technique involves the placement of a cell-occlusive barrier membrane to protect the blood clot and to create a secluded space around the bone defect to allow bone regeneration without competition from other tissues. Schenk et al[2] demonstrated how the newly regenerated bone progresses in a programmed sequence through a series of biologic steps that closely parallel the pattern of normal bone growth and development.

Horizontal deficiencies such as fenestrations and/or dehiscence type defects around dental implants have been successfully treated; however, severe loss of alveolar bone often results in the absence of bone in both the horizontal and vertical dimensions. Vertical bone loss in partially edentulous patients constitutes a major challenge because of anatomic limitations and technical difficulties in implant placement. The presence of the nasal cavity, the maxillary sinus, and the alveolar nerve limits the bone height available for proper implant placement. Moreover, a large interarch space alters coronal length and form and produces an unfavorable crown-root ratio in the final prosthetic reconstruction.[3]

In 1994 Simion et al[4] reported the first human and histologic study of vertical bone regeneration of the atrophic edentulous ridge with the GBR technique. In five partially edentulous patients, 10 implants were inserted, protruding 4 to 7 mm from the original cortical bone level, and covered with expanded polytetrafluoroethylene (e-PTFE) membranes secured with fixation screws. In addition, titanium miniscrews were placed for later histologic evaluation. The results demonstrated that vertical bone regeneration was possible, to an extent of 4 mm in height. The histologic examination revealed that all retrieved miniscrews were in direct contact with bone and that regenerated bone was able to osseointegrate with commercially pure titanium implants. The mean percentage of direct contact between the titanium surface and the newly regenerated bone was approximately 42%.

Jovanovic et al[5] achieved supracrestal bone regeneration in five dogs with a submerged membrane technique in 1995. Renvert et al[6] later supported these findings in a dog model, demonstrating the potential of alveolar bone to grow in a protected space around screw implants with exposed threads.

Tinti et al[7] tested this model in a clinical study in which six patients received 14 implants; the membrane technique was augmented with autogenous bone chips at all sites. The results demonstrated vertical bone regeneration extending to 7 mm. This technique for vertical augmentation was later confirmed by Simion et al[8] when 20 patients received 56 implants. The patients were divided into two groups of 10; in one group the space under the membrane was filled with demineralized freeze-dried bone, and in the other the space was filled with autogenous bone chips. The study demonstrated highly successful and predictable vertical bone regeneration. The percentage of bone-to-implant contact varied from 39.1% to 63.2% regardless of whether the allograft or the autograft was used.

A year earlier, an unsuccessful attempt was made to use a resorbable polylactic membrane for vertical ridge augmentation in a dog model.[9] Histologic and morphometric analyses performed after 3 and 5 months revealed that the membrane group did not exhibit greater bone-to-implant contact than the untreated controls. Thus, the resorbable membrane did not provide the space maintenance requisite for vertical ridge augmentation. In 1999 another human study[10] analyzed six experimental implants placed in vertical bone defects and allowed to protrude 5 to 7 mm above the bone crest. The exposed implant threads were completely covered by autogenous bone chips, and a titanium-reinforced e-PTFE membrane was secured on top. After a 12-month healing phase, the implants were removed. Histomorphometry indicated that the regenerated bone had a mean bone density of 43.2%.

These studies indicated that a substantial amount of new bone is formed underneath titanium-reinforced nonresorbable membranes. Studies performed in the 1990s

were useful for clinicians to verify the efficacy and safety of the procedure. At that time, the results were encouraging, but insufficient data existed about long-term implant stability and the resorption pattern of bone regenerated with this technique. A retrospective multicenter study[11] of 1 to 5 years of prosthetic loading evaluated 123 implants inserted in atrophic alveolar ridges either after bone augmentation or coincident with bone augmentation procedures. Three techniques were included in the study; the implants were allowed to protrude 2 to 7 mm from the bone crest, and a titanium-reinforced e-PTFE membrane was positioned to protect either the blood clot (group A), an allograft (group B), or an autograft (group C). The mean bone loss for groups A, B, and C of 1.35 mm, 1.87 mm, and 1.71 mm, respectively, are in accordance with previous long-term studies on implants placed in horizontally regenerated bone[12–14] or in native bone.[15–17] Only 1 of 123 implants failed, and 2 demonstrated greater bone loss than normal, leading to an overall success rate of 97.5% according to the criteria described by Albrektsson et al.[18] On the basis of these results, the authors concluded that bone vertically regenerated with GBR techniques responds to implant placement like native, nonregenerated bone.[11] Hence, the success and predictability of the technique have been shown.

Graft materials

Autografts

Autogenous bone has long been considered as the gold standard for bone regeneration procedures. It is thought to be osteoconductive and capable of providing vital osteogenic cells and signaling molecules[19,20] Autogenous bone harvesting is invasive and presents with issues of morbidity when harvested from an extraoral site.

Xenografts

Deproteinized bovine bone mineral is a xenogeneic graft material that has been widely used as a bone substitute in implant dentistry[21–24] and periodontology.[25,26] Deproteinized bovine bone mineral has osteoconductive properties[27]; it promotes cellular adhesion and the formation of new bone tissue. It has physical and chemical structures similar to those of human cancellous bone, such as the

Fig 10-1a Clinical image of the left side of the atrophic mandible (*outlined*).

Fig 10-1b Radiograph of the same patient revealing a bilaterally atrophic posterior mandible.

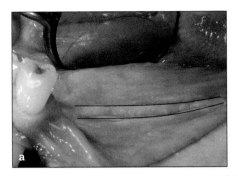
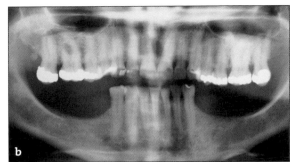

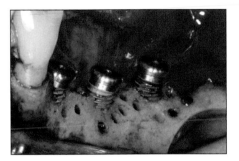

Fig 10-1c Three titanium dental implants placed in the correct prosthetic position, protruding from the bone crest, after elevation of a full-thickness flap, exposure of the crest, and cortical perforation.

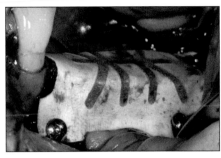

Fig 10-1d Mixture of autogenous bone graft and deproteinized bovine bone particles in a 1:1 ratio, positioned under a titanium-reinforced expanded polytetrafluoroethylene membrane.

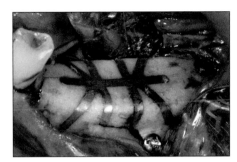

Fig 10-1e Clinical image at reopening. The membrane has perfectly maintained the correct position, and no signs of inflammation are evident.

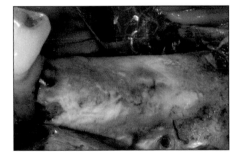

Fig 10-1f Removal of the membrane. A thin layer of connective tissue is interposed between the newly formed bone and the membrane.

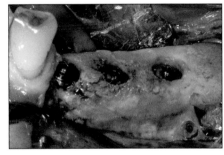

Fig 10-1g Implants completely covered with newly formed bone.

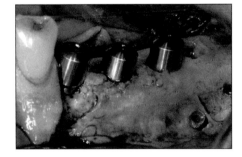

Fig 10-1h Healing abutment connection. The flaps are sutured.

(Fig 10-1 continued on next page.)

calcium phosphorus index (2.03) and the isomeric crystalline dimension.[28]

Combination grafts

A combination of autogenous bone and a xenograft would allow a reduction of the amount of autogenous bone harvesting, subsequently decreasing the invasiveness of the technique and postoperative discomfort of the patient.[26] Simion et al[29] recently used a mixture of autogenous bone chips harvested from an intraoral site and deproteinized bovine mineral in the vertical ridge augmentation technique (Fig 10-1). Besides minimizing bone harvesting, the rationale for mixing autogenous bone with the deproteinized bovine mineral is to add the osteoconductive properties of the xenograft to the osteogenic properties of the autograft.

The mixture was applied under a titanium-reinforced e-PTFE membrane in a 1:1 ratio (see Fig 10-1d). After a healing period of 6 to 9 months, the sites were reopened, the membrane was removed, and healing abutments were secured to the underlying implants (see Figs 10-1e to 10-1h). All the biopsy specimens from the study

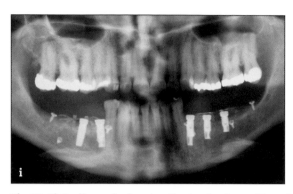

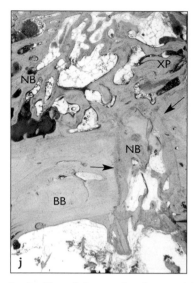

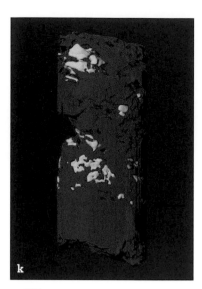

Fig 10-1i Radiograph showing the implants positioned on both sides of the previously atrophic mandible.

Fig 10-1j Histologic image of the specimen. The xenograft particles (XP) are well integrated with newly regenerated lamellar bone. The arrows indicate a groove in the basal bone (BB), where newly formed bone (NB) and xenograft particles are present. This was a cortical perforation performed with a round diamond bur to expose the medullary spaces and increase bleeding in the area (toluidine blue/pyronine G stain; original magnification ×25).

Fig 10-1k Microtomogram of the bone biopsy specimen. The xenograft is represented by gray and the bone by red. (*arrows*) Base of the original defect.

demonstrated mineralized bone with different degrees of maturation and mineralization. In the apical portion, native lamellar bone was evident in direct continuity with the overlying regenerated bone (see Figs 10-1j and 10-1k). In the middle and coronal portions of the specimens, both the autogenous bone particles and the xenograft demonstrated an intimate contact with varying amounts of new mineralized bone. Hence, the findings from this clinical and histologic study supported the use of a deproteinized bovine mineral in a 1:1 ratio with autogenous bone chips as a composite graft for vertical ridge augmentation of atrophic ridges. The regenerated bone may allow proper osseointegration of a dental implant inserted at the time of the regenerative procedure or after a healing period of at least 6 months.

Tissue Engineering with Recombinant Growth Factors

The aforementioned study protocol[29] reached the end point goal of decreasing the invasiveness of the GBR pro-cedure by reducing the required volume of autogenous bone. However, the technique still requires use of a titanium-reinforced e-PTFE membrane and a second surgical site for bone harvesting. Eliminating the need for the membrane and the autogenous bone harvesting would sensibly simplify and reduce the invasiveness of vertical ridge augmentation procedures.

In addition, the current technique of GBR for vertical ridge augmentation poses another challenge: The technique requires excellent soft tissue management, because the major complication is premature membrane exposure, resulting in bacterial contamination.[30,31] This complication is generally due to insufficient use of periosteal releasing incisions and excessive tension in the sutures at closure and is particularly evident when nonresorbable membranes are used.

To overcome these problems, researchers and clinicians are striving to develop less invasive surgical modalities that are less demanding technically and promote faster bone regeneration.

Advances in tissue engineering may offer solutions that resolve bone volume deficits and periodontal defects while at the same time eliminating some of the concerns posed by current techniques. One signaling wound-healing molecule that has been extensively studied in preclinical models and humans is platelet-derived growth factor (PDGF), contained in the alpha granules of blood platelets and bone matrix[32] and now recombinantly produced and recently approved by the US Food and Drug Administration in combination with β-tricalcium phosphate (GEM 21S, BioMimetic Therapeutics) for the treatment of periodontally related defects.[33] PDGF is a natural hormone produced by the body at sites of soft tissue and bone injury. It is both chemotactic and mitogenic for osteoblasts and helps initiate osteogenesis by promoting capillary budding into the graft site.

The use of purified recombinant human PDGF-BB (rhPDGF-BB) mixed with bone allograft results in robust periodontal regeneration in both class II furcation invasions and intrabony defects. Histologic evidence demonstrates that the combination of demineralized freeze-dried bone allograft with 0.5 mg/mL of rhPDGF-BB results in periodontal regeneration.[34,35] In addition, no unfavorable tissue reaction or other safety concern was associated with the treatment throughout the course of the studies. Hence, evidence of periodontal regeneration in humans has been reported after the use of PDGF.

Animal studies

The only data available concerning the use of PDGF for three-dimensional alveolar bone augmentation in association with dental implants are reported in a recent study by Simion et al.[36] The main purpose of this study was to evaluate the outcome of vertical ridge augmentation in a standardized dog model[37] by combining purified rhPDGF-BB and a deproteinized bovine bone block. The secondary objective of this study was to determine the value of a resorbable barrier membrane when used with this tissue-engineered approach to bone regeneration.

Six adult fox hounds presented bilateral severely atrophic ridges following extraction of all four premolars. The edentulous ridge was then surgically reduced with rotary and hand instruments under copious saline irrigation, resulting in an apicocoronal defect of 10 mm and a mesiodistal defect of 30 mm. The buccal and lingual bone plates were removed to mimic a flat atrophic ridge. Primary wound closure was achieved and sutured by means of interrupted 4-0 e-PTFE sutures.

Following a healing period of 3 months, full-thickness mucoperiosteal flaps, extending from the distal aspect of the canine to the mesial aspect of the first molar, were

carefully elevated. All soft tissue remnants were carefully removed from the defect surface. Cortical perforations were made with a carbide round bur, exposing the underlying medullary spaces (Fig 10-2a). A deproteinized bovine block was then closely adapted to the bony defect site and stabilized by means of two titanium implants (MKIII, 3.3 × 10.0 mm, machined-surface implants, Nobel Biocare; Ti-Unite biomaterial, Nobel Biocare) placed 10 mm apart (Fig 10-2b).

Three cohorts were included in the study design. Group A used a deproteinized bovine block (Bio-Oss cancellous [spongiosa] block, 20 × 10 × 10 mm, Osteohealth) in combination with a resorbable bilayer collagen membrane (Bio-Gide, Osteohealth). Group B used a deproteinized bovine block infused with rhPDGF-BB (Gem 21S). Group C used a deproteinized bovine block saturated with rhPDGF-BB and covered with a resorbable collagen barrier membrane. Four sites were randomly assigned and included in each group. The bovine cancellous block used in groups B and C was inserted in an empty sterile syringe, infused with rhPDGF-BB under pressure, and left to sit for 5 minutes (Fig 10-2c). The aforementioned implants were used to fix the fragile cancellous blocks in all three groups to the atrophic ridge. As noted, a resorbable collagen membrane was placed over the grafted sites in groups A and C.

Primary tension-free wound closure was achieved by using periosteal releasing incisions with e-PTFE horizontal mattress and interrupted sutures (Fig 10-2d). The sutures were removed 2 weeks postoperatively. The dogs were maintained on a soft diet throughout the study. After a period of 4 months, the animals were sacrificed. Two sites were reentered clinically for macroscopic evaluation (Fig 10-3).

The results revealed uneventful healing for 7 of 12 sites. Four sites exhibited soft tissue dehiscence and another site had a fistula. Of these five failures, three were in sites that received a deproteinized bovine block and a resorbable membrane without rhPDGF-BB (group A). These demonstrated fistulas and flap dehiscences shortly after suture removal, probably because of the extreme size of the defect and the significant volume of supracrestal regeneration necessary, which had been intended to test the potential of the growth factor. The management of severe atrophic alveolar ridges is the major challenge in daily clinical practice. These defects were created to mimic severe mandibular atrophy.

Inspection of two sites (groups B and C) reentered 4 months after surgery, before the dogs were killed, revealed that the implants were completely covered by

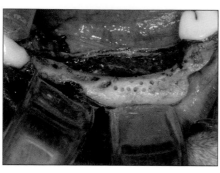

Fig 10-2a Elevation of a full-thickness mandibular flap, followed by cortical perforation to encourage bleeding. The defect measures 30 mm mesiodistally and 10 mm apicocoronally.

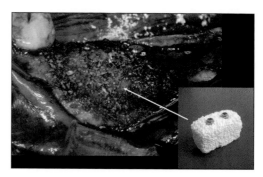

Fig 10-2b Deproteinized bovine block (*inset*) placed over the atrophic mandible and secured with two titanium dental implants in mesial and distal positions. In eight sites (groups B and C), the block was infused with rhPDGF-BB. (From Simion et al.[36] Reprinted with permission.)

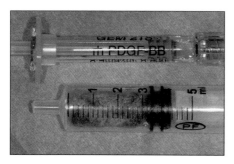

Fig 10-2c Deproteinized bovine block inserted in a sterile syringe and infused with rhPDGF under vacuum conditions.

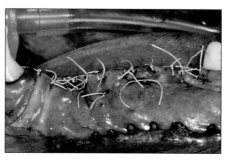

Fig 10-2d Tension-free flap closure with horizontal mattress and interrupted sutures.

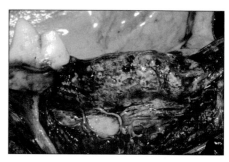

Fig 10-3 Reentry after 4 months of submerged healing of the deproteinized bovine block with rhPDGF-BB. The implants are covered with tissue that resembles bone. Note the hard bleeding surface and the volume regenerated. Residual deproteinized bovine bone is visible at the surface.

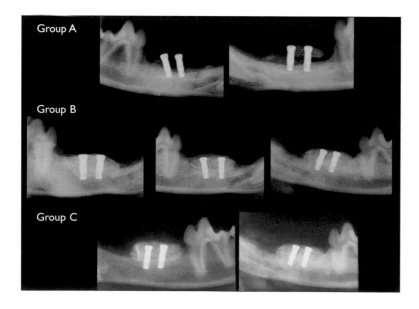

Fig 10-4 Periapical radiographs of all the specimens in the three groups at the time of sacrifice. In group A, absence of new bone formation is indicated by the radiolucent image between the implants. The block appears to be integrated with the surrounding bone in group B. A radiographic distinction between the block and the native bone is apparent in group C. (From Simion et al.[36] Reprinted with permission.)

Fig 10-5 Histologic image of a control specimen (group A; deproteinized bovine block plus membrane). Overview of the mesiodistal ground section. No bone regeneration is evident (toluidine blue/pyronine G stain; original magnification ×8). (From Simion et al.[36] Reprinted with permission.)

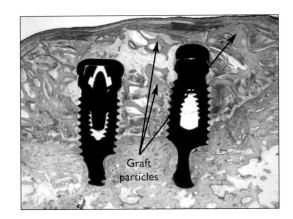

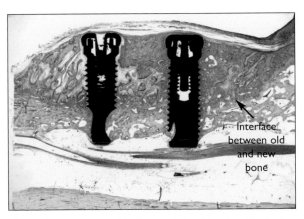

Fig 10-6 Specimen with deproteinized bovine block plus rhPDGf-BB (group B). Overview of the mesiodistal ground section. Note the formation of new bone around the two implants and the bovine block replacement (toluidine blue/pyronine G stain; original magnification ×12.5). (From Simion et al.[36] Reprinted with permission.)

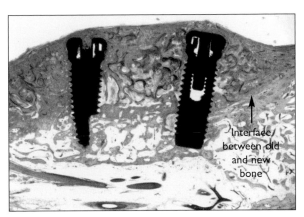

Fig 10-7 Another specimen with deproteinized bovine block plus rhPDGF-BB (group B). Overview of the mesiodistal ground section. Bone has regenerated over the implant cover screws and integrated with the native bone (toluidine blue/pyronine G stain; original magnification ×12.5). (From Simion et al.[36] Reprinted with permission.)

tissue resembling bone tissue (see Fig 10-3). Radiographs were taken before the animals died. Group A showed a large area of radiolucency, indicating that no bone regeneration had occurred. In the sites receiving the deproteinized bovine block infused with rhPDGF-BB (group B), the block had perfectly integrated with the underlying basal bone, evidenced by a radiopaque appearance of the radiograph. In contrast, sites receiving the deproteinized bovine block infused with rhPDGF-BB and a resorbable membrane showed a radiographic distinction between the block and the alveolar ridge (Fig 10-4).

Histologic results of the group A specimen revealed that there was no bone regeneration in the whole bovine block area. The block appeared embedded in healthy connective tissue, and there were no signs of inflammation (Fig 10-5).

On the other hand, a significant amount of new bone formation was demonstrated by an overview of the mesiodistal ground sections of group B specimens (Figs 10-6 and 10-7), particularly at the coronal portion of the regenerated tissue facing the periosteum and the soft tissues. Bone formation was also evident at the apical third of the specimens, in direct continuity with the native lamellar bone. In the middle portion, a relatively small area without new bone formation was present. In this area, remnants of the deproteinized bovine block structure appeared embedded in healthy connective tissue.

Microtomographic images (Micro-CT, SkyScan) highlighted the significant new bone formation in the defect site (Fig 10-8). Evidence of ongoing bone formation is supported by the presence of typical bright seams of demineralization and numerous resorption lacunae adja-

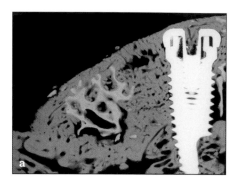
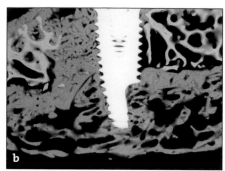

Fig 10-8a Microtomogram of the specimen with deproteinized bovine block plus rhPDGF-BB (Fig 10-7). The image reflects the significant amount of regenerated hard tissue along the side and over the implant.

Fig 10-8b Apical portion of the same implant. The regenerated bone closely resembles the native bone in terms of density. No demarcation limit is visible between the base of the defect and the new tissue. The distal aspect shows a small area of trabecular xenograft embedded in loose connective tissue.

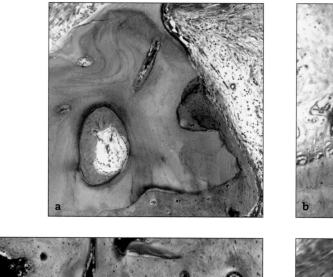
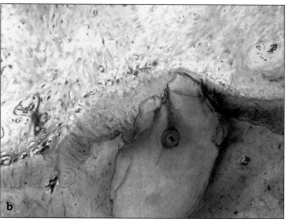
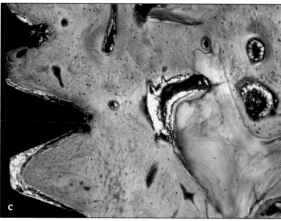
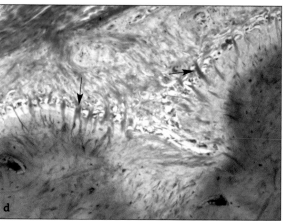

Fig 10-9a Ongoing bone formation at the periphery and in the central portion of deproteinized bovine bone trabeculae. Osteoblast linings are evident on the regenerated bone surface (toluidine blue/pyronine G stain; original magnification ×160).

Fig 10-9b Higher magnification of an osteoblastic lining depositing osteoid tissue (toluidine blue/pyronine G stain; original magnification ×160).

Fig 10-9c Intense remodeling activity is evident in the regenerated bone. Resorption of the xenograft and substitution with new bone is apparent. Abundant bone remodeling units are present (toluidine blue/pyronine G stain; original magnification ×100).

Fig 10-9d Collagen fibers embedded in woven bone (*arrows*), indicating ongoing woven bone formation (toluidine blue/pyronine G stain; original magnification ×160).

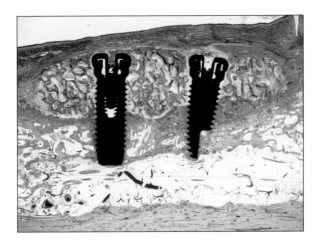

Fig 10-10 Specimen with deproteinized bovine block plus rhPDGF-BB plus membrane. Overview of the mesiodistal ground section. Only a thin layer of new bone is visible at the coronal aspect of the specimen (toluidine blue/pyronine G stain; original magnification ×8). (From Simion et al.[36] Reprinted with permission.)

cent to areas with the xenograft particles embedded in bone (Fig 10-9). This feature indicated that, in augmented areas, intense physiologic remodeling was ongoing with alternately occurring demineralization and remineralization steps.

Intense osteoblastic activity and an unusually large number of bone-remodeling units, together with the forming of mature osteons, were evidence of physiologic remodeling (see Fig 10-9). A high rate of bone-to-implant contact was visible in the areas of bone regeneration, extending over the top of the implant cover screw. The positive effect of PDGF on bone formation was highlighted by the large number of osteoblastic seams present in all the sections and by the finding of a higher density of the regenerated bone in comparison with the residual alveolar ridge.

Equally noteworthy was the intense remodeling of the bovine deproteinized block that occurred in group B, in which xenograft particles, embedded in newly formed bone, exhibited numerous resorption lacunae and bright seams of demineralization, evidence of intense physiologic remodeling. Such accelerated remodeling of xenograft particles is normally not observed, suggestive of further influence of the rhPDGF-BB on the original graft.

The mesiodistal ground sections of the sites in group C showed some new bone formation in both the coronal portion facing the periosteum and at the apical portion in continuity with the native bone (Fig 10-10). However, the amount of regenerated bone observed when the resorbable membrane was used was obviously less than that in the sites not covered by a membrane.

This proof-of-principle research utilized a dog model and investigated the potential of a xenograft infused with

PDGF to achieve vertical bone enhancement in a surgically created atrophic mandible. In addition, the role and potential of a resorbable membrane were studied. The end point goals of this research were accomplished in the specimens treated by means of a deproteinized bovine block infused with rhPDGF-BB. The infused specimens treated with a barrier membrane demonstrated significantly less bone regeneration, which is consistent with findings found in studies of recombinant bone morphogenetic protein.[38,39] Tissue-occlusive barrier membranes seem not to provide additional value to growth factors; in contrast, it appears that membranes may complicate wound healing.

A possible explanation for this finding derives from the observation that rhPDGF-BB seemed to have strongly stimulated more bone formation from the periosteal surface than from the residual native bone.[36,37] Therefore, the use of a membrane could have impeded the osteoblastic differentiation stimulated by the periosteum.[40–42] The role of the periosteum in osteogenesis, serving as a source for pluripotential mesenchymal cells and osteoblasts, especially at fracture sites, is well documented.[23–25] The chemotactic effects of PDGF, to be effective in bone regenerative procedures, require an adequate supply of locally available osteoblastic type cells, which are found in the undersurface of an intact periosteum. Interposing a barrier membrane between the periosteum and graft, as used in current GBR procedures, appears to block the penetration of periosteally derived osteogenic cells into the wound area and therefore appears contraindicated in PDGF-mediated regenerative procedures.

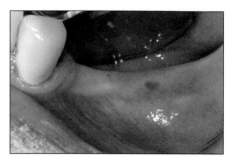

Fig 10-11a Preoperative view of the mandibular left edentulous site.

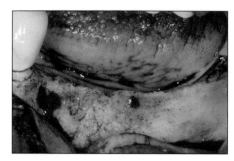

Fig 10-11b Deficient alveolar ridge, evidenced after full-thickness flap elevation.

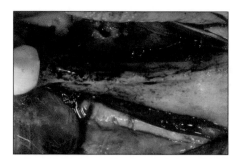

Fig 10-11c Occlusal view of the atrophic alveolar ridge. The very thin bone crest does not allow proper implant placement.

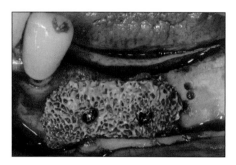

Fig 10-11d Deproteinized bovine block placed over the buccal wall of the atrophic mandible and secured by means of two fixation screws in mesial and distal positions. The block was previously infused with rhPDGF-BB. (From Simion et al.[43] Reprinted with permission.)

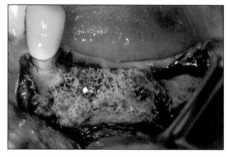

Fig 10-11e Clinical appearance during reopening after 5 months of submerged healing. The deproteinized bovine block appears well integrated with the native alveolar crest. Remnants of the xenograft are also visible. Note the hard bleeding surface of the regenerated tissue.

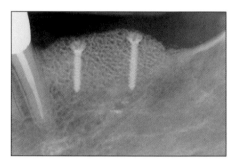

Fig 10-11f Radiographic appearance at reopening of the site.

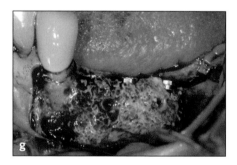

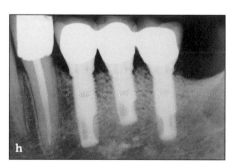

Fig 10-11g Three implants placed in the left side of the mandible.

Fig 10-11h Radiographic appearance of the three implants. (Figs 10-11f to 10-11h from Simion et al.[43] Reprinted with permission.)

Case studies

The next step in the development of these techniques is to apply these encouraging results to severe atrophic human alveolar defects. Two patients with deficient posterior mandibular defects were selected.[43] The defects developed because of the loss of periodontally compromised premolars and molars in one case and the failure of two implants in the other. The treatment plan consisted of three-dimensional alveolar bone reconstruction to allow proper implant placement. The goal was to eliminate the need for a membrane and intraoral bone harvesting.

The first patient was a woman who had lost the two mandibular left premolars and molars because of untreated periodontal disease (Fig 10-11a). The residual alveolar ridge appeared inadequate in height and thickness to allow effective implant placement. Local anesthetic was administered, and a full-thickness incision within the keratinized mucosa was made from the distal aspect of the

Fig 10-11i Microtomogram of a specimen obtained from a trephine biopsy. Red represents the regenerated bone, and the xenograft trabeculae appear in gray. New bone formation is present through the whole bovine bone block trabeculae.

Fig 10-11j Microtomogram of the same specimen. The image of the xenograft trabeculae has been subtracted to highlight the regenerated bone.

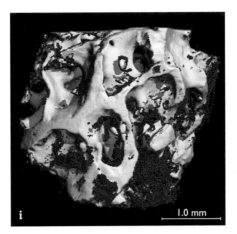

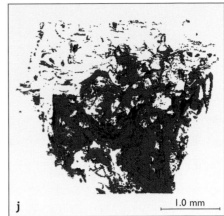

Fig 10-11k Histologic overview of the specimen. New bone is visible throughout the whole specimen. Resorption lacunae, associated with ongoing bone formation, are detectable in the xenograft trabeculae (toluidine blue/pyronine G stain; original magnification ×12.5).

Fig 10-11l Higher magnification of xenograft trabeculae embedded in regenerated bone. A lacuna in the central portion of the xenograft, filled with new bone and an osteoblastic lining, indicates ongoing bone formation in the central portion of the deproteinized bovine bone trabeculae (toluidine blue/pyronine G stain; original magnification ×160). (Figs 10-11k and 10-11l from Simion et al.[43] Reprinted with permission.)

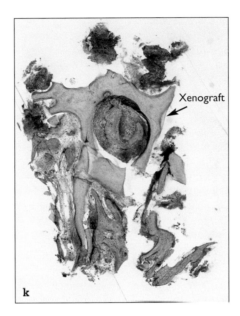

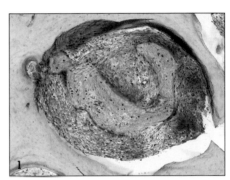

canine to the ascending ramus of the mandible. The incision was extended intrasulcularly to the mesial aspect of the canine. A vertical releasing incision was made at the mesiobuccal angle and at the distal aspect of crestal incision. The exposed atrophic alveolar ridge measured 2 mm in thickness, and at least 3 mm of vertical height was lacking (Figs 10-11b and 10-11c).

Soft tissue remnants were carefully removed from the bone crest and cortical perforations were performed to allow and encourage bleeding in the area. A deproteinized bovine block (Bio-Oss) infused with rhPDGF-BB (Fig 10-11d) was then adapted to the buccal bone of the defect and stabilized by means of two fixation screws. The wound was closed with horizontal mattress and interrupted sutures after the flaps were abundantly released by buccal and lingual releasing incisions of the periosteum.

Reopening was scheduled after 5 months. Healing was uneventful, and the exposed tissue was hard and resem-

bled bone (Fig 10-11e). The radiographic appearance at the time of reopening suggested the cancellous bovine block had correctly integrated with the basal bone (Fig 10-11f). The fixation screws were removed and replaced by three titanium dental implants (Figs 10-11g and 10-11h).

A core biopsy was taken for histologic and microtomographic evaluation. The microtomograms evidenced new bone formation through the entire arrangement of bovine bone block trabeculae (Figs 10-11i and 10-11j). The histologic analysis demonstrated the presence of woven bone with ongoing bone formation through the whole specimen (Fig 10-11k). The xenograft particles were embedded in bone, presenting resorption lacunae close to areas with ongoing bone formation (Fig 10-11l). This indicated that in augmented areas intense physiologic bone remodeling was present, evidenced by the anticipated demineralization and remineralization.

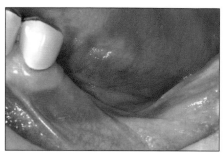

Fig 10-12a Preoperative view of the edentulous site in a patient with a deep vertical bone defect in the left side of the posterior mandible.

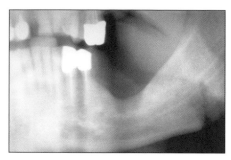

Fig 10-12b Radiographic appearance of the severe defect prior to surgery.

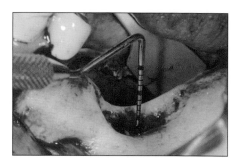

Fig 10-12c Vertical bone defect visible after elevation of a full-thickness flap. The defect extends to a depth of 11 mm.

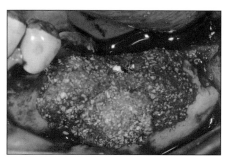

Fig 10-12d Placement of deproteinized bovine bone particles, which are embedded in a collagen matrix and infused with rhPDGF-BB, on top of the defect. The material is retained with a fixation screw.

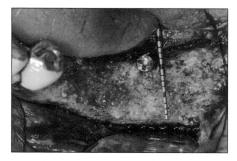

Fig 10-12e Appearance after 5 months' healing. The bone defect appears to be completely filled with a hard tissue clinically resembling bone. The site exhibits a total vertical gain of about 8 mm.

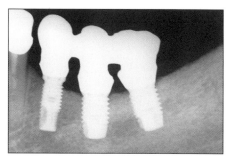

Fig 10-12f Radiograph of three titanium dental implants, 8 months after their placement in the regenerated site.

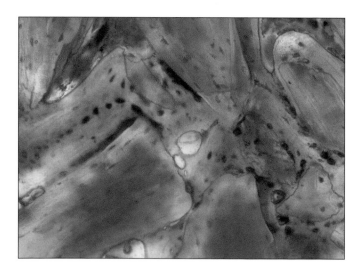

Fig 10-12g Overview of the specimen. Mature lamellar regenerated bone is visible in contact with the xenograft (acid fuchsin stain; original magnification ×200). (Figs 10-12b to 10-12g from Simion et al.[43] Reprinted with permission.)

The second patient was a man whose dental implants failed, resulting in an extreme vertical mandibular defect (Fig 10-12a and 10-12b). A full-thickness crestal incision was made in the keratinized mucosa of the edentulous ridge. The crestal incision was extended intrasulcularly along the adjacent natural tooth. Two vertical releasing incisions were made at the mesial and distal ends of the crestal incision. The defect was exposed, and the vertical bone deficiency measured 11 mm (Fig 10-12c).

The crestal bone and the defect were carefully curetted and perforated with a round bur to create bleeding. Deproteinized bovine bone particles embedded in a collagen matrix (Bio-Oss Collagen) were infused with rhPDGF-BB, positioned on top of the defect, and supported with a fixation screw (Fig 10-12d). The flaps were released and closed with horizontal mattress and interrupted sutures.

At 5 months, during the reopening, the screw was removed and the amount of defect fill was assessed. The 11-mm-long fixation screw could be considered as a reference point, because it protruded 3 mm from the new bone crest. The bone defect appeared completely filled with a hard tissue that clinically resembled bone and exhibited a total vertical gain of 8 mm (Fig 10-12e).

Three implants and the healing abutments were positioned in the sites of the mandibular left second premolar, first molar, and second molar (Fig 10-12f).

Bone biopsy specimens were taken in the regenerated bone with a 3-mm trephine and processed for histologic examination. The formation of mature, well-mineralized trabecular bone with lamellar parallel-fibered structure was found in these specimens. The bovine bone particles were surrounded by newly formed bone that seemed to have been fully integrated. A high level of cellular activity was found in the histologic sections (Fig 10-12g).

Conclusion

The future of ridge augmentation procedures is moving toward an era in which less invasive treatment regimens will be available to minimize the complications and side effects of a surgical procedure, decrease morbidity, increase success rates, and decrease technical difficulties. The maturation of tissue engineering and its application to clinical surgical procedures has helped create a new paradigm. Efforts have been made by clinicians and researchers to study the effects of a well-documented growth factor,

rhPDGF-BB, in three-dimensional bone augmentation procedures. The results of preclinical canine studies and of clinical application in humans are extremely promising, and sufficient volumes of bone have been successfully regenerated in previously deficient alveolar ridges. This will allow placement of dental titanium implants in an ideal position for correct esthetic and functional prosthetic rehabilitation.

References

1. Nyman S, Karring T, Lindhe J, Planten S. Healing following implantation of periodontitis-affected roots into gingival connective tissue. J Clin Periodontol 1980;7:394–401.
2. Schenk RK, Buser D, Hardwick WR, Dahlin C. Healing pattern of bone regeneration in membrane-protected defects: A histologic study in the canine mandible. Int J Oral Maxillofac Implants 1994;9:13–29.
3. Mecall RA, Rosenfield AL. The influence of residual ridge resorption patterns on fixture placement and tooth position. I. Int J Periodontics Restorative Dent 1991;11:9–23.
4. Simion M, Trisi P, Piattelli A. Vertical ridge augmentation using a membrane technique associated with osseointegrated implants. Int J Periodontics Restorative Dent 1994;14:496–511.
5. Jovanovic SA, Schenk RK, Orsini M, Kenney EB. Supracrestal bone formation around dental implants: An experimental dog study. Int J Oral Maxillofac Implants 1995;10:23–31.
6. Renvert S, Claffey N, Orafi H, Albrektsson T. Supracrestal bone growth around partially inserted titanium implants in dogs. A pilot study. Clin Oral Implants Res 1996;7:360–365.
7. Tinti C, Parma-Benfenati S, Polizzi G. Vertical ridge augmentation: What is the limit? Int J Periodontics Restorative Dent 1996;16:220–229.
8. Simion M, Jovanovic SA, Trisi P, Scarano A, Piattelli A. Vertical ridge augmentation around dental implants using a membrane technique and autogenous bone or allografts in humans. Int J Periodontics Restorative Dent 1998;18:8–23.
9. Schliephake H, Kracht D. Vertical ridge augmentation using polylactic membranes in conjunction with immediate implants in periodontally compromised extraction sites: An experimental study in dogs. Int J Oral Maxillofac Implants 1997;12:325–334.
10. Parma-Benfenati S, Tinti C, Albrektsson T, Johansson C. Histologic evaluation of guided vertical ridge augmentation around implants in humans. Int J Periodontics Restorative Dent 1999;19:424–437.
11. Simion M, Jovanovic SA, Tinti C, Parma-Benfenati S. Long-term evaluation of osseointegrated implants inserted at the time or after vertical ridge augmentation. A retrospective study on 123 implants with 1-5 year follow-up. Clin Oral Implants Res 2001;12:35–45.
12. Dahlin C, Lekholm U, Linde A. Membrane-induced bone augmentation at titanium implants. A report on ten fixtures followed from 1 to 3 years after loading. Int J Periodontics Restorative Dent 1991;11:273–281.
13. Dahlin C, Lekholm U, Becker W, et al. Treatment of fenestration and dehiscence bone defects around oral implants using the guided tissue regeneration technique: A prospective multicenter study. Int J Oral Maxillofac Implants 1995;10:312–318.
14. Fugazzotto PA. Success and failure rates of osseointegrated implants in function in regenerated bone for 6 to 51 months: A preliminary report. Int J Oral Maxillofac Implants 1997;12:17–24.
15. Adell R, Lekholm U, Rockler B, Brånemark PI. A 15-year study of osseointegrated implants in the treatment of the edentulous jaw. Int J Oral Surg 1981;10:387–416.
16. Lekholm U, Adell R, Lindhe J, et al. Marginal tissue reactions at osseointegrated titanium fixtures. 2. A cross-sectional retrospective study. Int J Oral Maxillofac Surg 1986;15:53–61.

17. Nevins M, Langer B. The successful application of osseointegrated implants to the posterior jaw: A long-term retrospective study. Int J Oral Maxillofac Implants 1993;8:428–432.
18. Albrektsson T, Zarb G, Worthington P, Eriksson B. The long-term efficacy of currently used dental implants: A review and proposed criteria of implant success. Int J Oral Maxillofac Implants 1986;1:11–25.
19. Szpalski M, Gunzburg R. Recombinant human bone morphogenetic protein-2: A novel osteoinductive alternative to autogenous bone graft? Acta Orthop Belg 2005;71:133–148.
20. Ito K, Yamada Y, Nagasaka T, Baba S, Ueda M. Osteogenic potential of injectable tissue-engineered bone: A comparison among autogenous bone, bone substitute (Bio-Oss), platelet-rich plasma, and tissue-engineered bone with respect to their mechanical properties and histological findings. J Biomed Mater Res A 2005;73:63–72.
21. Valentini P, Abensur D. Maxillary sinus floor elevation for implant placement with demineralized freeze-dried bone and bovine bone (Bio-Oss): A clinical study of 20 patients. Int J Periodontics Restorative Dent 1997;17:232–241.
22. Zitzmann NU, Naef R, Schärer P. Resorbable versus nonresorbable membranes in combination with Bio-Oss for guided bone regeneration. Int J Oral Maxillofac Implants. 1997;12:844–852.
23. Zitzmann NU, Schärer P, Marinello CP. Long-term results of implants treated with guided bone regeneration: A 5-year prospective study. Int J Oral Maxillofac Implants 2001;16:355–366.
24. Hammerle CH, Lang NP. Single stage surgery combining transmucosal implant placement with guided bone regeneration and bioresorbable materials. Clin Oral Implants Res 2001;12:9–18.
25. Camelo M, Nevins ML, Schenk RK, et al. Clinical, radiographic, and histologic evaluation of human periodontal defects treated with Bio-Oss and Bio-Gide. Int J Periodontics Restorative Dent 1998;18:321–331.
26. Camelo M, Nevins ML, Lynch SE, Schenk RK, Simion M, Nevins M. Periodontal regeneration with an autogenous bone–Bio-Oss composite graft and a Bio-Gide membrane. Int J Periodontics Restorative Dent 2001;21:109–119.
27. Hammerle CH, Karring T. Guided bone regeneration at oral implant sites. Periodontol 2000 1998;17:151–175.
28. Peetz M. Characterization of xenogeneic bone material. In: Boyne PJ (ed). Osseous Reconstruction of the Maxilla and the Mandible: Surgical Techniques Using Titanium Mesh and Bone Mineral. Chicago: Quintessence, 1997:87–100.
29. Simion M, Fontana F, Rasperini G, Maiorana C. Vertical ridge augmentation by e-PTFE membrane and a combination of intraoral autogenous bone graft and deproteinized anorganic bovine bone (Bio-Oss). Clin Oral Implant Res (in press).
30. Simion M, Trisi P, Maglione M, Piattelli A. A preliminary report on a method for studying the permeability of expanded polytetrafluoroethylene membrane to bacteria in vitro: A scanning electron microscopic and histological study. J Periodontol 1994;65:755–761.
31. Simion M, Trisi P, Maglione M, Piattelli A. Bacterial contamination in vitro through GTAM membrane with and without topical chlorhexidine application. A light and scanning electron microscopic study. J Clin Periodontol 1995;22:321–331.
32. Lynch SE. Introduction. In: Lynch SE, Genco RJ, Marx RE (eds). Tissue Engineering: Applications in Maxillofacial Surgery and Periodontics, ed 1. Chicago: Quintessence, 1999: xi–xviii.
33. Nevins M, Giannobile WV, McGuire MK, et al. Platelet-derived growth factor stimulates bone fill and rate of attachment level gain: Results of a large multicenter randomized controlled trial. J Periodontol 2005;76:2205–2215.
34. Nevins M, Camelo M, Nevins ML, Schenk RK, Lynch SE. Periodontal regeneration in humans using recombinant human platelet-derived growth factor-BB (rhPDGF-BB) and allogenic bone. J Periodontol 2003;74:1282–1292.
35. Camelo M, Nevins ML, Schenk RK, Lynch SE, Nevins M. Periodontal regeneration in human Class II furcations using purified recombinant human platelet-derived growth factor-BB (rhPDGF-BB) with bone allograft. Int J Periodontics Restorative Dent 2003;23:213–225.
36. Simion M, Rocchietta I, Kim D, Nevins M, Fiorellini J. Vertical ridge augmentation by means of deproteinized bovine bone block and recombinant human platelet-derived growth factor-BB. A histologic study in a dog model. Int J Periodontics Restorative Dent 2006;26:415–423.
37. Simion M, Dahlin C, Rocchietta I, Stavropoulos A, Sanchez R, Karring T. Vertical ridge augmentation with guided bone regeneration in association with dental implants: An experimental study in dogs. Clin Oral Implants Res 2007;18:86–94.
38. Hunt DR, Jovanovic SA, Wikesjö UME, Wozney JM, Bernard GW. Hyaluronan supports rh-BMP-2 induced bone reconstruction of advanced alveolar defects in dogs. A pilot study. J Periodontol 2001;72:651–658.
39. Zellin G, Linde A. Importance of delivery systems for growth-stimulatory factors in combination with osteopromotive membranes. An experimental study using rh-BMP-2 in rat mandibular defects. Biomed Mater Res 1997;35:181–190.
40. Weng D, Hurzeler MB, Quinones CR, Ohlms A, Caffesse RG. Contribution of the periosteum to bone formation in guided bone regeneration. A study in monkeys. Clin Oral Implants Res 2000;11:546–554.
41. Shimizu T, Sasano Y, Nakajo S, Kagayama M, Shimauchi H. Osteoblastic differentiation of periosteum-derived cells is promoted by the physical contact with the bone matrix in vivo. Anat Rec 2001;264:72–81.
42. Li M, Amizuka N, Oda K, et al. Histochemical evidence of the initial chondrogenesis and osteogenesis in the periosteum of a rib fractured model: Implications of osteocyte involvement in periosteal chondrogenesis. Microsc Res Tech 2004;64:330–342.
43. Simion M, Rocchietta I, Dellavia C. Three-dimensional ridge augmentation with xenograft and recombinant human platelet-derived growth factor-BB in humans: Report of two cases. Int J Periodontics Restorative Dent 2007;27:109–115.

11

rhBMP-2: Biology and Applications in Oral and Maxillofacial Surgery and Periodontics

John M. Wozney, PhD

Ulf M. E. Wikesjö, DDS, PhD, DMD

An assortment of devices, biomaterials, bioactive factors, and combinations thereof are available to the oral and maxillofacial and periodontal surgeon for various craniofacial and dentoalveolar indications. These include allogenic or xenogeneic cadaver-sourced as well as synthetic bone biomaterials; bioresorbable or nonresorbable occlusive or porous membranes of synthetic or tissue-derived origin; and matrix, growth, and differentiation factors. All of these materials are commonly compared with autogenous bone grafts, which are considered the gold standard for bone regeneration. The availability of recombinant human bone morphogenetic protein 2 (rhBMP-2), the bone-inductive component in several tissue engineering constructs, has allowed it to be extensively studied for its bone-forming capacity in a broad range of preclinical models as well as controlled clinical studies.

Using rodent models, Urist[1] observed that devitalized bone, and subsequently bone extracts, induced bone formation when implanted subcutaneously or intramuscularly. Because of the histologic observation of transformation of soft tissue into bone, he named this activity *bone morphogenetic protein* (BMP), although it was unclear whether a single or unique protein was responsible for the observed bone formation. Once this bone-inductive activity was extensively purified from bovine bone extracts,[2] and the component proteins were molecularly cloned and expressed in a recombinant system, it became apparent that the activity was the result of a family of proteins collectively called the *BMPs*.[3–5]

The BMP family of proteins sequestered in bone includes several subfamilies. BMP-2 and BMP-4 are closely related molecules with more than 90% amino acid identity. BMP-5, BMP-6, and BMP-7 (also called *osteogenic protein 1*) constitute a subfamily that shares approximately 70% amino acid identity with the BMP-2 and BMP-4 subfamily. BMP-3, probably the most abundant protein in the purified bone-inductive extract, shares about 50% amino acid identity with the other BMP family members. Each of the BMP molecules is unique biochemically and biologically; however, each also presents some redundancy.

BMP-2 has been characterized as a bone-inductive molecule because it is a single bioactive factor demonstrating the same inductive activity present in bone and bone extracts. rhBMP-2 has been evaluated in preclinical studies emulating many potential clinical applications and has been developed through controlled clinical studies into a marketed product. A unique aspect to the development of osteoinductive factors is the contribution of the carrier or matrix material, used to apply the BMP at the desired site of action, to the biology of bone induction. This chapter discusses the biology of BMP-2, from the molecular mechanism of action, through preclinical studies evaluating how it induces bone in vivo and the many clinical settings in which it may be applied, to clinical studies supporting its use clinically.

Biology

Cellular mechanism of action

By amino acid sequence homology, BMP-2 is a member of the transforming growth factor β (TGF-β) superfamily of growth and differentiation factors. Like other members of this family, it is a dimeric protein with three intrachain disulfide bonds forming a cysteine knot structure and one interchain disulfide bond forming the covalent dimer.[6] This highly disulfide-bonded structure results in high stability of the BMP-2 molecule. Because of the dimeric nature of the proteins, TGF-β family members may form homodimers or heterodimers. rhBMP-2 is a homodimeric protein consisting of two BMP-2 protein subunits. It has been found that BMP-2 subunits can heterodimerize with other family members, for example BMP-6 and BMP-7, at least in recombinant expression systems.[7]

rhBMP-2 is produced in a recombinant expression system using mammalian cells overexpressing the BMP-2 coding sequence.[8] Using a batch fermentation process, the rhBMP-2 in the conditioned medium is purified through a series of biochemical steps and lyophilized in vials. It is a glycosylated molecule, with a single site per chain containing high-mannose–type glycans.

rhBMP-2 is a locally acting bioactive factor that binds to receptors on the surface of responsive cell types. The receptors for rhBMP-2 consist of several types of heteromeric serine-threonine kinases.[9] For the molecule to signal, it must bind both type I and type II kinase receptors. Type I receptors for rhBMP-2 include the molecules BMPR-IA (ALK-3) and BMPR-IB (ALK-6), and may also use the activin type I receptor (ACVR1). Interestingly it has recently been found that a (presumably activating) mutation in the ACVR1 gene results in the hereditary dis-

order fibrodysplasia ossificans progressiva.[10] This condition is characterized by progressive cartilage and bone formation in the musculature of affected individuals, eventually resulting in fusion of the joints. Only one type II receptor (BMPR-II) has been shown to transduce the rhBMP-2 signal.

The crystal structure of BMP-2 complexed with the ligand-binding domains of type I and both type I and type II receptors has been determined.[11–13] The receptor complex consists of a single dimeric BMP with two type I and two type II receptors. It has been reported that BMPs can either sequentially bind the receptors or bind preformed multimeric receptor complexes; the downstream signaling pathways may be affected by the mode of binding.[14,15] In the former case, BMP-2 first binds the high-affinity (K_D approximately 1 nM) type I receptor and then recruits the low-affinity (K_D approximately 100 nM) type II receptor into the complex (Fig 11-1). The type II receptor then phosphorylates the type I receptor, which then gains the ability to transmit the BMP signal by phosphorylating intermediary intracellular signal transduction proteins called *SMADs*.[9,16–18] BMP receptors phosphorylate SMADs 1, 5, and 8; other members of the TGF-β superfamily, such as TGF-β1 signal through SMADs 2 and 3. Thus there are two separate and competing intracellular signaling pathways for the TGF-β superfamily of proteins. Phosphorylated SMADs 1, 5, and 8 subsequently dimerize with the co-SMAD, SMAD 4. This complex then translocates into the nucleus, where it can activate the various BMP-2–responsive genes. In addition to the receptor-binding SMADs and co-SMADs, there are inhibitory or anti-SMADs (SMADs 6 and 7) that interfere with recruitment of the co-SMADs and thus inhibit signaling. Transcription of the SMAD 6 gene in fact is greatly stimulated by BMP-2, resulting in an inherent negative feedback loop that attenuates BMP-2 signaling.

Bioactive factors may affect cells in several different ways. Growth factors such as platelet-derived growth factor, insulin-like growth factor, epidermal growth factor, and so on stimulate cells to divide.[19] In contrast, BMP-2 is a differentiation factor, which changes the phenotype of precursor cells such as mesenchymal stem cells into osteoblasts (bone cells) and chondroblasts (cartilage cells). This has been demonstrated by examining the effects of BMP-2 on cell types in vitro. For example, BMP-2 has been shown to induce expression of markers of the osteoblastic phenotype such as bone alkaline phosphatase and osteocalcin in murine osteoprogenitor cells, including W-20 cells,[20] the multipotential embryonic stem cells 10T1/2,[21] and embryonic limb bud cell lines such as

Fig 11-1 rhBMP-2 signal transduction pathway, from binding of rhBMP-2 to its cell surface receptors through activation of BMP-responsive genes in the nucleus of the cell. See text for details. (R-SMAD) Receptor-activated SMAD; (P) phosphate.

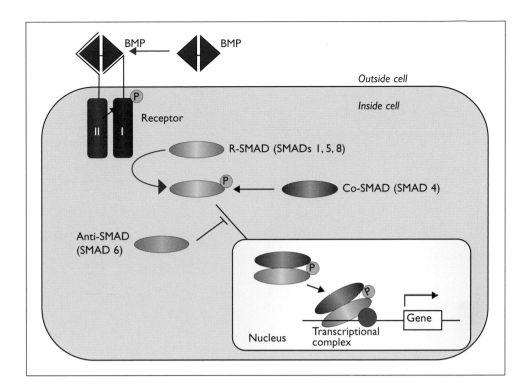

C14 cells.[22] In addition, it can change the differentiation potential of the myoblast precursor cell line, C2C12, which forms myotubes on serum withdrawal, to cells that express osteoblastic markers including osteocalcin and alkaline phosphatase.[23]

Taken together, these and other studies suggest that in vivo, multiple types of cells and tissue respond to rhBMP-2 by differentiating into bone cells. These likely include bone cells such as periosteal cells, bone marrow stromal cells, cells from the soft tissues including muscle and gingival cells, and perivascular cells. Depending on the site of application, the relative contribution of these cell types to the bone-forming process may differ depending on their availability.

The in vivo mechanism by which BMP-2 functions is therefore distinct from that of the true growth factors. Growth factors can act on existing bone cells or bone cell progenitors to expand the cellular population. Thus, they may stimulate bone growth when applied locally at a bony site. Alternatively, rhBMP-2 differentiates precursor cells into bone-forming cells and thus may act at bony or soft tissue sites to induce local bone formation.

In vivo bone induction

A locally acting factor, rhBMP-2, induces bone formation at the site of application. Based on a large number of pre-clinical studies (some described later in this chapter), rhBMP-2 initially induces woven trabecular bone formation whether applied at bony or soft tissue sites; this new bone then remodels into lamellar trabecular and/or cortical bone, consistent with the anatomic location and the associated biomechanical environment.

For example, rhBMP-2 has been evaluated for its ability to repair a 3-cm segmental critical-sized defect in the dog mandible.[24,25] Radiographically evident bone formation was visible at 4 weeks (Fig 11-2). Longer time points demonstrated remodeling of the bone and integration with the surrounding bone, returning function to the mandible and enabling the removal of the fixation plate used to stabilize the surgically created defect. While the bone continued to remodel and corticalize, the height and width of the ridge remained stable over the 20-month observation interval. Thus, as rhBMP-2 caused the

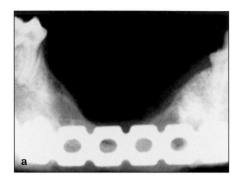

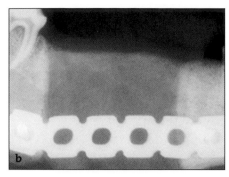

Fig 11-2a Induction of bone by rhBMP-2 and bone remodeling in a canine model. A mandibular critical-sized defect (3-cm full-thickness defect) is shown 12 weeks after creation of the defect.

Fig 11-2b Treated mandibular defect 4 weeks after implantation of rhBMP-2.

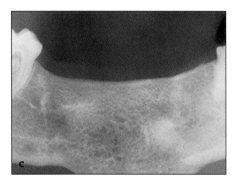

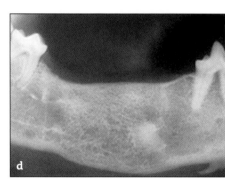

Fig 11-2c Mandibular defect 9 months after implantation of rhBMP-2.

Fig 11-2d Mandibular defect 20 months after implantation of rhBMP-2. (For further details of this case, see Toriumi et al.[24,25])

animal to induce its own normal bone, the bone remodeled in response to the physiologic forces placed on it.

At the cellular level, bone induction by rhBMP-2 occurs both through the endochondral bone formation pathway and by direct intramembranous bone induction. These processes were initially characterized in the rat ectopic system, where rhBMP-2 was implanted subcutaneously in rats in combination with rat bone matrix that had been demineralized and extracted (to remove endogenous BMPs).[26] The cellular series of events is essentially indistinguishable from those observed by Urist[1] and others with devitalized bone and bone extracts. Initial events include chemotaxis, during which numerous undifferentiated mesenchymal cells infiltrate the implant site, and proliferation of these cells.

Whether the proliferative effect is directly or indirectly caused by rhBMP-2 remains unclear, because in vitro most cell types respond by differentiating (and hence arrest growth) rather than proliferating. The mesenchymal cells then differentiate into chondrocytes in response to the presence of rhBMP-2. Numerous blood vessels infiltrate the area, and the cartilage begins to be removed and replaced with bone. This robust angiogenic response on application of rhBMP-2 is likely an indirect effect via

induction of vascular endothelial cell growth factor in the BMP-responsive cells.

Eventually the implant converts entirely to bone, and bone marrow elements populate the bone. With the presence of these elements, including osteoclasts, the implant remodels into an ossicle of bone, and the hematopoietic bone marrow matures toward more adipogenic marrow. Over time, because ectopic bone is not biomechanically loaded, the induced bone will remodel away. Clearly, the observed cellular events are quite complex; they are initiated by administration of rhBMP-2 but undoubtedly involve contributions of many other locally acting growth factors and hormones.

With the availability of rhBMP-2, a dose response to the factor could be examined. With higher doses of rhBMP-2, bone and cartilage formed at the same time in the ectopic system,[26] suggesting that rhBMP-2 also induces intramembranous bone formation. This finding is consistent with the histologic observation of condensation of mesenchymal cells and their subsequent differentiation into bone trabeculae. Subsequent animal studies have indicated that the relative contributions of the endochondral and intramembranous process to rhBMP-2 depend on dose, the nature of the carrier, and the site of implantation (with the associated contributions of different responsive cell populations and local bioactive factors). For example, early histologic evaluation of bone induction in the dog mandible showed only direct bone formation without evidence of cartilage formation. On the other hand, application in long-bone site or sites of fracture revealed both endochondral and direct bone formation.[27,28]

Carriers and matrices

For optimal bone induction, rhBMP-2 is administered in a carrier or matrix. Desirable characteristics of the matrix may vary with the clinical indication.[27,29,30] For example, different matrix characteristics would be needed for surgical implantation of rhBMP-2 to reconstruct large mandibular resection defects or for alveolar ridge augmentation than would be needed for a minimally invasive percutaneous injection to accelerate repair of a closed fracture. From a practical perspective, the matrix allows application of rhBMP-2 and the ability to distribute rhBMP-2 over a defined volume, delineating the geometry of the bone to be induced. While onlay indications often call for structural integrity of the matrix, this may not be critical for inlay indications or when supportive devices are available to maintain a space for bone formation.

The matrix also provides key components to the way in which bone is induced by rhBMP-2. A critical role of the matrix is to maintain rhBMP-2 at the site of application so that a pharmacologically relevant concentration or dose is sufficiently present to initiate migration and proliferation of responsive mesenchymal cells into the matrix and differentiation into bone- and cartilage-forming cells. In rodent systems, rhBMP-2 in aqueous formulation buffer can be effective, for example, in accelerating fracture repair.[31] However, it will not form bone in ectopic soft tissue sites.[32] In addition, application without a matrix appears less effective in higher animals, likely because of the slower rate at which cells infiltrate the area and the lower bone formation rate. Because rhBMP-2 is generally applied once, the longer it remains at the site, the greater the rate and quantity of bone formed, within the limits of spatial restrictions by the site or the carrier. However, the optimal characteristics of release and retention of the rhBMP-2 are still obscure and may differ from indication to indication.

The matrix should allow cellular access so that precursor cells and vascular elements may enter or invade the implant. This can be accomplished by using a porous material, a material that disperses, or one that degrades as bone is formed. Other valuable qualities of the matrix include osteoconductivity, that is, promotion of bone formation directly on its surfaces.

While a number of nonresorbable materials have been evaluated with rhBMP-2, and indeed support rhBMP-2–induced bone induction, resorbable materials seem to be preferable. In this way, the bone formed is allowed to function as the normal host bone, unimpeded by residual foreign material that may compromise biomechanics or the biologic response of the bone. This may be particularly critical for immediately load-bearing bone and bone intended to support fixation and retention of metallic implants, including dental implants.

Polymers

A number of biomaterials have been evaluated as carriers or matrices for rhBMP-2. Broadly these can be divided into tissue-sourced or synthetic polymers, tissue-sourced or synthetic ceramics, and composites of these categories.[33] Tissue-sourced polymers include collagen, the major organic constituent of bone and most soft tissues. Type I collagen is a heteromeric triple helical molecule, typically sourced from bone, skin, or tendon. Demineralized bone matrix, the carrier used in the rat ectopic assay during the purification of BMP from bone, is primarily type I collagen. Collagen-based biomaterials are derived in a variety of formats, including particulates, sponges, and sheets. Advantages of collagen include biocompatibility (because it is a major protein component of the native extracellular matrix), the ability to bind rhBMP-2 and retain it at the site of application, and flexibility in formulation. Disadvantages include the potential for immunogenicity and disease transmission.

Hyaluronic acid, another ubiquitous constituent of the extracellular matrix, has also been used in combination with rhBMP-2. Hyaluronans can be derived from avian or microbial sources. Natural forms of hyaluronan are relatively soluble and have short in vivo residence times; however, esterification can be used to decrease hydrophilicity and prolong residence time. Hyaluronan can be manufactured into a variety of pads, sponges, or sheets.

Other tissue-sourced polymers include the polysaccharides chitosan and alginate. Fibrin (eg, fibrin glue) has also been used as a carrier system for BMPs.

Synthetic polymers have been extensively studied as drug delivery systems. The most commonly used materials are the poly-α-hydroxyacids, including polylactic acid, polyglycolic acid, and the copolymer poly(lactic-co-glycolic acid) (PLGA). Advantages of these materials are the elimination of risk of disease transmission, the ability to control degradation rate by varying the chemical composition of the polymer, and the previous experience of regulatory agencies with these polymers. Disadvantages include hydrolytic degradation, which results in bulk erosion of the material; fragmentation (of some poly-α-hydroxyacids), which results in undesirable foreign-body reactions, including accumulation of foamy macrophages and osteoclasia; and the possibility of a locally acidic environment generated by the degradation products.

PLGA microspheres, in combination with a blood clot, have been used in combination with rhBMP-2 in several preclinical studies.[25,34,35] The rhBMP-2 can also be incorporated directly into PLGA microspheres.

Other polymeric materials have also been evaluated as BMP delivery systems, including polyanhydrides, polyphosphazenes, polypropylene fumarate, poloxamers, and polyethylene glycol–polylactic acid combinations.

Ceramics

Inorganic calcium phosphate–based materials have also been used as carriers for rhBMP-2. These materials include tricalcium phosphate (TCP) and hydroxyapatite (HA), the latter being the predominant mineral component of bone. The ceramics can be in particulate or block form, and many are available as bone void fillers. Porosity can be provided either by virtue of the particulate nature of the material or by manufacturing methods that generate interconnected pores within the ceramic blocks.

Depending on the chemical composition of the calcium phosphate material and the crystallinity, these materials may be resorbable; however, the ceramics can have very long residence times and remain resident within the newly formed bone. Advantages of these biomaterials again are their synthetic nature and the ability of rhBMP-2 to bind tightly to HA.

Several calcium phosphate cements have also been evaluated with rhBMP-2.[28,36–40] These cements harden following addition of liquid either in an exothermic or endothermic reaction; the latter is less likely to damage a bioactive protein. An endothermically setting material that forms a poorly crystalline HA similar to that in bone has been evaluated in combination with rhBMP-2 in a series of animal models. An advantage of using a cementing material is that the rhBMP-2 is incorporated within the

material as it hardens, rather than merely binding to the surface. It can then be released as the material is resorbed or becomes fragmented, resulting in an extended residence of the rhBMP-2 at the site of application.

Composites

Combinations of these classes of materials can combine properties of the various classes. Many such composites have been used with BMPs. For example, a gelatin sponge impregnated with PLGA has been tested with rhBMP-2 in preclinical studies emulating a range of clinical applications.[41–45] Other examples include collagen-HA-TCP composites (discussed later in the chapter), collagen-PLGA composites, and hyaluronic acid–impregnated polylactic acid sponges.

For clinical applications, an absorbable collagen sponge (ACS) has been developed as a carrier for use with rhBMP-2. The lyophilized rhBMP-2 is reconstituted with sterile water that is then applied to the sponge. The rhBMP-2 rapidly binds to the collagen so that any liquid that is expressed from the sponge during surgical manipulation contains little rhBMP-2. The ACS retains the rhBMP-2 at the surgical site of application for a period of weeks, during which bone formation occurs. The ACS is resorbed by foreign-body giant cells as the bone is induced, leaving only the host's normal bone, free of any residual biomaterials.

The ACS sponge itself has been a marketed product (as a hemostatic sponge) and thus has an extended safety record showing biocompatibility. The rhBMP-2/ACS combination has been tested in a wide variety of preclinical models successfully showing bone induction and repair in oral and maxillofacial and orthopedic applications, as detailed in the following section.

Although the ACS can provide an area in which bone is formed, under some circumstances it does not resist compression from muscles or other soft tissues. This can be observed, for example, in a monkey model of intertransverse process spinal fusion.[46] In this study, the addition of a rigid plastic shield to protect the rhBMP-2/ACS resulted in large fusion masses; without this additional device, only a small volume of bone induction was observed. Rigid materials such as HA/TCP granules or allogeneic material can be added to the rhBMP-2/ACS to enhance its ability to resist soft tissue compression.[47,48] A compression-resistant matrix, consisting of HA/TCP granules within a collagen sponge, has also been used successfully with rhBMP-2 in spinal fusion models.[49]

The endothermically setting calcium phosphate cement cited earlier, α-BSM (Etex), has been used in combination with rhBMP-2 as a percutaneously injectable material for acceleration of closed fracture repair in rabbit and canine models.[37,38] When modified to better granulate and disperse around a fracture site by the addition of sodium bicarbonate, α-BSM is called *calcium phosphate matrix* and has been evaluated in combination with rhBMP-2 in fracture repair models, including monkey fibular osteotomies.[28,39] In these studies, rhBMP-2 with calcium phosphate matrix was shown to accelerate dramatically (by up to 50%) the healing of osteotomy defects, treated either acutely or in a delayed fashion, as evaluated by biomechanics, radiographs, and histologic evaluation.

Applications in Oral and Maxillofacial Surgery and Periodontics

As rhBMP-2 was developed for indications in the axial and appendicular skeleton, many of the same evaluations and considerations occurred in parallel in its development for indications in the craniofacial skeleton. Particular focus was placed on alveolar augmentation, dental implant osseointegration, and periodontal regeneration, but research also included congenital malformations, resection defects, orthognathic surgery gap defects, and plastic procedures.[50] A large number of studies, mainly using canine and nonhuman primate models, have been performed to evaluate rhBMP-2 combined with various carrier technologies and devices for alveolar augmentation and dental implant osseointegration. The following discussion focuses on some critical advances that demonstrate the remarkable biologic and clinical potential that rhBMP-2 may bring to dentoalveolar rehabilitation, including osseointegration of dental implants.

Combined rhBMP-2/ACS

An initial report demonstrating that a BMP construct has potential to induce clinically relevant bone formation and dental implant osseointegration was presented in 1997.[51] In a canine model, 10-mm machined, threaded endosseous implants were inserted 5 mm into the surgically reduced edentulous mandibular ridge, creating critical-sized, 5-mm, supra-alveolar peri-implant defects (Fig 11-3a). Either rhBMP-2/ACS or buffer/ACS (control) was draped to cover the implants in contralateral jaw quadrants (Fig 11-3b). The defect sites were closed by advancing and suturing the mucoperiosteal flaps over the implants to achieve healing by primary intention (Fig 11-3c).

The defect sites were subjected to histometric evaluation following a 16-week healing interval. Sites receiving rhBMP-2/ACS revealed significantly more bone formation along the exposed implant surface than did the ACS control (Figs 11-3d to 11-3f). The newly formed bone exhibited significant osseointegration (see inset in Fig 11-3d). Nevertheless, there was considerable variability in bone formation. Apparently, as discussed earlier in this chapter, the ACS carrier was ineffective in consistently producing room for adequate rhBMP-2–induced bone formation.

Nevertheless, the aforementioned observations were even more notable when compared with those made when the same preclinical model was used to evaluate demineralized freeze-dried bone allograft (DFDBA) combined with guided bone regeneration (GBR) or GBR alone,[52] both treatment concepts that are significant to today's clinical practice. Contralateral critical-sized, 5-mm, supra-alveolar peri-implant defects, each of which included two endosseous implants, received either a space-providing expanded polytetrafluoroethylene (e-PTFE) membrane for GBR and DFDBA rehydrated in autologous blood or the e-PTFE membrane alone (Figs 11-4a to 11-4c).

The defect sites were subjected to histometric evaluation following a 16-week healing interval (Figs 11-4d to 11-4f). The type I collagen DFDBA biomaterial remained apparently unaltered in all sites receiving this treatment, exhibiting no signs of biodegradation. Rather, the DFDBA particles appeared solidified within a dense connective tissue matrix and in close contact with the titanium implant surface without evidence of bone formation and osseointegration.

Overall, bone formation along the implant surface was limited and clinically irrelevant for both treatments, GBR with DFDBA and GBR alone. Notably, physiologic concentrations of bone growth factors and BMPs sequestered in the DFDBA matrix apparently had no relevant effect on alveolar bone formation, given that the DFDBA particles were invested in fibrous connective tissue without evidence of any bone metabolic activity. In contrast with those observed for the rhBMP-2 protocol described earlier, the results from this study suggest that DFDBA has no relevant osteoinductive, osteoconductive, or other ad-

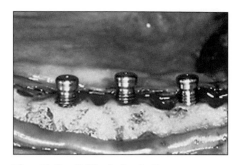

Fig 11-3a Critical-sized, 5-mm, supra-alveolar peri-implant defect, to be treated with rhBMP-2/ACS or with an ACS alone.

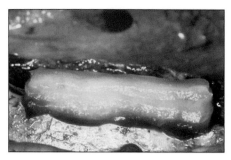

Fig 11-3b Defect treated with rhBMP-2/ACS, shown before wound closure.

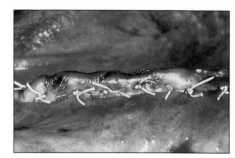

Fig 11-3c Defect after wound closure for healing by primary intention.

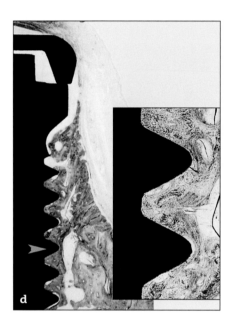

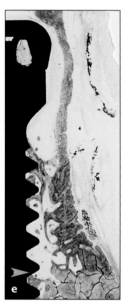

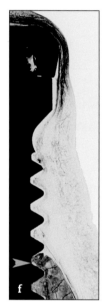

Figs 11-3d and 11-3e Bone formation reaches the implant platform 16 weeks after treatment with rhBMP-2/ACS (Stevenel blue and van Gieson picro fuchsin stain). *(arrowhead)* Level of the surgically reduced alveolar crest. *(inset)* The newly formed bone shows osseointegration to the titanium implant surface.

Fig 11-3f Control site receiving ACS without rhBMP-2. There is limited, if any, bone formation at 16 weeks. *(arrowhead)* Level of the surgically reduced alveolar crest (Stevenel blue and van Gieson picro fuchsin stain). (Figs 11-3a to 11-3f from Sigurdsson et al.[51] Reprinted with permission.)

junctive effect on GBR and that GBR technologies have limited potential to support osteogenesis (augment alveolar bone), at least for onlay indications.

Subsequent studies evaluated a space-providing, porous e-PTFE device to support rhBMP-2/ACS–induced bone formation.[53,54] The concept behind the design was to provide an unobstructed space to prevent compression of the rhBMP-2/ACS and, at the same time, allow vascularity from the gingival connective tissue to support rhBMP-2–induced bone formation. Bilateral critical-sized, 5-mm, supra-alveolar peri-implant defects were created in the canine model, each defect site including two turned and one acid-etched endosseous implant (Fig 11-5a). Four animals received the space-providing, dome-shaped, porous e-PTFE device alone or combined with rhBMP-2/ACS in contralateral jaw quadrants, and four animals re-

ceived rhBMP-2/ACS alone versus rhBMP-2/ACS combined with the porous e-PTFE device in contralateral jaw quadrants (Figs 11-5b to 11-5d).

The defect sites were subjected to histometric evaluation following an 8-week healing interval (Figs 11-5e to 11-5h). Similar to the findings of the previously described study of GBR using occlusive e-PTFE membranes,[52] this study showed that GBR as a stand-alone therapy had limited ability to enhance alveolar bone formation. Furthermore, as observed in other studies,[51,55] jaw quadrants receiving rhBMP-2/ACS alone showed significant augmentation of the alveolar ridge; however, the height and volume of the induced bone varied considerably.

In contrast, the combination of the dome-shaped, space-providing, porous e-PTFE device and rhBMP-2/ACS predictably resulted in formation of large volumes of bone,

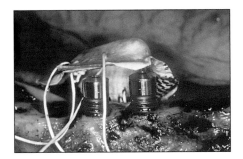

Fig 11-4a Critical-sized, 5-mm, supra-alveolar peri-implant defect, to be treated with a GBR technique using an occlusive, space-providing e-PTFE membrane with or without DFDBA.

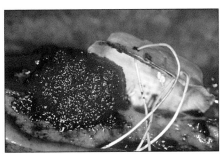

Fig 11-4b Supra-alveolar defect with the e-PTFE membrane and DFDBA rehydrated in autologous blood.

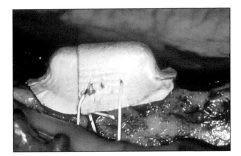

Fig 11-4c Membrane in place prior to wound closure for healing by primary intention.

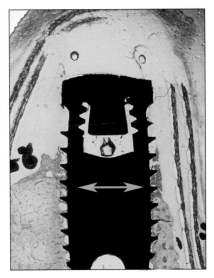

Fig 11-4d Result of GBR alone after 16 weeks' healing. There is limited regeneration of alveolar bone, suggesting that the innate regenerative potential of alveolar bone is limited (Stevenel blue and van Gieson picro fuchsin stain). *(green arrows)* Level of the surgically reduced alveolar crest.

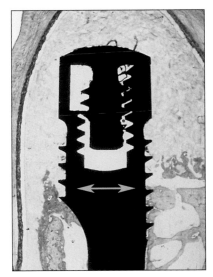

Fig 11-4e Result of GBR with DFDBA after 16 weeks' healing. There is limited regeneration of alveolar bone in the presence of DFDBA, suggesting that DFDBA has limited, if any, osteoinductive or osteoconductive properties to support bone regeneration (Stevenel blue and van Gieson picro fuchsin stain). *(green arrows)* Level of the surgically reduced alveolar crest.

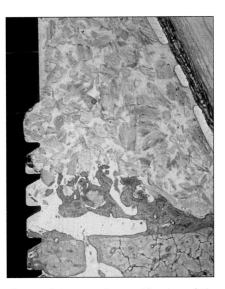

Fig 11-4f Increased magnification of Fig 11-4e. (Figs 11-4a to 11-4f from Caplanis et al.[52] Reprinted with permission.)

consistently filling the space provided by the e-PTFE device. The newly formed bone provided osseointegration without remarkable differences between turned and acid-etched titanium implants. This study provides important insight about tissue engineering principles using BMPs. BMP bone formation follows the outline of a space or matrix; in other words, the geometry of the newly formed bone may be outlined already in the design of the matrix.

Still other studies evaluating rhBMP-2/ACS for inlay indications showed rhBMP-2/ACS to be an effective treatment when implanted into space providing alveolar ridge defects.[56] Combining rhBMP-2/ACS with GBR provided no additional value. In a canine model, full-thickness

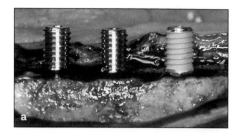

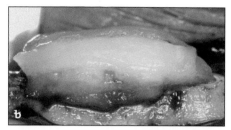

Fig 11-5a Critical-sized, 5-mm, supra-alveolar peri-implant defect, to be treated with rhBMP-2/ACS alone, GBR alone, or rhBMP-2/ACS at one of two volumes combined with a space-providing e-PTFE membrane.

Fig 11-5b Supra-alveolar defect covered with rhBMP-2/ACS.

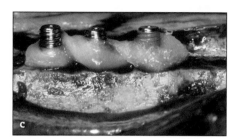

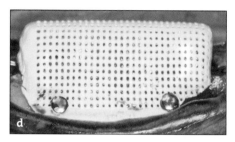

Fig 11-5c rhBMP-2/ACS at smaller volume but same dosage compared with Fig 11-5b, placed at a supra-alveolar defect. It will not fill the space underneath the e-PTFE membrane that will be placed.

Fig 11-5d Defect covered with the porous, space-providing e-PTFE membrane prior to wound closure for healing by primary intention.

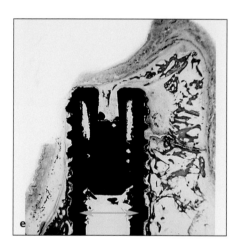

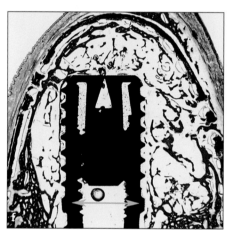

Fig 11-5e Healing of a site with rhBMP-2/ACS alone at 8 weeks. Treatment with rhBMP-2/ACS in the absence of a space-providing membrane provides very irregular bone formation (Stevenel blue and von Gieson picro fuchsin stain). *(green arrows)* Level of the surgically reduced alveolar crest.

Fig 11-5f Healing of a site with large-volume rhBMP-2/ACS with an e-PTFE membrane at 8 weeks. The rhBMP-2–induced bone fills the large space provided by the membrane (Stevenel blue and von Gieson picro fuchsin stain). *(green arrows)* Level of the surgically reduced alveolar crest.

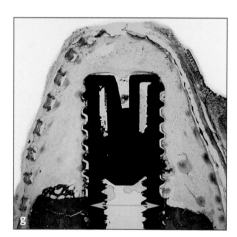

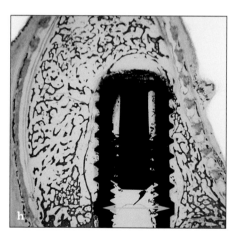

Fig 11-5g Healing of a GBR only site at 8 weeks. Despite the space provided by the membrane, the result of GBR alone is limited, if any, regeneration of alveolar bone in this onlay indication (Stevenel blue and von Gieson picro fuchsin stain). *(green arrows)* Level of the surgically reduced alveolar crest.

Fig 11-5h Healing of a site with small-volume rhBMP-2/ACS with an e-PTFE membrane at 8 weeks. The rhBMP-2/ACS–induced bone fills the large space provided by the membrane. Apparently it is the space provided by the membrane, rather than the volume of rhBMP-2/ACS, that determines the shape of the new bone (Stevenel blue and von Gieson picro fuchsin stain). *(green arrows)* Level of the surgically reduced alveolar crest. (Figs 11-5a to 11-5h from Wikesjö et al.[53,54] Reprinted with permission.)

Fig 11-6a Mandibular alveolar ridge before surgery to create a saddle-type defect, which will be treated with rhBMP-2/ACS, GBR, rhBMP-2/ACS combined with GBR, or a control treatment.

Fig 11-6b Surgical outline of the alveolar ridge defect.

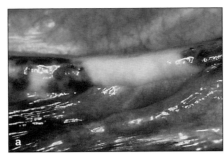
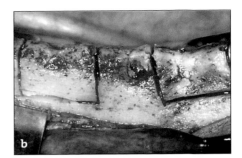

Fig 11-6c Saddle-type 10 × 15–mm alveolar ridge defect.

Fig 11-6d Application of rhBMP-2/ACS and GBR membranes.

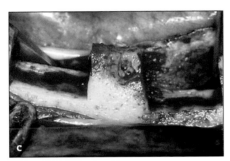
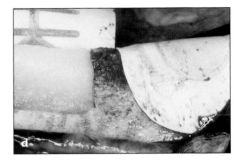

Fig 11-6e Clinical observation of a site implanted with rhBMP-2/ACS alone after 12 weeks of healing. Note the considerable swelling of the site.

Fig 11-6f Clinical observation of a site treated with GBR alone after 12 weeks of healing. Note a commonly observed membrane exposure/wound failure. (Figs 11-6a to 11-6f from Jovanovic et al.[56] Reprinted with permission.)

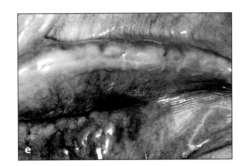
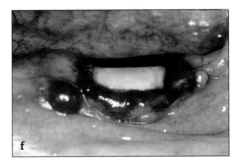

15 × 10–mm saddle-type defects were surgically created in the mandibular alveolar ridge and randomly assigned to receive rhBMP-2/ACS, rhBMP-2/ACS combined with GBR, GBR alone, or a control treatment (Fig 11-6). The GBR protocol used traditional occlusive e-PTFE membranes.

The defect sites were subjected to histometric evaluation following a 12-week healing interval (Fig 11-7). Postsurgery complications included wound failure in as many as 44% of the sites receiving the e-PTFE membrane, with or without rhBMP-2. Histologic analysis revealed bone fill averaging 101% for defects receiving rhBMP-2/ACS or rhBMP-2/ACS combined with GBR (without wound failure), and 92% for defects receiving GBR alone (without wound failure). Bone fill for the surgical control averaged only 60% of the original defect volume.

These observations demonstrate that rhBMP-2 may be used to augment alveolar bone when used as an onlay and as an inlay. The observations also point to the importance of space provision for rhBMP-2–induced bone formation. Supra-alveolar defects (onlay indications) such as the critical-sized peri-implant defect model may require rhBMP-2 constructs that exhibit structural integrity to provide space for alveolar augmentation or may have to be combined with suitable space-providing devices for optimal bone formation. In contrast, space-providing intrabony defects (inlay indications), such as the saddle-type defect, may be treated successfully using rhBMP-2 constructs of lesser structural integrity. The addition of GBR devices does not provide additional value to the rhBMP-2 technology in these defects. Furthermore, occlusive GBR devices may readily become exposed, thereby compromising overall wound healing.

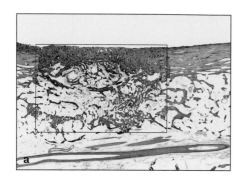

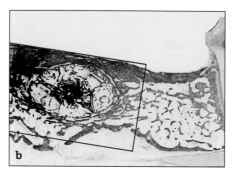

Figs 11-7a and 11-7b Photomicrographs of defect sites receiving rhBMP-2/ACS alone. *(red frame)* Approximate size and location of the original defect site. *(a)* The site exhibits cortex formation and complete trabecular bone fill. *(b)* Cortex formation and a resolving seroma filled with trabecular bone can be observed.

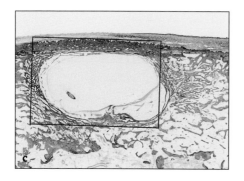

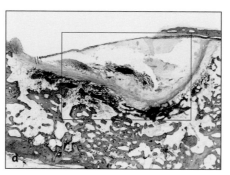

Figs 11-7c and 11-7d Photomicrographs of defect sites receiving rhBMP-2/ACS with a GBR membrane. *(red frame)* Approximate size and location of the original defect site. *(c)* Cortex formation and a large seroma are evident. *(d)* Wound failure and membrane exposure have occurred. Note the cortex formation over part of the GBR barrier.

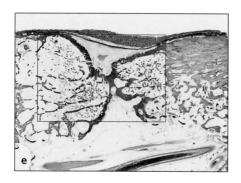

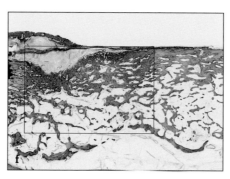

Figs 11-7e and 11-7f Photomicrographs of defect sites receiving a GBR membrane only. *(red frame)* Approximate size and location of the original defect site. *(e)* Cortex formation can be observed. *(f)* The site exhibits limited membrane exposure resulting in local bone loss. Note the cortex formation over part of the GBR barrier.

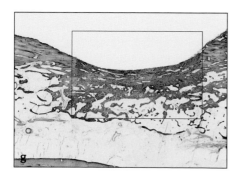

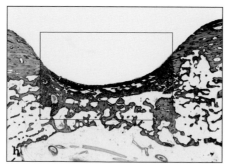

Figs 11-7g and 11-7h Photomicrographs of surgical controls. *(red frame)* Approximate size and location of the original defect site. *(g)* The site received ACS alone and shows limited bone fill. *(h)* The site received a sham surgery, which also resulted in limited bone fill. (Figs 11-7a to 11-7h from Jovanovic et al.[56] Reprinted with permission.)

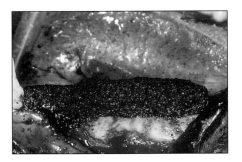

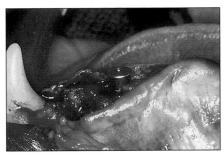

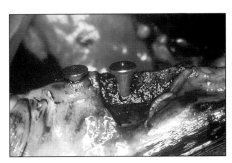

Fig 11-8a Surgically created horizontal alveolar ridge defect, implanted with rhBMP-2 combined with DFDBA rehydrated in autologous blood.

Fig 11-8b Transmucosal dental implant placed in the rhBMP-2–induced alveolar ridge 8 weeks postsurgery.

Fig 11-8c Second transmucosal dental implant placed in the rhBMP-2–induced alveolar ridge 16 weeks postsurgery.

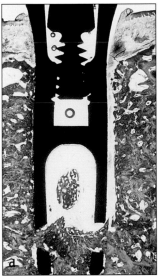

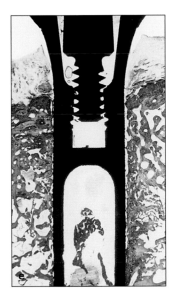

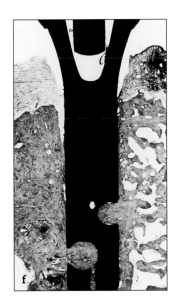

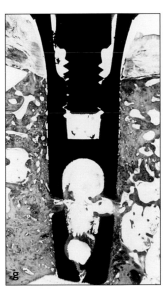

Figs 11-8d to 11-8g Implants placed at week 8 and allowed to osseointegrate for 16 weeks (*d and e*); implants placed at week 16 and allowed to osseointegrate for 8 weeks (*f and g*). Approximately 90% of the bone-anchoring surface of the implants is housed in rhBMP-2–induced bone that exhibits limited evidence of crestal resorption. There is no significant difference in bone density between rhBMP-2–induced bone and the contiguous resident bone. Osseointegration (approximately 55%) is similar in induced and resident bone, irrespective of whether the implants were placed at week 8 or 16 (Stevenel blue and von Gieson picro fuchsin stain). (Figs 11-8a to 11-8g from Sigurdsson et al.[57] Reprinted with permission.)

Alternative delivery technologies

Two recent studies have evaluated BMP technologies that exhibit structural integrity for dentoalveolar onlay indications.[57,58] In one study, it was shown that rhBMP-2 in a DFDBA/fibrin clot carrier might have substantial clinical utility to augment demanding alveolar ridge defects, allowing placement and osseointegration of endosseous dental implants.[57] In a canine model, bilateral critical-sized horizontal alveolar ridge defects were surgically created and received an rhBMP-2/DFDBA/fibrin onlay (Fig 11-8a). Nonsubmerged 10-mm dental implants were placed in the rhBMP-2–induced alveolar ridge 8 and 16 weeks after placement of the onlay (Figs 11-8b and 11-8c).

The defect sites were subjected to histometric evaluation following a 24-week healing interval (Figs 11-8d to 11-8g). Approximately 90% of the bone-anchoring surface of the implants was invested in rhBMP-2 induced bone. Similar levels of bone-to-implant contact (approximately 55%) were observed in induced and resident bone, irrespective of the osseointegration interval (8 or

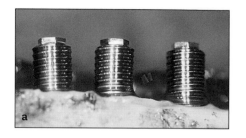

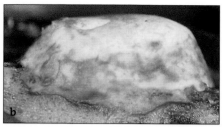

Fig 11-9a Critical-sized, 5-mm, supra-alveolar peri-implant defect, to be treated with rhBMP-2 in a calcium phosphate cement (α-BSM, Etex) or with α-BSM without rhBMP-2 (control).

Fig 11-9b Defect after application of rhBMP-2/α-BSM and prior to wound closure.

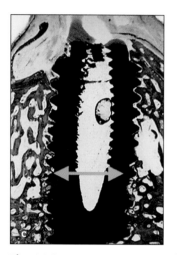

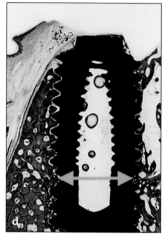

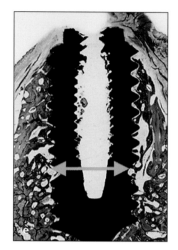

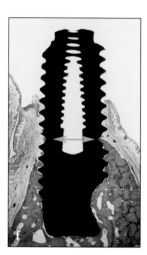

Figs 11-9c to 11-9e Representative observations at 16 weeks for jaw quadrants receiving rhBMP-2/α-BSM, with rhBMP-2 at 0.40 mg/mL or 0.75 mg/mL. The rhBMP-2–induced bone exhibits trabeculation, osseointegration, and cortex formation similar to the contiguous resident bone. There is no evidence of residual biomaterial. There are no appreciable differences in bone formation based on rhBMP-2 concentrations (Stevenel blue and von Gieson picro fuchsin stain). *(arrows)* Apical extension of the supra-alveolar peri-implant defects.

Fig 11-9f Control site at 16 weeks, exhibiting limited, if any, evidence of new bone formation (Stevenel blue and von Gieson picro fuchsin stain). *(arrows)* Apical extension of the supra-alveolar peri-implant defects. (Figs 11-9a to 11-9f from Wikesjö et al.[58] Reprinted with permission.)

16 weeks). There was no significant difference in bone density between rhBMP-2–induced and resident bone. Nonetheless, the use of cadaver-sourced biomaterials such as DFDBA may have difficulty receiving public acceptance; thus, synthetic carrier technologies for alveolar indications must be explored.

In a separate study, rhBMP-2 in a calcium phosphate cement matrix (α-BSM) was shown to be an effective protocol for alveolar ridge augmentation and immediate dental implant osseointegration.[58] Critical-sized supra-alveolar peri-implant defects were created in dogs (Fig 11-9a). Contralateral jaw quadrants received rhBMP-2/α-BSM using two concentrations of rhBMP-2, 0.40 and 0.75 mg/mL (Fig 11-9b). Control defects received α-BSM without rhBMP-2.

The defect sites were subjected to histometric evaluation following a 16-week healing interval. The combination of rhBMP-2 and α-BSM induced clinically relevant augmentation of the alveolar ridge (Figs 11-9c to 11-9e). Control sites exhibited limited bone formation (Fig 11-9f). Vertical bone augmentation encompassed almost the entire 5-mm exposed implant; the newly formed bone exhibited bone density of approximately 60% (type II bone), an established cortex, and bone-to-implant contact of approximately 27%.

This novel technology shows considerable promise for a number of clinical indications, because α-BSM may easily be shaped to desirable contour before setting to provide space for rhBMP-2–induced bone formation. Moreover, as discussed previously, α-BSM is injectable for inlay and minimally invasive indications. The material may well prove to be a significant technology for augmentation of the maxillary sinus in conjunction with placement of dental implants in the posterior maxilla, predictably pinpointing bone formation to the implant body.

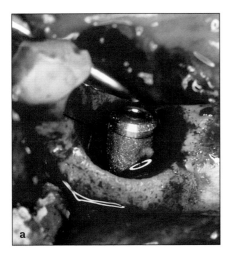 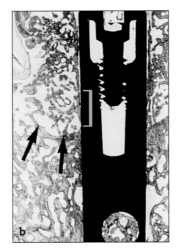 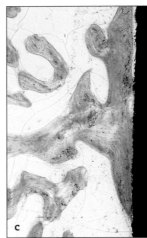

Fig 11-10a Debrided peri-implantitis defect prior to treatment with rhBMP-2/ACS. *(arrow)* Aspect of the implant shown in Figs 11-10b and 11-10c.

Fig 11-10b Healing at 16 weeks. *(arrows)* Apical aspect of the peri-implantitis defect. *(green bracket)* Area depicted in Fig 11-10c.

Fig 11-10c Higher magnification (polarized light) showing reosseointegration. The rhBMP-2–induced bone exhibits qualities of the contiguous resident bone. (Figs 11-10a to 11-10c from Hanisch et al.[59] Reprinted with permission.)

Peri-implantitis and reosseointegration

It has also been shown that rhBMP-2 supports significant reosseointegration of endosseous implants exposed to peri-implantitis.[59,60] The application of rhBMP-2/ACS resulted in bone fill and reosseointegration in advanced bone defects resulting from peri-implantitis. Ligature-induced peri-implantitis lesions were created around hydroxyapatite-coated titanium implants in the posterior mandible and maxilla over 11 months in a nonhuman primate model. Induced peri-implantitis lesions exhibited a microbiota similar to that of advanced human peri-implantitis and periodontal disease as well as a complex, vertical-horizontal defect morphology. At reconstruction, the defects were surgically debrided and the implant surfaces were properly cleaned prior to surgical placement of rhBMP-2/ACS (Fig 11-10a). Control defects received buffer/ACS.

Histometric analysis following a 16-week healing interval revealed that vertical bone gain was three-fold greater in rhBMP-2–treated sites than in control sites. Sites treated with rhBMP-2 exhibited convincing evidence of reosseointegration (Figs 11-10b and 11-10c). The results of this challenging nonhuman primate model suggest that surgical implantation of rhBMP-2 may have considerable clinical utility in the reconstruction of peri-implantitis defects and alveolar defects of lesser complexity.

Functional loading of rhBMP-2–induced bone

Functional loading is a decisive test for any technology aimed at alveolar augmentation in support of the osseointegration of dental implants. A recent study indeed established that rhBMP-2 induces normal physiologic bone, allowing the installation, osseointegration, and long-term functional loading of endosseous dental implants.[61] Mandibular full-thickness, 15 × 10–mm, saddle-type defects were surgically created in canine alveolar ridges (Fig 11-11a). The defects were immediately treated with rhBMP-2/ACS (Fig 11-11b). Healing was allowed to progress for 12 weeks, when endosseous dental implants were placed into rhBMP-2–induced and adjacent resident bone (Figs 11-11c and 11-11d). After 16 weeks of osseointegration,

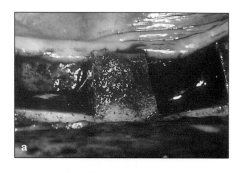

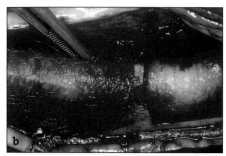

Fig 11-11a Surgically induced mandibular, saddle-type (approximately 15 × 10–mm) alveolar ridge defects. The defects are to be treated with rhBMP-2/ACS and restored with implants subjected to 12 months of functional loading.

Fig 11-11b Defect immediately treated with rhBMP-2/ACS.

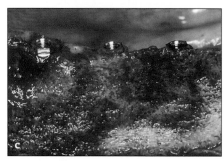

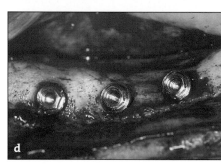

Figs 11-11c and 11-11d Healing at 3 months, when endosseous dental implants were placed in the rhBMP-2/ACS–induced bone and in the resident bone between the defect sites (control).

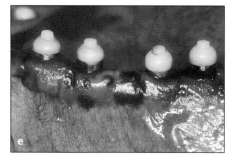

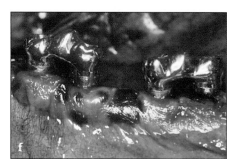

Fig 11-11e Placement of abutments following 4 months of osseointegration.

Fig 11-11f Implants with prosthetic reconstruction.

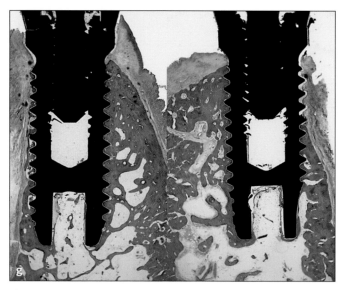

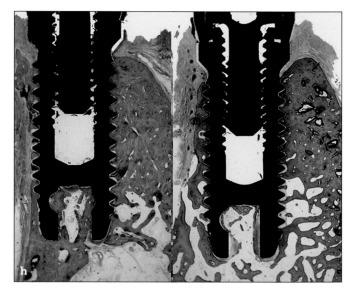

Figs 11-11g and 11-11h Implants placed in rhBMP-2–induced (*left*) and resident bone (*right*) following 12 months of functional loading. There is no discernable difference in bone formation or osseointegration between rhBMP-2–induced and resident bone. (Figs 11-11a to 11-11h from Jovanovic et al.[61] Reprinted with permission.)

the implants received abutments and prosthetic reconstruction (Figs 11-11e and 11-11f).

The reconstructed implants were then exposed to functional loading over 12 months, at which time the defect sites were subjected to a histometric analysis (Figs 11-11g and 11-11h). The rhBMP-2–induced bone exhibited features of the resident bone, including an established cortex. Implants placed in rhBMP-2–induced or resident bone and exposed to functional loading for 12 months all exhibited some crestal resorption. All implants exhibited clinically relevant osseointegration. There were no significant differences between implants placed in rhBMP-2–induced and those placed in resident bone, for any parameter evaluated. Although previous preclinical studies convincingly demonstrated clinically relevant alveolar bone augmentation following surgical implantation of rhBMP-2 and implant osseointegration, this study first showed the functional utility of rhBMP-2–induced bone in implant dentistry.

Clinical Evaluations

Large, controlled clinical studies evaluating rhBMP-2/ACS have resulted in its approval as InFuse bone graft (Medtronic Sofamor Danek) in the United States and as InductOs (Medtronic Sofamor Danek) in Europe for particular indications. Clinical studies evaluating rhBMP-2/ACS for sinus floor augmentation and extraction socket defect repair are detailed in chapter 13 of this volume as well as in the literature.[62–64] As a basis for these clinical programs, preclinical studies demonstrated the ability of rhBMP-2/ACS to induce clinically relevant amounts of bone for sinus floor augmentation[65,66] as well as in extraction sockets.[67] In addition, as discussed earlier, several preclinical studies demonstrated the ability of the bone induced by rhBMP-2/ACS to allow placement and loading of endosseous dental implants as well as to achieve successful osseointegration.[56,59,61,68,69]

The efficacy of rhBMP-2/ACS in interbody spinal fusion has been evaluated in several clinical studies.[70–74] In this application, the off-the-shelf rhBMP-2/ACS material is placed within titanium spinal fusion cages to generate bone that creates the arthrodesis; this eliminates the need for autogenous bone grafts, commonly harvested from the iliac crest. These studies demonstrated that the fusion rates are at least equivalent between patients treated with InFuse and those treated with autogenous bone grafts. The rhBMP-2/ACS treatment group required significantly shorter operating room time, experienced less blood loss, and reported less hip pain; these results could be expected because they did not experience a second surgery site to harvest autogenous bone. These studies led to approval for the use of InFuse for interbody spinal fusions in combination with fusion cages.

An international study with 450 patients evaluated the ability of rhBMP-2/ACS to accelerate and assure fracture healing in open tibial shaft fractures.[75] Compared with standard of care, InFuse resulted in a more than 40% reduction in the number of secondary interventions needed because of nonunions as well as less invasive procedures and significantly faster fracture healing. This study resulted in its approval for treatment of acute open tibial shaft fractures. InFuse has also been studied in combination with allograft in tibial fractures associated with segmental bone loss.[76] In this study, InFuse performed similarly to the current standard, autogenous bone graft, again eliminating the need for the secondary surgical procedure.

A clinical study has also been performed with rhBMP-2 combined with compression-resistant matrix (CRM) for posterolateral spinal fusion.[73] At 24 months, the fusion rate in the iliac crest bone graft control group was lower than that in the rhBMP-2/CRM group. Similar to the findings in other clinical studies, the operative time was shorter and there was less blood loss in the rhBMP-2/CRM group than in the autogenous bone graft group.

Conclusion

rhBMP-2, the recombinant form of a naturally occurring protein involved in bone formation and repair, is the bioactive component of several tissue engineering constructs. Extensive basic research has clarified the mechanisms of action of rhBMP-2 at the molecular, cellular, and organism levels. As a differentiation factor, it binds to cell surface receptors on responsive mesenchymal precursor cells, causing them to become bone- and cartilage-forming cells. This activity translates in vivo to the ability of rhBMP-2 to induce the formation of host bone, whether placed in bone or soft tissue sites, in inlay or onlay applications, or in small or large defects.

Through applied preclinical research, the potential applications of rhBMP-2 have been evaluated, and practical use of this technology has been optimized. Comparison with current bone regenerative technologies such as DFDBA and barrier membranes has revealed the substantial capacity of rhBMP-2 to generate bone.

The carrier or matrix used with rhBMP-2 contributes practically and biologically to where the tissue engineering construct may be best used. For example, resorbable materials allow the induced bone to function as normal bone without hindrance from nonbiologic residual materials. An absorbable collagen sponge has many advantageous qualities as a carrier for rhBMP-2, and many studies evaluating rhBMP-2/ACS in inlay and onlay applications where soft tissue compression is minimized have demonstrated successful bone induction, ability to place dental implants, and osseointegration that allows functional loading of the implants. In other applications, it may compress and require the use of devices or additional materials to provide sufficient space for an optimal volume of bone to be formed. However, while barrier membranes may aid in definition of the shape of the bone that is formed, occlusive membranes appear to provide limited benefit to the use of rhBMP-2. Additional carriers continue to be developed to expand the clinical utility of rhBMP-2.

Clinical studies, including dose-ranging and large, controlled pivotal studies, have demonstrated the ability of rhBMP-2/ACS (InFuse/InductOs) to induce bone, repair tooth extraction socket defects, augment the maxilla in sinus augmentation procedures, successfully induce spinal arthrodesis in interbody spinal procedures, and accelerate and ensure acute tibial fracture repair. In aggregate, studies indicate that rhBMP-2/ACS is an alternative or replacement for bone graft. Additional clinical studies continue to evaluate rhBMP-2 in combination with other materials for further potential applications.

References

1. Urist MR. Bone: Formation by autoinduction. Science 1965;150:893–899.
2. Wang EA, Rosen V, Cordes P, et al. Purification and characterization of other distinct bone-inducing factors. Proc Natl Acad Sci U S A 1988;85:9484–9488.
3. Wozney JM, Rosen V, Celeste AJ, et al. Novel regulators of bone formation: Molecular clones and activities. Science 1988;242:1528–1534.
4. Özkaynak E, Rueger DC, Drier EA, et al. OP-1 cDNA encodes an osteogenic protein in the TGF-β family. EMBO J 1990;9:2085–2093.
5. Celeste AJ, Iannazzi JA, Taylor RC, et al. Identification of transforming growth factor β family members present in bone-inductive protein purified from bovine bone. Proc Natl Acad Sci U.S.A 1990;87:9843–9847.
6. Scheufler C, Sebald W, Hulsmeyer M. Crystal structure of human bone morphogenetic protein-2 at 2.7. A resolution. J Mol Biol 1999;287:103–115.
7. Israel DI, Nove J, Kerns KM, et al. Heterodimeric bone morphogenetic proteins show enhanced activity in vitro and in vivo. Growth Factors 1996;13:291–300.
8. Israel DI, Nove J, Kerns KM, Moutsatsos IK, Kaufman RJ. Expression and characterization of bone morphogenetic protein-2 in Chinese hamster ovary cells. Growth Factors 1992;7:139–150.
9. Miyazono K, Kusanagi K, Inoue H. Divergence and convergence of TGF-beta/BMP signaling. J Cell Physiol 2001;187:265–276.
10. Shore EM, Xu M, Feldman GJ, et al. A recurrent mutation in the BMP type I receptor ACVR1 causes inherited and sporadic fibrodysplasia ossificans progressiva. Nat Genet 2006;38:525–527 [erratum 2007;39:276].
11. Kirsch T, Sebald W, Dreyer MK. Crystal structure of the BMP-2-BRIA ectodomain complex. Nat Struct Biol 2000;7:492–496.
12. Nickel J, Dreyer MK, Kirsch T, Sebald W. The crystal structure of the BMP-2:BMPR-IA complex and the generation of BMP-2 antagonists. J Bone Joint Surg Am 2001;83A(suppl 1):S7–14.
13. Allendorph GP, Vale WW, Choe S. Structure of the ternary signaling complex of a TGF-beta superfamily member. Proc Natl Acad Sci U S A 2006;103:7643–7648.
14. Hassel S, Schmitt S, Hartung A, et al. Initiation of Smad-dependent and Smad-independent signaling via distinct BMP-receptor complexes. J Bone Joint Surg Am 2003;85A(suppl 3):44–51.
15. Nohe A, Hassel S, Ehrlich M, et al. The mode of bone morphogenetic protein (BMP) receptor oligomerization determines different BMP-2 signaling pathways. J Biol Chem 2002;277:5330–5338.
16. Miyazono K. Signal transduction by bone morphogenetic protein receptors: Functional roles of Smad proteins. Bone 1999;25:91–93.
17. Miyazono K, Maeda S, Imamura T. BMP receptor signaling: Transcriptional targets, regulation of signals, and signaling cross-talk. Cytokine Growth Factor Rev 2005;16:251–263.
18. Feng XH, Derynck R. Specificity and versatility in TGF-beta signaling through Smads. Annu Rev Cell Dev Biol 2005;21:659–693.
19. Cochran DL, Wozney JM. Biological mediators for periodontal regeneration. Periodontol 2000 1999;19:40–58.
20. Thies RS, Bauduy M, Ashton BA, et al. Recombinant human bone morphogenetic protein-2 induces osteoblastic differentiation in W-20-17 stromal cells. Endocrinology 1992;130:1318–1324.
21. Katagiri T, Yamaguchi A, Ikeda T, et al. The non-osteogenic mouse pluripotent cell line, C3H10T1/2, is induced to differentiate into osteoblastic cells by recombinant human bone morphogenetic protein-2. Biochem Biophys Res Commun 1990;172:295–299.
22. Rosen V, Nove J, Song JJ, et al. Responsiveness of clonal limb bud cell lines to bone morphogenetic protein 2 reveals a sequential relationship between cartilage and bone cell phenotypes. J Bone Miner Res 1994;9:1759–1768.
23. Katagiri T, Yamaguchi A, Komaki M, et al. Bone morphogenetic protein-2 converts the differentiation pathway of C2C12 myoblasts into the osteoblast lineage. J Cell Biol 1994;127:1755–1766.
24. Toriumi DM, Kotler HS, Luxenberg DP, Holtrop ME, Wang EA. Mandibular reconstruction with a recombinant bone-inducing factor. Arch Otolaryngol Head Neck Surg 1991;117:1101–1112.
25. Toriumi DM, O'Grady K, Horlbeck DM, et al. Mandibular reconstruction using bone morphogenetic protein 2: Long-term follow-up in a canine model. Laryngoscope 1999;109:1481–1489.
26. Wang EA, Rosen V, D'Alessandro JS, et al. Recombinant human bone morphogenetic protein induces bone formation. Proc Natl Acad Sci U S A 1990;87:2220–2224.
27. Seeherman H. The influence of delivery vehicles and their properties on the repair of segmental defects and fractures with osteogenic factors. J Bone Joint Surg Am 2001;83A(suppl 1):S79–S81.
28. Seeherman H, Li R, Bouxsein M, et al. rhBMP-2/calcium phosphate matrix accelerates osteotomy-site healing in a nonhuman primate model at multiple treatment times and concentrations. J Bone Joint Surg Am 2006;88:144–160.
29. Seeherman H, Wozney J, Li R. Bone morphogenetic protein delivery systems. Spine 2002;27:S16–S23.
30. Seeherman H, Wozney JM. Delivery of bone morphogenetic proteins for orthopedic tissue regeneration. Cytokine Growth Factor Rev 2005;16:329–345.
31. Einhorn TA, Majeska RJ, Mohaideen A, et al. A single percutaneous injection of recombinant human bone morphogenetic protein-2 accelerates fracture repair. J Bone Joint Surg Am 2003;85A:1425–1435.

32. Hsu HP, Zanella JM, Peckham SM, Spector M. Comparing ectopic bone growth induced by rhBMP-2 on an absorbable collagen sponge in rat and rabbit models. J Orthop Res 2006;24:1660–1669.

33. Li RH, Wozney JM. Delivering on the promise of bone morphogenetic proteins. Trends Biotechnol 2001;19:255–265.

34. Kenley R, Marden L, Turek T, et al. Osseous regeneration in the rat calvarium using novel delivery systems for recombinant human bone morphogenetic protein-2 (rhBMP-2). J Biomed Mater Res 1994;28:1139–1147.

35. Smith JL, Jin L, Parsons T, et al. Osseous regeneration in preclinical models using bioabsorbable delivery technology for recombinant human bone morphogenetic protein 2 (rhBMP-2). J Control Release 1995;36:183–195.

36. Bragdon CR, Doherty AM, Rubash HE, et al. The efficacy of BMP-2 to induce bone ingrowth in a total hip replacement model. Clin Orthop Relat Res 2003;Dec(417):50–61.

37. Edwards RB, III, Seeherman HJ, Bogdanske JJ, et al. Percutaneous injection of recombinant human bone morphogenetic protein-2 in a calcium phosphate paste accelerates healing of a canine tibial osteotomy. J Bone Joint Surg Am 2004;86A:1425–1438.

38. Li RH, Bouxsein ML, Blake CA, et al. rhBMP-2 injected in a calcium phosphate paste (α-BSM) accelerates healing in the rabbit ulnar osteotomy model. J Orthop Res 2003;21:997–1004.

39. Seeherman HJ, Bouxsein M, Kim H, et al. Recombinant human bone morphogenetic protein-2 delivered in an injectable calcium phosphate paste accelerates osteotomy-site healing in a nonhuman primate model. J Bone Joint Surg Am 2004;86A:1961–1972.

40. Seeherman HJ, Azari K, Bidic S, et al. rhBMP-2 delivered in a calcium phosphate cement accelerates bridging of critical-sized defects in rabbit radii. J Bone Joint Surg Am 2006;88:1553–1565.

41. Takahashi D, Odajima T, Morita M, Kawanami M, Kato H. Formation and resolution of ankylosis under application of recombinant human bone morphogenetic protein-2 (rhBMP-2) to class III furcation defects in cats. J Periodontal Res 2005;40:299–305.

42. Ueki K, Takazakura D, Marukawa K, et al. The use of polylactic acid/polyglycolic acid copolymer and gelatin sponge complex containing human recombinant bone morphogenetic protein-2 following condylectomy in rabbits. J Craniomaxillofac Surg 2003;31:107–114.

43. Itoh T, Mochizuki M, Nishimura R, et al. Repair of ulnar segmental defect by recombinant human bone morphogenetic protein-2 in dogs. J Vet Med Sci 1998; 60:451–458.

44. Kokubo S, Mochizuki M, Fukushima S, et al. Long-term stability of bone tissues induced by an osteoinductive biomaterial, recombinant human bone morphogenetic protein-2 and a biodegradable carrier. Biomaterials 2004;25:1795–1803.

45. Marukawa E, Asahina I, Oda M, et al. Functional reconstruction of the non human primate mandible using recombinant human bone morphogenetic protein 2. Int J Oral Maxillofac Surg 2002;31:287–295.

46. Martin GJ Jr, Boden SD, Marone MA, Moskovitz PA. Posterolateral intertransverse process spinal arthrodesis with rhBMP-2 in a nonhuman primate: Important lessons learned regarding dose, carrier, and safety. J Spinal Disord 1999;12: 179–186.

47. Akamaru T, Suh D, Boden SD, et al. Simple carrier matrix modifications can enhance delivery of recombinant human bone morphogenetic protein-2 for posterolateral spine fusion. Spine 2003;28:429–434.

48. Barnes B, Boden SD, Louis-Ugbo J, et al. Lower dose of rhBMP-2 achieves spine fusion when combined with an osteoconductive bulking agent in non-human primates. Spine 2005;30:1127–1133.

49. Suh DY, Boden SD, Louis-Ugbo J, et al. Delivery of recombinant human bone morphogenetic protein-2 using a compression-resistant matrix in posterolateral spine fusion in the rabbit and in the non-human primate. Spine 2002;27: 353–360.

50. Wikesjö UME, Sorensen RG, Wozney JM. Augmentation of alveolar bone and dental implant osseointegration: Clinical implications of studies with rhBMP-2. J Bone Joint Surg Am 2001;83A(suppl 1):S136–S145.

51. Sigurdsson TJ, Fu E, Tatakis DN, Rohrer MD, Wikesjö UME. Bone morphogenetic protein-2 for peri-implant bone regeneration and osseointegration. Clin Oral Implants Res 1997;8:367–374.

52. Caplanis N, Sigurdsson TJ, Rohrer MD, Wikesjö UME. Effect of allogeneic, freeze-dried, demineralized bone matrix on guided bone regeneration in supra-alveolar peri-implant defects in dogs. Int J Oral Maxillofac Implants 1997;12:634–642.

53. Wikesjö UME, Qahash M, Thomson RC, et al. Space-providing expanded polytetrafluoroethylene devices define alveolar augmentation at dental implants induced by recombinant human bone morphogenetic protein 2 in an absorbable collagen sponge carrier. Clin Implant Dent Relat Res 2003;5:112–123.

54. Wikesjö UME, Qahash M, Thomson RC, et al. rhBMP-2 significantly enhances guided bone regeneration. Clin Oral Implants Res 2004;15:194–204.

55. Tatakis DN, Koh A, Jin L, et al. Peri-implant bone regeneration using recombinant human bone morphogenetic protein-2 in a canine model: a dose-response study. J Periodontal Res 2002;37:93–100.

56. Jovanovic SA, Hunt DR, Bernard GW, Spiekermann H, Wozney JM, Wikesjö UME. Bone reconstruction following implantation of rhBMP-2 and guided bone regeneration in canine alveolar ridge defects. Clin Oral Implants Res 2007;8:224–230.

57. Sigurdsson TJ, Nguyen S, Wikesjö UM. Alveolar ridge augmentation with rhBMP-2 and bone-to-implant contact in induced bone. Int J Periodontics Restorative Dent 2001;21:461–473.

58. Wikesjö UME, Sorensen RG, Kinoshita A, Wozney JM. rhBMP-2/alphaBSM induces significant vertical alveolar ridge augmentation and dental implant osseointegration. Clin Implant Dent Relat Res 2002;4:174–182.

59. Hanisch O, Tatakis DN, Boskovic MM, Rohrer MD, Wikesjö UME. Bone formation and reosseointegration in peri-implantitis defects following surgical implantation of rhBMP-2. Int J Oral Maxillofac Implants 1997;12:604–610.

60. Hanisch O, Cortella CA, Boskovic MM, et al. Experimental peri-implant tissue breakdown around hydroxyapatite-coated implants. J Periodontol 1997;68: 59–66.

61. Jovanovic SA, Hunt DR, Bernard GW, et al. Long-term functional loading of dental implants in rhBMP-2 induced bone. A histologic study in the canine ridge augmentation model. Clin Oral Implants Res 2003;14:793–803.

62. Boyne PJ, Marx RE, Nevins M, et al. A feasibility study evaluating rhBMP-2/absorbable collagen sponge for maxillary sinus floor augmentation. Int J Periodontics Restorative Dent 1997;17:10–25.

63. Boyne PJ, Lilly LC, Marx RE, et al. De novo bone induction by recombinant human bone morphogenetic protein-2 (rhBMP-2) in maxillary sinus floor augmentation. J Oral Maxillofac Surg 2005;63:1693–1707.

64. Fiorellini JP, Howell TH, Cochran D, et al. Randomized study evaluating recombinant human bone morphogenetic protein-2 for extraction socket augmentation. J Periodontol 2005;76:605–613.

65. Nevins M, Kirker-Head C, Wozney JM, Palmer R, Graham D. Bone formation in the goat maxillary sinus induced by absorbable collagen sponge implants impregnated with recombinant human bone morphogenetic protein-2. Int J Periodontics Restorative Dent 1996;16:9–19.

66. Hanisch O, Tatakis DN, Rohrer MD, et al. Bone formation and osseointegration stimulated by rhBMP-2 following subantral augmentation procedures in nonhuman primates. Int J Oral Maxillofac Implants 1997;12:785–792.

67. Cochran DL, Schenk R, Buser D, Wozney JM, Jones AA. Recombinant human bone morphogenetic protein-2 stimulation of bone formation around endosseous dental implants. J Periodontol 1999;70:139–150.

68. Boyne PJ, Nakamura A, Shabahang S. Evaluation of the long-term effect of function on rhBMP-2 regenerated hemimandibulectomy defects. Br J Oral Maxillofac Surg 1999;37:344–352.

69. Boyne PJ, Salina S, Nakamura A, Audia F, Shabahang S. Bone regeneration using rhBMP-2 induction in hemimandibulectomy type defects of elderly sub-human primates. Cell Tissue Bank 2006;7:1–10.

70. Burkus JK, Heim SE, Gornet MF, Zdeblick TA. Is INFUSE bone graft superior to autograft bone? An integrated analysis of clinical trials using the LT-CAGE lumbar tapered fusion device. J Spinal Disord Tech 2003;16:113–122.

71. Burkus JK, Dorchak JD, Sanders DL. Radiographic assessment of interbody fusion using recombinant human bone morphogenetic protein type 2. Spine 2003; 28:372–377.

72. Burkus JK, Transfeldt EE, Kitchel SH, Watkins RG, Balderston RA. Clinical and radiographic outcomes of anterior lumbar interbody fusion using recombinant human bone morphogenetic protein-2. Spine 2002;27:2396 2408.

73. Dimar JR, Glassman SD, Burkus KJ, Carreon LY. Clinical outcomes and fusion success at 2 years of single-level instrumented posterolateral fusions with recombinant human bone morphogenetic protein-2/compression resistant matrix versus iliac crest bone graft. Spine 2006;31:2534–2539.

74. McKay B, Sandhu HS. Use of recombinant human bone morphogenetic protein-2 in spinal fusion applications. Spine 2002;27:S66–S85.

75. Govender S, Csimma C, Genant HK, et al. Recombinant human bone morphogenetic protein-2 for treatment of open tibial fractures: A prospective, controlled, randomized study of four hundred and fifty patients. J Bone Joint Surg Am 2002;84A:2123–2134.

76. Jones AL, Bucholz RW, Bosse MJ, et al. Recombinant human BMP-2 and allograft compared with autogenous bone graft for reconstruction of diaphyseal tibial fractures with cortical defects. A randomized, controlled trial. J Bone Joint Surg Am 2006;88:1431–1441.

12

Osseous Regeneration with rhBMP-2

Joseph P. Fiorellini, DMD, DMSc
N. Guzin Uzel, DMD, DMSc
Julio Sekler, DMD, MMSc

Over the past century, the evolution of medical and dental technologies has altered the practice of health care. Discoveries such as antibiotics and aseptic surgical techniques have extended the human life span and resulted in a better quality of life for many individuals. During the past several years, biotechnological developments have again begun to change the paradigm of patient care. One of these technologies has been the evolution of biomimetics, including devices that replace anatomic structures and compounds that promote the in vitro or in vivo development of organ systems.

In dentistry, the goal has been to develop effective substitutes or replacements for bone, dentin, enamel, cementum, and the periodontal ligament. Approaches to achieving this objective will likely involve three complementary strategies:

1. Utilization of stem cells and their linkages to regenerate missing or damaged tissues in vitro or in vivo. This has required research focused on isolating and characterizing the relevant progenitor cells and then devising methodologies for introducing such cells into the appro-

priate body site to replicate the developmental events and thereby reconstitute missing or damaged tissues.
2. Development of new classes of biomaterials that may be either biologically derived or wholly synthetic. In either case, the aim has been to provide a definitive tissue replacement or, alternatively, to provide a matrix to facilitate natural tissue ingrowth and remodeling by directing natural repair and regeneration.
3. Development of innovative physical and chemical stimuli to induce existing adult tissues to regenerate missing or damaged body parts.

Underlying all three strategies is a need to understand tissue structure and properties at cell, tissue, and organ levels, and most certainly at the molecular level. Especially important will be an improved understanding of interfaces between cells, between cells and matrices, between differing matrices and cells, and between matrix and mineral. Interfaces between organic and inorganic compounds must be more thoroughly elucidated to determine the environment needed for physiologic calcification and to achieve new approaches to tissue design. In addition to the biologic engineering considerations, an improved understanding of factors that affect regeneration and repair of tissues, including nutrients, hormones, age, and sex, is required.

The implications for dentistry are just being realized. The repair or regeneration of structures lost to disease has been one of the first applications of this technology. An example of this is regrowth of osseous and periodontal structures. Conventional procedures most often involve the use of barrier membranes to foster selective cell repopulation and regrowth of osseous structures. Because the predictability of these techniques may be limited to certain case types, efforts have begun to investigate the possibility of harnessing osseous regrowth potential via a molecular approach. Several potent biologic mediators that promote many of the events in wound healing have been identified; among these are the bone morphogenetic proteins (BMPs). The purpose of this chapter is to review published data about recombinant human BMP-2 (rhBMP-2), one of the most studied growth factor therapies to have a potential impact in clinical dentistry.

Evaluation of Delivery Systems

The therapeutic efficacy of growth factors seems to be affected by the carrier or delivery system. Ideally, a carrier should localize the protein spatially and temporally for regional requirements. In addition, carriers must be safe, bioresorbable, and not impair the effects of the proteins. At the same time, delivery materials should support angiogenesis.[1,2] Additional characteristics of the carrier should include structural integrity, absence of immunogenicity, and proper release kinetics. Although the carrier may not be essential for efficacy, it could provide the advantage of protein immobilization, define the shape of the resulting structures, and to a lesser extent reduce the total protein dose for efficacy by its localization effect.

In the majority of studies, insoluble matrices, including demineralized bone and hydroxyapatite, have been used.[3–6] Parallel with these investigations, several studies with absorbable collagen sponges (ACSs) and methylcelloluse gels have been completed.[7,8]

Specific studies on the influence of different carriers on the in vivo effects of rhBMP-2 have been completed.[9–12] In these studies, the pharmacokinetics of radiolabeled

rhBMP-2, in combination with ACS, human demineralized bone, bovine bone mineral, polyglycolic acid matrix, 100% tricalcium phosphate (TCP) matrix, and others were studied to determine their efficacy in protein retention and the relationship of this retention to bone induction activity in an ectopic site. The carriers were chosen based on their compositional similarities to materials that had been used in previous bone generation experiments.[9]

The carriers were soaked with rhBMP-2 obtained from Chinese hamster ovary cells 30 minutes prior to subcutaneous implantation in Long-Evans rats. The implant-retained radioactivity was used as a measure of rhBMP-2 within the implant. The results indicated that the amount of radioactivity retained within the implant after 3 hours was dependent on the matrix. The ACS appeared to retain the highest amount of radioactivity (75%), and the lowest radioactivity (10%) was retained in synthetic hydroxyapatite.[9]

In a study course of 14 days, the ACS also showed higher retention levels of rhBMP-2 than any other carrier.[9] The amount of retained protein was positively correlated to the amount of bone induced.[10]

Further in vitro studies were done on ACS as a carrier to determine the in vivo effects of certain changes inflicted, demonstrating that cross-linking of the sponge, or its succinylation and/or sterilization with ethylene oxide, affects the retention of protein within the carrier and the successful induction of bone.[11]

Evaluation in Animal Models

Defect repair

rhBMP-2 has been extensively studied at the preclinical level. In long-bone animal models, several experiments with nonunion fractures have been conducted. Yasko et al[13] created 5-mm segmental defects in the femurs of 45 adult male Sprague-Dawley rats to test the osteoinductive activity of rhBMP-2. Two doses of lyophilized rhBMP-2 in a collagenous matrix carrier were implanted in each defect, and results were compared with those in rats that received implantation of matrix only. Both doses of rhBMP-2 induced formation of endochondral bone in the osseous defects in a dose-related manner. In the defects treated with the matrix, no instances of union were observed. The same principle has been applied in other long-bone defect models in various animal species.[14]

In the craniofacial area, the majority of the animal models have been based on critical-sized defects, located mainly in the calvarial zone. These created or naturally occurring defects do not heal without intervention or treatment.

Urist et al[15] implanted a BMP/TCP composite in adult dogs with skull trephine defects of the critical size of 1.4 cm. The BMP/TCP implants induced 91% to 100% incorporation by deposits of new bone. In comparison, control implants of TCP impregnated with bovine serum albumin induced 0% to −8% incorporation, or only marginal host bed reactive bone formation.

Ferguson et al,[16] based on the knowledge that large cranial defects do not always heal spontaneously, especially in humans, created bilateral cranial trephine defects, measuring 14 to −20 mm in diameter, in three rhesus monkeys. The defects were treated with bovine BMP alone or with a carrier; control defects received no treatment. The results showed that BMP induced osteogenesis. Other species have been successfully employed with the same principles and results.[4,17,18]

Sinus augmentation

Subantral maxillary sinus augmentation in goats and non-human primates provided a different model that combined orthotopic and heterotopic conditions in one.[7,8,19] The maxillary sinus, besides its normal component turnover, does not create bone per se to fill the cavity; on the contrary, it has a tendency to resorb bone as part of a process called maxillary sinus pneumatization. The sinus membrane grows in a continuous fashion, filling the volume previously occupied by the floor and walls of the sinus osseous components. This study model permitted induced bone formation in the vicinity of native bone, allowing for evaluation of the integration between pre-existing bone and the newly created bone and the effects of loading the new bone with osseointegrated implants. Results showed that rhBMP-2 could be considered a good alternative to traditional bone grafts.

Evaluation in Humans

Defect repair

The success of the treatment in animal models led the way for human models of testing in long-bone segmental defects. Johnson et al[5] treated patients with traumatic segmental 3- to 17-cm tibial defects and developed solid union by implantation of human BMP, autogenous cancellous grafts, and stabilization. There were no allergic, infectious, or surgical complications. In a subsequent investigation, Johnson et al[6] treated different human nonunion defects of the tibia and femur with successful results.

In another early study, Sailer and Kolb[20] applied BMP in conjunction with lyophilized cartilage strips in patients with cranial defects or congenital malformations. Computerized tomography (CT) revealed calcification in the BMP layers as early as a few weeks after implantation. The reconstructed areas had solidified clinically within a few months. This represented an acceleration of the normal calcification process that occurs when lyophilized cartilage is applied alone.

Ridge and sinus augmentation

Over the past several years, two investigations have evaluated the safety and technical feasibility of using rhBMP-2 in humans. Howell et al[21] focused on localized bone regeneration. In this phase I study, a total of 12 patients were treated with a 0.43-mg/mL dose of rhBMP-2 in an absorbable collagen device, 6 for local ridge preservation and 6 for local ridge augmentation. The clinical results suggested that the device was well tolerated locally and systemically, with no adverse events. The absorbable collagen device treated with rhBMP-2 was easy to handle and could be adapted to the ridge or extraction site. Overall, bone fill was observed in all extraction sites treated with the rhBMP-2 device.

In a second study with the same 0.43-mg/mL dosage of rhBMP-2, maxillary sinus augmentations were performed in 12 patients.[22] All patients had insufficient alveolar bone height to support a dental implant. The total implanted dose of rhBMP-2 ranged from 1.77 to 3.40 mg. As in the other study,[21] no serious or unexpected immunologic or adverse events and no clinically significant changes in blood cell counts, blood chemistries, or urinalysis were noted. The overall mean sinus floor augmentation was 8.91 mm, as evaluated by CT. These results may indicate that rhBMP-2 represents an alternative to conventional bone-grafting methods for achieving adequate bone volume for dental implants in the posterior maxilla.

A pivotal investigation[23] studied 80 subjects requiring local alveolar ridge preservation and/or augmentation of buccal wall defects (50% or greater buccal bone loss of the extraction socket) following extraction of maxillary anterior teeth or premolars. Two sequential cohorts of 40 subjects each were randomized in a double-masked manner to receive 0.75 mg/mL (cohort 1) or 1.50 mg/mL (cohort 2) of rhBMP-2/ACS, placebo (ACS alone), or no treatment. In both cohorts, 20 subjects received rhBMP-2, 10 received placebo, and 10 received no treatment.

The efficacy of rhBMP-2/ACS was assessed by changes in alveolar bone height and bone width (three measurements). These measurements were taken from CT scans exposed at baseline (within 4 days following study treatment) and at 4 months following study treatment. In addition, CT scans were used to assess changes in bone density and to determine whether the treated ridge was adequate to support a dental implant. Adequate alveolar bone was defined as 6 mm or more in width at the narrowest point (buccal to palatal) and 12 mm or more in height.

The subjects in the study underwent the same surgical procedure, regardless of the treatment assignment. Following administration of local anesthesia, sulcular and vertical incisions were created to release full-thickness periosteal flaps. The teeth were extracted, and the extraction sockets were debrided. Four to eight perforations of the cortical plates were made with a No. 1/2 round bur. The placebo or rhBMP-2–soaked ACSs were cut into strips and placed to fill the defect sites. A larger strip of material was placed over the entire treatment site. A tension-free soft tissue wound closure was established. In patients who received no treatment, the procedure did not include placement of the rhBMP-2/ACS or ACS.

The results indicated that this novel method to recreate the alveolar ridge to support a dental implant was efficacious (Figs 12-1 and 12-2). The alveolar bone height measurements indicated that the palatal wall of the extraction socket was preserved in subjects in the 1.50-mg/mL group, whereas those in the placebo and no-treatment groups experienced decreases in height. In addition, the bone width near the top of the extraction site increased in all study groups except the no-treatment group. The increase was statistically significant for both active rhBMP-2 treatment groups. The differences in the increases between the 0.75-mg/mL and 1.50-mg/mL groups also were statistically significant.

There was no statistically significant difference in bone density according to treatment groups. Furthermore there was no difference between inducted bone and native bone.

When the adequacy of bone for the placement of a dental implant was analyzed, the number of sites achieving this goal was approximately twice as great in the rhBMP-2/ACS groups compared with the groups receiving no treatment or placebo. A comparison of patients who required a secondary augmentation to allow placement of a dental implant indicated that the group treated with 1.50 mL/mg of rhBMP-2/ACS had significantly fewer procedures.

The histologic cores revealed trabecular bone, the thickness of which was graded as moderate to large (Fig 12-3). Active remodeling was observed. Osteoblasts and osteoclasts were noted. There was normal vascularity, and no evidence of inflammation or residual collagen matrix from the absorbable sponge carrier was identified in any of the specimens.

Findings indicated that the buccal wall extraction defect model used to assess rhBMP-2 was effective. Partial healing was observed in sites treated with the ACS placebo, and no spontaneous bone healing was observed in the no-treatment group. Previous studies involving post-extraction bone resorption rates and histology after uncomplicated extractions indicate similar patterns to the data presented in this investigation.[23]

The rhBMP-2/ACS data in this investigation also indicates a significant enhancement in patient outcomes and several advantages over current therapies:

- Not only was the volume required to place a dental implant restored, but the quantity of bone regeneration at the top of the alveolar crest (75% of the extraction socket length) also optimized dental implant position. When the implant location approaches or is in the natural tooth root position, fabrication of the prosthesis is facilitated, which usually results in lower laboratory and patient costs.
- Current augmentation procedures require advanced surgical skills. The implantation of the rhBMP-2/ACS added no greater complexity to the surgical procedure than the tooth extraction itself.

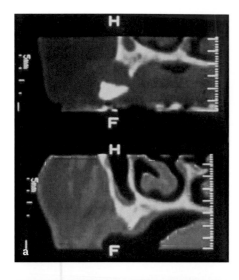

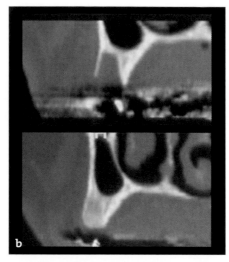

Fig 12-1a Baseline *(top)* and 4-month *(bottom)* CT scans of an extraction site receiving no treatment.

Fig 12-1b Baseline *(top)* and 4-month *(bottom)* CT scans of an extraction site receiving an ACS alone.

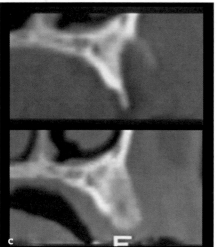

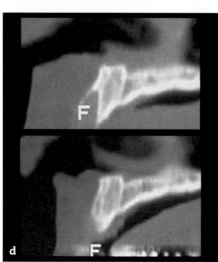

Figs 12-1c and 12-1d Baseline *(top)* and 4-month *(bottom)* CT scans of a site receiving 1.50 mg/mL of rhBMP-2/ACS.

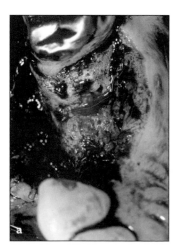

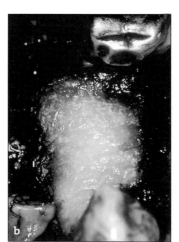

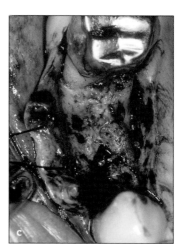

Fig 12-2a Extraction site exhibiting greater than 50% buccal bone height loss.

Fig 12-2b Treatment site with rhBMP-2/ACS contoured to reconstruct the alveolar ridge.

Fig 12-2c Extraction site following 4 months of healing.

Fig 12-3a Histologic section of a site 32 weeks after treatment with 0.75 mg/mL of rhBMP-2/ACS (hematoxylin-eosin stain; original magnification ×10).

Fig 12-3b Histologic section of a site 32 weeks after treatment with demineralized freeze-dried bone allograft (hematoxylin-eosin stain; original magnification ×10).

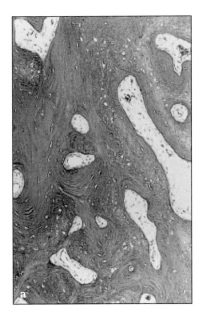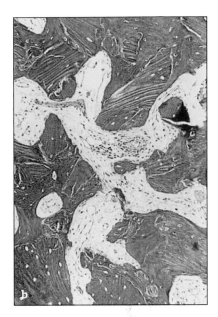

- The patients in this investigation did not experience the postsurgical exposures that can occur with a traditional membrane augmentation. The absence of such complications maximizes the restored bone volume and reduces the number of patient visits.
- The patients did not require harvesting of bone from a secondary site such as the iliac crest, which clearly reduced patient morbidity.
- Clinical safety profiles were similar for all treatment groups, indicating that the rhBMP-2/ACS implantation procedure was no different from a tooth extraction.

Evaluation of Wound-Healing Properties

BMPs of osteoinductive nature may be used to accelerate healing of bony defects. Several animal studies have been conducted to evaluate the osteoinductive effects of BMPs around implants. For instance, the interface between hip implant and bone may decrease implant fixation and eventually lead to loosening. The same issue is also critical in dental implant survival in terms of initial stability. The use of combined recombinant human transforming growth factor β2 (rhTGF-β2) and rhBMP-2 led to greater implant fixation strength in the presence of

interface gaps than the use of either growth factor alone, providing more secure mechanical fixation. The success of this combination reached the level of success obtained with autogenous bone graft.[24]

The osteoinductivity of growth factors and the delivery method of these factors have important effects on the outcome of treatment. Thus, different carriers and technologies have been tested. Once again, animal studies were used for initial evaluation. Histologic analysis of ectopic bone formation in association with implants with calcium phosphate coatings containing BMP-2 was performed. This combination not only induced bone formation but also established it with a very high potency at a low pharmacologic level. Moreover, as expected from an ideal carrier-cytokine combination, the osteogenic activity was sustained for an extended time, which is of great clinical importance for the osseointegration of dental implants.[25] Furthermore, depending on BMP-2 incorporation or adsorption in the calcium phosphate coatings, the osteoconductivity of implant surfaces can be increased.[26,27]

Another carrier of extracellular matrix origin, glycosaminoglycans, was used as implant surface coating in combination with collagen, with and without BMP-4, on miniature pigs that received dental implants. The highest stability was reached with collagen-coated, BMP-4–integrated implants, which were instrumental for peri-implant bone formation.[20] Hydroxyapatite-coated implants with BMP-2 were also used for the same goal. The BMP-2 coating significantly increased bone growth compared with hydroxyapatite-coated implants at 2 and 4 weeks.[29] In addition, the application of BMP-2 with a bioabsorbable bioceramic with fluid permeability characteristics enhanced osteogenic activity.[30] Meanwhile, the application of liposomal vectors carrying BMP-2–complementary DNA directly into freshly created peri-implant bone defects on pig calvaria, with or without autologous bone graft, showed great potential in terms of molecular initiation of bone formation.[31] In this study, the BMP-2 gene was efficiently introduced into osteogenic cells. After only 1 week, BMP-2 protein was detected in the peri-implant bone defect. This stimulation was still active at 4 weeks; BMP-producing cells were still present in the defect and peri-implant area. Therefore, direct application of the BMP-2 gene with a liposomal vector increased bone regeneration and stimulated an early phase of osseointegration of the bone-implant interface. This technique is certainly promising for future clinical applications.[31]

As far as the healing process goes, the addition of a synthetic bioabsorbable carrier for rhBMP-2 used in osseous defects around dental implants in the canine model demonstrated clinical and radiographic success.[32] Early healing at 4 weeks revealed that rhBMP-2–treated sites had a significantly higher percentage of contact, more new bone area, and a higher percentage of defect fill compared with control sites; this difference decreased after 12 weeks. Thus, the carrier for rhBMP-2 significantly stimulated bone formation around dental implants in this model in the early stages of healing, which may have important clinical relevance.[32]

Besides carriers, implant surface characteristics may be relevant. An earlier ossification process was observed when porous implants were placed in combination with BMP-4 and TGF-β1 than when machined implants were used with the same growth factors.[33]

With consideration of the aging population and increasing need for implant placement in osteoporotic individuals, another animal model evaluated osseointegration in these conditions. The healing process is severely compromised in bones affected by osteoporosis because of impaired healing. Nevertheless, implant placement with rhBMP-2 in osteoporotic, aged sheep was more successful than that in a control group that did not receive rhBMP-2. Furthermore, in mechanical tests, the rhBMP-2–coated implants displayed an average 50% higher stability. Thus, the application of an rhBMP-2 coating to solid implants may stimulate bone healing and regeneration even in aged and systemically compromised individuals.[34]

In addition, rhBMP-2 improves the quantity and quality of implant osseointegration, as shown through biomechanical testing and histomorphometric analysis performed with scanning electronic microscopic evaluation at the implant-bone interface.[35] As stated previously, the use of rhBMP-2 with implants is as effective as autologous bone. The induction of expression of BMP-2 at surgical sites at early stages has been shown in different animal models.[36]

Conclusion

Studies using animal models have indicated the osteogenic activity of rhBMP-2. These studies have evaluated the safety and efficacy of rhBMP-2 as well as the effects of different delivery vehicles on outcome. Successful results in animals have encouraged clinical trials in humans, which have also revealed the effectiveness of rhBMP-2 in repair of craniofacial defects and augmentation of the alveolar ridge and sinus cavity. Additional studies have indicated its ability to accelerate and improve wound healing. These promising results and ongoing developments in tissue engineering indicate the need for further clinical trials.

References

1. Ripamonti U, Reddi AH. Periodontal regeneration: Potential role of bone morphogenetic proteins. J Periodontal Res 1994;29:225–235.
2. Lee M. Bone morphogenetic proteins: Background and implications for oral reconstruction. A review. J Periodontol 1997;24:355–365.
3. Reddi AH, Weintroub S, Muthukumaran N. Biologic principles of bone induction. Orthop Clin North Am 1987;18:207–212.
4. Lindholm TC, Lindholm TS, Alitalo I, Urist MR. Bovine bone morphogenetic protein (bBMP) induced repair of skull trephine defects in sheep. Clin Orthop Relat Res 1988;227:265–268.
5. Johnson EE, Urist MR, Finerman GA. Bone, morphogenetic protein augmentation grafting of resistant femoral nonunions. A preliminary report. Clin Orthop Relat Res 1988;230:257–265.
6. Johnson EE, Urist MR, Finerman GA. Distal metaphyseal tibial nonunion. Deformity and bone loss treated by open reduction, internal fixation, and human bone morphogenetic protein (hBMP). Clin Orthop Relat Res 1990;250:234–240.
7. Nevins M, Kirker-Head C, Nevins M, Wozney JA, Palmer R, Graham D. Bone formation in the goat maxillary sinus induced by absorbable collagen sponge implants impregnated with recombinant human bone morphogenetic protein-2. Int J Periodontics Restorative Dent 1996;16:8–19.

8. Kirker-Head CA, Nevins M, Palmer R, Nevins ML, Schelling SH. A new animal model for maxillary sinus floor augmentation: Evaluation parameters. Int J Oral Maxillofac Implants 1997;12:403–411.

9. Uludag H, D'Augusta D, Palmer R, Timony G, Wozney J. Characterization of rhBMP-2 pharmacokinetics implanted with biomaterial carriers in the rat ectopic model. J Biomed Mater Res 1999;46:193–202.

10. Uludag H, Friess W, Williams D, et al. rhBMP-collagen sponges as osteoinductive devices: Effects of in vitro sponge characteristics and protein pI on in vivo rhBMP pharmacokinetics. Ann N Y Acad Sci 1999;875:369–378.

11. Uludag H, D'Augusta D, Golden J, et al. Implantation of recombinant human bone morphogenetic proteins with biomaterial carriers: A correlation between protein pharmacokinetics and osteoinduction in the rat ectopic model. J Biomed Mater Res 2000;50:227–238.

12. Riedel GE, Valentin-Opran A. Clinical evaluation of rhBMP-2/ACS in orthopedic trauma: a progress report. Orthopedics 1999;22:663–665.

13. Yasko AW, Lane JM, Fellinger EJ, Rosen V, Wozney JM, Wang EA. The healing of segmental bone defects, induced by recombinant human bone morphogenetic protein (rhBMP-2). A radiographic, histological, and biochemical study in rats. J Bone Joint Surg Am 1992;74:659–670 [erratum 1992;74:1111].

14. Ripamonti U, Duneas N, Van Den Heever B, Bosch C, Crooks J. Recombinant transforming growth factor-beta-1 induces endochondral bone in the baboon and synergizes with recombinant osteogenic protein-1 (bone morphogenetic protein-7) to initiate rapid bone formation. J Bone Miner Res 1997;12:1584–1595.

15. Urist MR, Nilsson O, Rasmussen J, et al. Bone regeneration under the influence of a bone morphogenetic protein (BMP) beta tricalcium phosphate (TCP) composite in skull trephine defects in dogs. Clin Orthop Relat Res 1987;214:295–304.

16. Ferguson D, Davis WL, Urist MR, Hurt WC, Allen EP. Bovine bone morphogenetic protein (bBMP) fraction-induced repair of craniotomy defects in the rhesus monkey (Macaca speciosa). Clin Orthop Relat Res 1987;219:251–258.

17. Lindholm TC, Lindholm TS, Martinnen A, Urist MR. Bovine bone morphogenetic protein (bBMP/NCP)-induced repair of skull trephine defects in pigs. Clin Orthop Relat Res 1994;301:263–270.

18. Marden LJ, Hollinger JO, Chaudhari A, Turek T, Schaub RG, Ron E. Recombinant human bone morphogenetic protein-2 is superior to demineralized bone matrix in repairing craniotomy defects in rats. J Biomed Mater Res 1994;28:1127–1138.

19. Hanisch O, Tatakis DN, Rohrer MD, Wohrle PS, Wozney JM, Wikesjö UM. Bone formation and osseointegration stimulated by rhBMP-2 following subantral augmentation procedures in nonhuman primates. Int J Oral Maxillofac Implants 1997;12:403–411.

20. Sailer H, Kolb E. Application of purified bone morphogenetic protein (BMP) preparations in cranio-maxillo-facial surgery. Reconstruction in craniofacial malformations and post-traumatic or operative defects of the skull with lyophilized cartilage and BMP. J Craniomaxillofac Surg 1994;22:191–199.

21. Howell TH, Fiorellini J, Jones A, et al. A feasibility study evaluating rhBMP-2/absorbable collagen sponge device for local alveolar ridge preservation of augmentation. Int J Periodontics Restorative Dent 1997;17:125–139.

22. Boyne PH, Marx RE, Nevins M, et al. A feasibility study evaluating rhBMP-2/absorbable collagen sponge for maxillary sinus floor augmentation. Int J Periodontics Restorative Dent 1997;17:11–25.

23. Fiorellini JP, Howell TH, Cochran D, et al. Randomized study evaluating recombinant human bone morphogenetic protein-2 for extraction socket augmentation. J Periodontol 2005;76:605–613.

24. Sumner DR, Turner TM, Urban RM, Virdi AS, Inoue N. Additive enhancement of implant fixation following combined treatment with rhTGF-β2 and rhBMP-2 in a canine model. J Bone Joint Surg Am 2006;88:806–817.

25. Liu Y, de Groot K, Hunziker EB. BMP-2 liberated from biomimetic implant coatings induces and sustains direct ossification in an ectopic rat model. Bone 2005;36:745–757.

26. Liu Y, Huse RO, de Groot K, Buser D, Hunziker EB. Delivery mode and efficacy of BMP-2 in association with implants. J Dent Res 2007;86:84–89.

27. Liu Y, Enggist L, Kuffer AF, Buser D, Hunziker EB. The influence of BMP-2 and its mode of delivery on the osteoconductivity of implant surfaces during the early phase of osseointegration. Biomaterials 2007;28:2677–2686.

28. Stadlinger B, Pilling E, Huhle M, et al. Influence of extracellular matrix coatings on implant stability and osseointegration: An animal study. J Biomed Mater Res B Appl Biomater 2007;83:222–231.

29. Aebli N, Stich H, Schawalder P, Theis JC, Krebs J. Effects of bone morphogenetic protein-2 and hyaluronic acid on the osseointegration of hydroxyapatite-coated implants: An experimental study in sheep. J Biomed Mater Res A 2005;73:295–302.

30. Murata M, Akazawa T, Tazaki J, et al. Blood permeability of a novel ceramic scaffold for bone morphogenetic protein-2. J Biomed Mater Res B Appl Biomater 2006;81B:469–475.

31. Park J, Lutz R, Felszeghy E, et al. The effect on bone regeneration of a liposomal vector to deliver BMP-2 gene to bone grafts in peri-implant bone defects. Biomaterials 2007;28:2772–2782.

32. Jones AA, Buser D, Schenk R, Wozney J, Cochran DL. The effect of rhBMP-2 around endosseous implants with and without membranes in the canine model. J Periodontol 2006;77:1184–1193.

33. Schierano G, Canuto RA, Navone R, et al. Biological factors involved in the osseointegration of oral titanium implants with different surfaces: A pilot study in minipigs. J Periodontol 2005;76:1710–1720.

34. Sachse A, Wagner A, Keller M, et al. Osteointegration of hydroxyapatite-titanium implants coated with nonglycosylated recombinant human bone morphogenetic protein-2 (BMP-2) in aged sheep. Bone 2005;37:699–710.

35. Lan J, Wang ZF, Shi B, Xia HB, Cheng XR. The influence of recombinant human BMP-2 on bone-implant osseointegration: biomechanical testing and histomorphometric analysis. Int J Oral Maxillofac Surg 2007;36:345–349.

36. Alam S, Ueki K, Marukawa K, et al. Expression of bone morphogenetic protein 2 and fibroblast growth factor 2 during bone regeneration using different implant materials as an onlay bone graft in rabbit mandibles. Oral Surg Oral Med Oral Pathol Oral Radiol Endod 2007;103:16–26.

13

Bone Augmentation of the Maxillary Sinus Floor with rhBMP-2

R. Gilbert Triplett, DDS, PhD

Patients with an edentulous posterior maxilla frequently exhibit a loss of alveolar bone from both the clinical alveolus as well as the maxillary sinus floor. The sinus enlarges after posterior teeth are extracted. The result is an inadequate amount of alveolar bone to allow an implant-supported prosthesis. Various surgical procedures have been devised to overcome this problem. Bone augmentation of the maxillary sinus floor (maxillary sinus lift) has become popular and predictable because it increases alveolar bone height in the lower third of the maxillary sinus.[1,2] This procedure allows dental restoration of missing teeth through the use of endosseous dental implants placed in the augmented bone.[3]

Various bone-grafting materials are currently being used in maxillary sinus floor augmentation procedures; these include autogenous bone (from the iliac crest, tibia, mandible, or maxilla), allogeneic bone (radiated and non-radiated), and bone graft substitutes (xenografts).[4,5] All of these materials have their disadvantages, which include the morbidity associated with harvesting from a secondary site, limitation in bone quantity, noninductive properties, marginal predictability, and high cost. It is generally agreed that autologous bone grafts are the gold standard and the benchmark against which other materials are judged.

Bone morphogenetic proteins (BMPs) are a family of osteoinductive proteins that stimulate endochondral and intramembranous bone formation from the patient's mesenchymal cells (in situ). Urist[6] first described bone morphogenetic activity after observing ectopic bone formation in rabbits. Currently, several BMPs have been purified and cloned. This recombinant material has provided a powerful tool to test osteoinductive activity.[7–9] Studies of large mandibular defects in dogs and nonhuman primates verify that recombinant human BMP-2 (rhBMP-2) induces rapid new bone growth sufficient to restore mandibular defects without the addition of a bone graft.[10–14] This recombinant material (rhBMP-2), carried on an absorbable collagen sponge (ACS), has demonstrated success in regenerating bone on the maxillary sinus floor of goats.[13]

Based on these studies and further preclinical studies showing local and systemic safety and pharmacology of rhBMP-2, a clinical pilot study was initiated to determine the feasibility of using rhBMP-2 to induce bone growth in patients who required two-stage maxillary sinus floor reconstruction. Subsequently, additional studies were designed to establish the correct concentration of rhBMP-2 that would be safe and effective, and these results in turn were used to design a pivotal trial to compare rhBMP-2/ACS with an autograft for sinus floor grafting. Following completion of these studies, rhBMP-2/ACS received approval from the US Food and Drug Administration (FDA) for use in dental applications and is marketed as InFuse (Medtronic Sofamor Danek) bone graft.

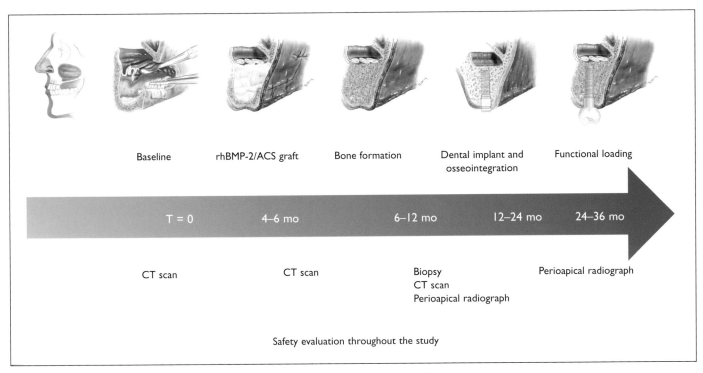

Fig 13-1 Treatment scheme for augmentation of the maxillary sinus floor with rhBMP-2/ACS.

Feasibility Study of rhBMP-2/ ACS for Maxillary Sinus Floor Augmentation

A 16-week open-label study assessed the safety and technical feasibility of implanting human rhBMP-2/ACS for two-stage maxillary sinus augmentation. The first use of rhBMP-2/ACS in human clinical maxillary sinus floor augmentation included 12 patients with inadequate bone height in the posterior maxilla to support a dental implant–borne fixed partial denture. In this study, the total dose of rhBMP-2 that was delivered to the sinus floor was absorbed onto a commercially available collagen sponge (Fig 13-1). Inclusion and exclusion criteria were established. This included safety precautions such as excluding pregnant and nursing women as well as patients with acute or chronic sinus disease, untreated periodontal disease, and medical conditions such as uncontrolled insulin-dependent diabetes, malignancy, and metabolic bone disease.[14]

The rhBMP-2/ACS device consisted of two components: rhBMP-2 and an ACS (Helistat absorbable collagen hemostatic agent, Integra). The rhBMP-2 portion is the osteoinductive factor that stimulates host bone formation. The carrier component, the ACS, consists of bovine type I collagen (from bovine tendons) and provides the matrix for delivery of rhBMP-2.

A dry 7.5 × 10.0–cm collagen sponge was saturated with 8 mL of rhBMP-2 solution (0.43-mg/mL concentration) (Fig 13-2). After saturation, each complete sponge contained 3.4 mg of rhBMP-2. The sponge was then layered into the prepared maxillary sinus, and the mucoperiosteal flap was reapproximated and closed (Figs 13-3 and 13-4). Standard preoperative and postoperative medications were routinely prescribed to prevent infection, control pain, and minimize swelling.[14]

Evaluation

The rhBMP-2/ACS treatment sites were monitored for erythema, exudate, edema, oroantral fistulas, and wound dehiscence. Patient complaints concerning the surgically treated sinus were recorded.

Blood and urine specimens were collected at baseline (prior to surgery) and 2 days and 4 weeks postoperatively to evaluate serum chemistries, register complete blood

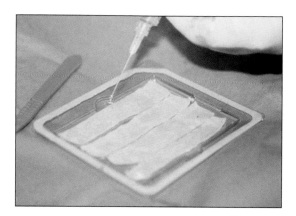

Fig 13-2 Soaking of ACS with reconstituted rhBMP-2.

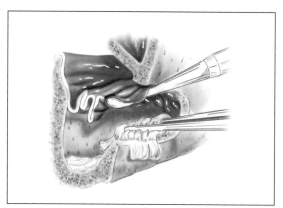

Fig 13-3 Placement of the ACS in the sinus floor.

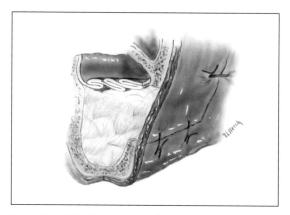

Fig 13-4 rhBMP-2-saturated sponge in the lower third of the sinus.

cell count, and perform urinalysis to monitor the effects of rhBMP-2/ACS on organ function. Blood and urine specimens were also collected 5 days and 4, 8, and 16 weeks postoperatively to assess immune responses to rhBMP-2/ACS. Serum samples were analyzed by enzyme-linked immunosorbent assay for immunoglobulin G, immunoglobulin M, and immunoglobulin A antibodies to rhBMP-2, bovine collagen type I, and human collagen type I.

Periapical radiographs were taken at baseline and 4 weeks postoperatively and computerized tomographic (CT) scans were taken at baseline and at 16 weeks postoperatively.

The rhBMP-2/ACS device was evaluated during surgical implantation for its cohesiveness, form, handling, volume, placement, ease of use, and time of preparation. These seven characteristics were rated on a scale of 1 to 4, with 4 being the most favorable.

For measurement of bone induction, all three dimensions of the alveolar ridge (width, length, and height) were measured. The radiographs and CT scans were performed by an independent dental radiology center, and analyses were performed by three different radiologists (raters) using the same images. For CT scans, the height,

width, and density measurements were obtained from two abutting 2-mm cross-sectional multiplanar reformatted images for each proposed endosseous dental implant site. Bone height was measured along a vertical line drawn parallel to the long axis of the cross section of the maxillary ridge, starting at the alveolar crest and ending at the antral floor (Fig 13-5). Postoperatively, the measurements were taken along the same vertical line to the most superior portion of the augmented bone.

The quality of new bone detected in the CT scan was assessed by measuring bone density in Hounsfield units. Values measured in Hounsfield units were converted to milligrams per milliliter using the known density of the standard by linear regression. Density in the adjacent area of native bone was measured in an area of interest box that was as large as possible but that did not include cortical bone (Fig 13-6).

Full-thickness core bone biopsy specimens were obtained from all patients at the time of endosseous dental implant placement. Standard histologic fixative procedures and preparation with a hematoxylin-eosin stain were used. Both native and newly induced bone were evaluated for the presence of cortical and trabecular

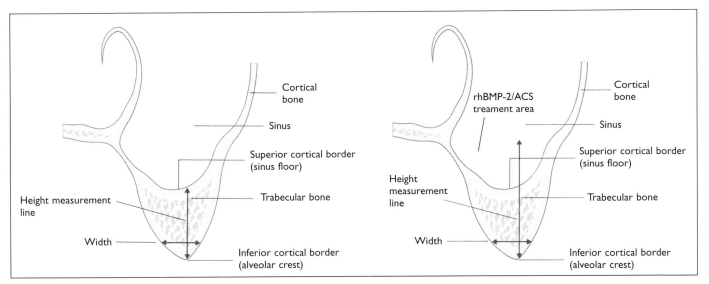

Fig 13-5 Measurement technique for calculation of new bone formation in the maxillary sinus. *(left)* Before augmentation; *(right)* after augmentation.

Fig 13-6 Sites for measurement of density of regenerated bone in the maxillary sinus. (AOI) Area of interest.

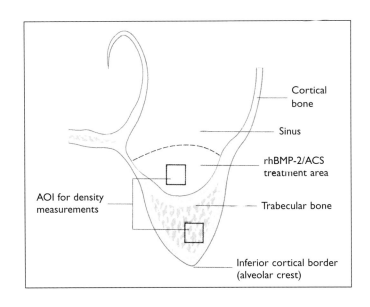

bone, the amount and thickness of osseous trabeculae, the location and amount of woven bone, the proportional amount of woven bone remodeling into lamellar bone, and the number of active bone cells (osteoblasts and osteoclasts). Fibrosis, vascularity, mononuclear cell infiltration, and/or mixed inflammatory cell infiltration were graded in the bone marrow. The extent of all changes was rated on a scale of 0 (absent) to 3 (large) by an independent pathologist.

The local and systemic toxicity of the rhBMP-2/ACS device was evaluated by reviewing results from oral examinations, radiographic images, adverse effects (severity and frequency), and laboratory test results.

The technical feasibility was evaluated by calculating the minimum, maximum, mean, and median scores for each of the seven handling characteristics mentioned previously.

Findings

Twelve patients (4 males and 8 females) were enrolled. One patient withdrew from the study after surgery; therefore, 11 patients could be evaluated for response to rhBMP-2/ACS.

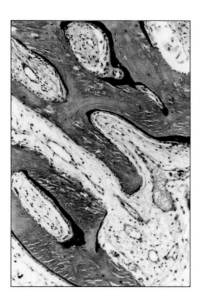

Fig 13-7 Histologic specimen showing de novo bone formation in the maxillary sinus at the time of implant placement (hematoxylin-eosin stain; original magnification ×20).

The patients were exposed to a mean rhBMP-2 dose/concentration of 2.89 mg (1.77 to 3.40 mg). There were no clinically significant changes in the vital signs of any of the patients. A total of 28 adverse effects were recorded. None of these was serious, and only five were considered to be related to rhBMP-2/ACS treatment.

The most common adverse effects were mouth pain (8 events) and facial edema (6 events). None of the patients developed antibody titers to rhBMP-2 or human type I collagen. One patient developed an antibody titer to bovine type I collagen but did not exhibit clinical symptoms. Technical feasibility scores indicated that the device (rhBMP-2/ACS) was easy to use (range, 3.7 to 4.0 on a scale of 1.0 to 4.0).[14]

Periapical radiographs did not prove useful for assessing bone induction because they could not capture the entire field. However, CT scans were available for 11 of the 12 patients and were assessed by three independent raters. They indicated that the device induced new bone in each of the 11 patients and resulted in a mean bone height response of 8.51 ± 4.13 mm (range, 2.28 to 15.73 mm).

Five of 11 patients (45%) met the optimal bone height criteria for dental implant placement. An additional three patients (27%) met the minimum bone requirement for dental implant placement. Overall, 8 of 11 (75%) of the patients treated with rhBMP-2/ACS had adequate bone for the placement of dental implants.

Biopsy specimens were obtained 4 months after graft placement from 7 of 8 patients who had adequate bone for dental implant placement. No residual collagen matrix was observed in any of the biopsy specimens harvested.

The amount of woven bone was moderate to large, and there were a moderate to large number of osteoblasts and capillaries in the bone marrow in the newly induced bone. The amount of osseous trabecular bone ranged from moderate to large, and the amount of woven bone was highly variable (Fig 13-7). The investigators rated the bone quality to be poor to marginal, although the histologic specimens revealed far more bone activity and maturity than was judged by the tactile rating of the biopsy specimens. Several sites were judged as having no bone by the surgeons after trephine biopsy; however, the histologic specimen revealed a moderate response.

Conclusions

This clinical study met its desired objective of evaluating the short-term safety and technical feasibility of device implantation and various methods of measurement. CT scans were determined to be the best available method to obtain reproducible quantitative measures of the treatment area. The rhBMP-2/ACS treatment induced bone in this anatomic site in 100% of the patients available for evaluation, and eight (73%) had adequate bone for placement of dental implants. This study proved to be the basis for a dosing study to evaluate the ability of higher concentrations of rhBMP-2/ACS to accelerate bone formation in patients requiring maxillary sinus floor augmentation procedures.

Comparison of Two Concentrations of rhBMP-2

Because of the encouraging results of bone formation in response to an increased dose of rhBMP-2 in animal models and the marginally satisfactory results that were obtained from a 0.43-mg/mL dose in the phase I safety and efficacy study, this phase II randomized, parallel group evaluation of escalating concentrations of rhBMP-2 (0.75 and 1.50 mg/mL) was designed.[15] These doses were compared with a standard bone graft for augmentation of the maxillary sinus floor.

The materials and methods for this phase II study follow those in the phase I trials. The objective was to induce adequate bone for endosseous dental implant placement (following a maxillary sinus floor augmentation procedure) in order to select one concentration for investigation in a future pivotal study. A secondary objective was to estimate success rates for patients and dental implants following 36 months of functional loading of dental implants placed and loaded in the newly induced bone within the grafted sinuses. The bone graft with which these escalating concentrations were compared was defined as the bone-grafting material used at each investigative site. The materials that could be used were limited to autogenous bone or a combination of autogenous bone and allogeneic bone.

Study protocol

Six investigative sites were selected to enroll a total of 48 patients in two cohorts of 24 patients each; within each cohort, patients were to be randomized in a 2:1 ratio to receive either rhBMP-2/ACS (16 patients) or a bone-grafting material (8 patients). Patients in the first cohort were treated with either rhBMP-2 at 0.75 mg/mL or a bone graft. Patients in the second cohort were treated with either rhBMP-2 at 1.50 mg/mL or a bone graft.

The treatment course was about 52 months in duration and comprised several phases: short-term safety and bone induction (4 months), dental implant placement and osseointegration, and a 36-month functional loading phase. A standardized surgical procedure was established. No concurrent extraneous materials (ie, barrier membranes) were to be used. The evaluations were the same as those used in the feasibility study.[15]

Findings

The volume of the rhBMP-2 implanted depended on the estimated size of the patient's sinus, the procedure type (unilateral versus bilateral), and the sinus void created by the surgeon. The mean volume of material implanted was 6.9, 11.9, and 13.8 cm^3 in bone graft, 0.75-mg/mL rhBMP-2/ACS, and 1.50-mg/mL rhBMP-2/ACS treatment groups, respectively. The mean total dose of rhBMP-2 per sinus was 8.9 mg/mL (5.2 to 12.0 mg) for the 0.75-mg/mL dose and 20.8 mg/mL (10.8 to 24.0 mg) for the 1.50-mg/mL dose.

The mean increases in alveolar ridge height 4 months after treatment were similar among groups: 11.3, 9.5, and 10.2 mm for bone graft, 0.75-mg/mL rhBMP-2/ACS, and 1.50-mg/mL rhBMP-2/ACS, respectively. The mean increase in buccolingual width at the crest of the alveolar ridge was significantly greater in the bone graft group than in the rhBMP-2/ACS groups: 4.6, 2.0, and 1.9 mm for bone graft, 0.75-mg/mL rhBMP-2/ACS, and 1.50-mg/mL rhBMP-2/ACS groups, respectively.

As expected, a significant difference in new bone density in favor of the bone graft was observed: 350, 84, and 134 mg/mL in bone graft, 0.75-mg/mL rhBMP-2/ACS, and 1.50-mg/mL rhBMP-2/ACS groups, respectively. The 1.50-mg/mL rhBMP-2/ACS treatment group also showed a significantly greater bone density than the 0.75-mg/mL group. It is theorized that the higher concentration of rhBMP-2 resulted in faster bone formation, which was manifested by greater radiographic density, that is, mineralized bone, 4 months postoperatively.

The histologic analysis from the specimens obtained at the time of dental implant placement (mean, 6.9 months after treatment; range, 5.9 to 11.5 months) indicated unambiguous bone induction of rhBMP-2. There were no differences in the histologic parameters that were evaluated among the treatment groups.

All 13 patients (100%) in the bone graft treatment group received a total of 63 dental implants in the newly induced bone within the grafted sinus. In these 13 patients, a total of 53 dental implants (84%) were functionally loaded with prostheses. The dental implant survival rate was 81% (51 of 63 implants). The majority of the failures (67%) occurred before functional loading. The cause of dental implant failures was primarily inadequate bone quality (92%); one dental implant failed because of infection.

Fifteen of 18 patients (83%) randomized to the 0.75-mg/mL rhBMP-2/ACS treatment group received a total of 83 dental implants in the newly induced bone in the grafted sinus. Two of the three patients who did not receive dental implants were considered treatment failures following their maxillary sinus floor augmentation procedures. The third patient withdrew from the study 16 weeks postsurgery, despite a good bone induction response. In 13 of 18 patients (72%), a total of 65 dental implants (78%) were functionally loaded with implant-borne prostheses. Twelve of 18 patients (67%), accounting for 59 dental implants (71%), were in function 24 through 36 months after functional loading. The dental implant survival rate, regardless of loading status, was 88% (73 of 83 implants). The cause of dental implant failures was primarily inadequate bone quality (90%).

Fifteen of 17 patients (88%) in the 1.50-mg/mL rhBMP-2/ACS treatment group received a total of 73 dental implants in the newly induced bone within the grafted sinus. Two patients were considered treatment failures following their procedures and required reaugmentation procedures for dental implant placement. In 14 of the 15 successfully augmented patients (82%), a total of 60 dental implants (82%) were functionally loaded with implant-borne prostheses and remained functionally loaded 6, 12, and 18 months after loading. The dental implant survival rate was 79% (58 of 73 dental implants). The etiologies of dental implant failure were primarily inadequate bone quality (57%) and peri-implantitis (27%).

Conclusions

This study was designed to determine the most effective concentration of rhBMP-2/ACS for maxillary sinus floor augmentation procedures and to estimate the efficacy rates (for patients and dental implants) of rhBMP-2/ACS and bone graft in these procedures.

The higher of the two rhBMP-2 concentrations was deemed the most effective for maxillary sinus floor augmentation procedures. Furthermore, the patient and dental implant success rates were estimated and found to be comparable among the three treatment groups following 36 months of functional loading.

It was anticipated that one of the two concentrations of rhBMP-2 would generate more bone than the other and have higher patient and dental implant success rates. This was not the case. Both concentrations were equally effective in terms of bone quantity. However, the difference between the two doses appeared to be in the rate of bone formation, as evidenced by the CT scans, densi-

ty data, and the investigators' assessments of the bone quality at the time of dental implant placement. This finding led the investigators to delay prosthesis placement by approximately 2 months in the 0.75-mg/mL rhBMP-2/ACS group, compared with the bone graft and 1.50-mg/mL rhBMP-2/ACS treatment groups, to allow the soft bone a longer interval to mature.

The results of the CT density data 6 months following functional loading showed the same phenomenon as had been observed in the rhBMP-2 pilot study. An increase in density in newly induced bone following the functional loading of dental implants placed in that bone would be expected. The increase in density suggests that the bone is responding to the mechanical forces placed on it and is consistent with Wolff's law.[16]

This study was based on intent to treat, and the patient, as opposed to dental implants, was the primary unit of analysis. As a result, it is difficult to compare the data generated with the nonrandomized case studies reported in the literature. At best, the results from this study can be compared with those of retrospective and prospective studies conducted in patients with two-stage maxillary sinus floor augmentation procedures using autograft alone or autograft combined with allograft as the bone-grafting material. Fifteen such studies were examined and found generally not to report success in terms of the number of patients with successful grafting procedures. However, a study reported by Blomqvist et al[17] evaluated autologous bone grafts harvested from the iliac crest in a two-stage maxillary sinus floor augmentation. The patient success rate (the number of patients who received a prosthesis) was 76% (38 of 50 patients), and the dental implant survival rate was 84% after an average of 16 months (0 to 34 months) following prosthesis placement. The remaining studies consistently reported dental implant survival rates (the number of implants that were not removed) of 57% to 100%.[15]

The dental implant survival rates in these studies are comparable with the survival rates reported in this study after 36 months of functional loading: 81%, 88%, and 79% in the bone graft, 0.75-mg/mL rhBMP-2/ACS, and 1.50-mg/mL rhBMP-2/ACS treatment groups, respectively.

Based on these data, it is concluded that (1) both concentrations of rhBMP-2 are safe and have a safety profile similar to that of bone graft; (2) both concentrations of rhBMP-2 induce a similar amount of bone, which is similar to that induced by bone graft; (3) the higher concentration of rhBMP-2 induces bone formation more rapidly than does the lower concentration; and (4) a maxillary sinus floor augmentation procedure using rhBMP-2/ACS is effective in inducing bone that can support the placement and long-term functional loading of dental implants in approximately 75% to 80% of patients treated. These study results support the use of rhBMP-2/ACS at a concentration of 1.50 mg/mL in future studies of maxillary sinus floor augmentation.[15]

Comparison of rhBMP-2 and Bone Graft

Data from the previously discussed study suggest that rhBMP-2/ACS at 1.50 mg/mL has efficacy and safety profiles that are similar to those of bone graft.[15] This pivotal study was designed as a multicenter, open-label, stratified (partially versus totally edentulous), randomized (1:1), parallel evaluation of rhBMP-2/ACS and bone graft. The patient population was the same as in the previous studies. Prior to randomization, patients were stratified based on dentate status to control for possible confounding effects of this variable on functional loads (that is, loads on a complete-arch prosthesis as opposed to loads placed on smaller units supported by dental implants).

Twenty-one investigative sites enrolled a total of 160 patients into two cohorts, rhBMP-2/ACS or bone graft, consisting of 80 patients each. During the procedure, 8.0 mL of 1.50-mg/mL rhBMP-2 was uniformly expressed onto a 7.5 × 10.0–cm absorbable collagen sponge to deliver a total of 12.0 mg per sponge. Up to two rhBMP-2/ACS implant grafts could be placed in each maxillary sinus. Bone grafts were limited to either autogenous bone alone (from the iliac crest, tibia, or oral cavity) or a combination of autogenous and allogeneic bone. The volume of either rhBMP-2/ACS or bone graft implanted was determined by the size of the patient's maxillary sinus and the surgical antral void created by the surgeon.

The patient was considered a treatment failure if he or she did not receive dental implants within 12 months postoperatively and prosthetics within 24 months following dental implant placement or required additional augmentation. Efficacy was measured as the proportion of rhBMP-2/ACS–treated patients who had a successful dental implant–borne restoration after 6 months of functional loading. Safety was monitored as in previous studies.

Evaluation methods

Bone induction

Bone induction was quantified by CT scans performed within 6 weeks before (baseline) and 6 months after implantation of rhBMP-2/ACS or bone graft at the location where the dental implants were placed. Measurements of all CT scans were performed by three independent radiologists who were masked from the study treatment used.

The amount of new bone formation was determined by measuring alveolar bone height (one measurement) as previously described. Measurement of the 6-month postoperative CT scan was performed first to establish points of measurement.

The same reference points were then used to measure the baseline CT scan (Fig 13-8a). The sites to be measured were determined by the investigators from the 6-month CT scan (Fig 13-8b). This was achieved by reformatting the 6-month CT scan and sending it to the investigator to identify the locations where the dental implants were to be placed. All measurements were then taken at these locations within the maxillary sinus. Bone height, width, and density measurements were taken from one 2-mm-thick, cross-sectional multiplanar reformatted image for each proposed endosseous implant site identified by the investigator, as determined on the 6-month CT scan. Measurements of the corresponding sites were then obtained from the baseline CT scans.

Bone density

The quality of the newly induced bone was assessed by measuring bone density (units expressed in mg/mL) with the aid of a standard density block.

Histologic methods

In addition to hematoxylin-eosin stain, vital staining with tetracycline was used. Patients were given subtherapeutic doses of tetracycline to label the new bone that was formed, allowing a dynamic study of bone remodeling.

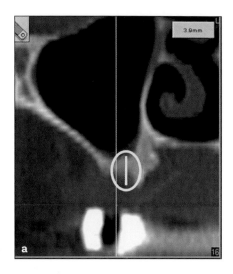 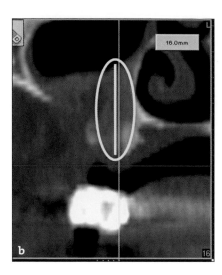

Fig 13-8a CT scan obtained preoperatively to plan the treatment. *Yellow circle and line* indicate available bone.

Fig 13-8b CT scan obtained 6 months after augmentation of the sinus floor with rhBMP-2. The height of the bone has increased from 3.9 mm to 16.0 mm at this point, prior to implant placement. *Yellow circle and line* indicate available bone.

Patient success

A patient was defined as having had a successful maxillary sinus floor augmentation procedure at 6, 12, 18, and 24 months after functional loading if he or she met the following criteria:

- A maxillary sinus floor augmentation procedure was performed with the study treatment.
- One or more dental implants were placed in the grafted sinus without an additional maxillary sinus floor augmentation procedure.
- Osseointegration of a sufficient number of dental implants placed in the grafted sinus (or sinuses) was achieved to allow placement of an implant-borne prosthetic device.
- The implants were loaded by functional use of a prosthesis.
- The functional use of the prosthesis was maintained.

For bilateral procedures, sufficient osseointegration of dental implants had to occur in both sinuses.

Dental implant success

A dental implant was defined as a success at 6, 12, 18, and 24 months after functional loading if it met the following criteria:

- It was immobile when tested clinically (providing it was unattached).
- There was no evidence of continuous peri-implant radiolucency.

- There were no chronic symptoms of pain, infection, or neuropathy.

A dental implant was considered to have survived if it was not removed following its placement.

Safety

Safety was evaluated, as previously described, through oral examinations, radiographs, and collection of blood samples to measure serum chemistry, hematology, and formation of antibody titers.

Statistical methods and analysis

This study was designed to compare the abilities of a recombinant human protein, rhBMP-2, and an autograft to induce bone formation in the maxillary sinus floor. Two analyses, based on both the intent to treat and the patient populations available for evaluation, were performed for both the primary and secondary efficacy and safety end points. The intent-to-treat population included all enrolled patients in their respective randomized treatment group, regardless of whether they actually received their assigned treatment, provided they had at least one documented outcome. The patient population available for evaluation was a subset of the intent-to-treat population and included patients who received the assigned treatment (in both sinuses for bilateral patients), had no major protocol violation, and had a verifiable outcome available for the analysis.

Table 13-1 Distribution of study patients

Treatment group	Enrolled, randomized	Discontinued*	Lost to follow-up	Completed
Bone graft	78	8	1	69
rhBMP-2/ACS	82	20	4	58 †
Total	160	28	5	127

*Discontinued includes treatment failures (5 in bone graft group and 16 in rhBMP-2/ACS group) and withdrawals.

†One patient in the rhBMP-2/ACS group was deemed a failure at the 24-month functional loading visit but is counted as having completed the study in this table.

The sample size for this pivotal study was calculated to generate a confidence interval of 12% to 13% around the observed success rate. The proportion of patients who were scored a success at the primary efficacy end point were summarized and evaluated with exact 95% confidence intervals for both treatment groups (rhBMP-2/ACS and bone graft). A sample size of 80 patients in each treatment group accommodated a patient dropout rate as high as 20% in this study (resulting in n = 64) and still generated confidence intervals within 12% to 13% around the estimate.

An overall comparison of changes among the treatment groups in bone measurements from baseline to 6 months postoperatively was carried out with an analysis of variance. If the overall *P* value was statistically significant, then pairwise comparisons were performed.

Findings

A total of 160 patients were randomized and enrolled over 5 years at 21 centers in the United States. Of those enrolled, 127 patients completed the study to 24 months after loading, including 69 patients in the bone graft and 58 patients in the rhBMP-2/ACS treatment groups (Table 13-1).

Study treatment

The mean total volume of material implanted per sinus was 8.3 mL (range, 1.0 to 30.0 mL) in the bone graft group and 12.9 mL (range, 1.1 to 16.0 mL) in the rhBMP-2/ACS group. Within the bone graft group, 77 of 78 patients received bone graft, while 1 patient received rhBMP-2/ACS because of a site randomization error. Of the 77 patients receiving grafts, 43 (56%) received unilateral sinus treatment, while 34 (44%) received bilateral sinus treatment.

Of the 83 patients who received rhBMP-2/ACS, 37 (45%) were treated unilaterally and 46 (55%) bilaterally. All patients randomized to the rhBMP-2/ACS group were treated. The mean total dose per patient was 28.3 mg (range, 6.4 to 48.0 mg), and the mean total dose implanted per sinus was 19.4 mg (range, 1.6 to 24.0 mg).

In the bone graft treatment group, 42 patients received autograft alone and 35 patients received autograft plus allograft (including one patient who received bilateral sinus treatment, in which one sinus received autograft alone and the other sinus received both autograft and allograft).

Bone induction

The amount of new bone formation following treatment with either rhBMP-2/ACS or bone graft is presented in Table 13-2. There was no statistically significant difference in the mean baseline bone heights in the two treatment groups. A statistically significant amount of new bone had formed 6 months postoperatively in each group. The bone graft group formed a mean of 1.63 mm more new bone than the rhBMP-2/ACS group, a statistically significant difference.

Bone density

A statistically significant difference in newly induced bone density (ie, mineralized bone) was observed 6 months postoperatively in favor of the bone graft treatment group (Table 13-3). However, subsequent to functional

Table 13-2 Change in bone height from baseline to 6 months postoperative

Variable	Bone graft (n = 78)	rhBMP-2/ACS (n = 82)	Comparability
Baseline height			
n	78	82	
Mean (mm)	5.51	5.44	$t = 0.1992$; $df = 158$
6-mo postoperative height			
n	76	82	
Mean (mm)	14.98	13.27	$t = 2.6434$; $df = 156$; $P = .009*$
SD (mm)	4.33	3.80	
Change in height			
n	76	82	
Mean (mm)	9.46	7.83	$t = 2.6977$; $df = 156$; $P = .008*$
SD (mm)	4.11	3.52	

*P value obtained from t test.

Table 13-3 Newly induced bone density

Variable	Intent to treat*		P[†]
	Bone graft	rhBMP-2/ACS	
Density 6 mo postoperative (visit 8)			
n (observed)	214	231	
Mean (mg/mL)	284	196	< .001
SD (mg/mL)	179	112	
Density 6 mo after dental implant placement (visit 10)			
n (observed)	166	151	
Mean (mg/mL)	311	350	.02
SD (mg/mL)	164	136	
Change in density from visit 8 to visit 10			
n (observed)	152	146	
Mean (mg/mL)	36	156	< .001
SD (mg/mL)	148	119	

*The intent-to-treat population included all enrolled patients in their respective randomized treatment group, regardless of whether they actually received their assigned treatment, provided they had at least one documented outcome.

[†]P value is from nonparametric Kruskal-Wallis test because results did not meet normal distribution.

loading (6 months after dental implant placement), the density of the newly induced bone increased significantly in the rhBMP-2/ACS treatment group and surpassed the increase in bone density observed in the bone graft treatment group.

Histologic methods

The quality of newly induced bone was evaluated by histologic analysis. Core bone biopsy specimens were obtained at the time of dental implant placement, approximately 8.6 months postoperatively, from newly induced bone within the grafted sinus. Histologic analysis of these specimens indicated no differences in parameters between treatment groups.

Exploratory analysis of responsive patients

In an exploratory analysis of responsive patients, an rhBMP-2/ACS responder was defined as any patient who, 6 months postoperatively, had an increase of more than 2 mm in alveolar ridge height. Based on these criteria, 99% (81 of 82) of the patients treated with 1.5 mg/mL rhBMP-2/ACS were considered responders to treatment. An example of one of the responders is shown in Fig 13-9.

Patient success

Analyses were based on the intent-to-treat population, which included all enrolled patients in their respective randomized treatment groups. Patients were deemed a success or failure at each functional loading visit. Patients who failed, withdrew, or were lost to follow-up during the postoperative treatment period were considered failures at all functional loading visits. Patients who successfully received prostheses but withdrew or were lost to follow-up anytime thereafter in the functional loading period were excluded from the intent-to-treat analysis. Patients and dental implants from patients in the intent-to-treat population were used as units of analysis.

Of the original 82 patients randomized to the rhBMP-2/ACS group, 1 patient was lost to follow-up after completing a successful postoperative treatment period and before the 6-month functional loading visit. Of the remaining 81 patients, 64 (79%) had successful dental implant–borne restorations after 6 months of functional loading.

A secondary analysis in the study was to compare the effectiveness of rhBMP-2/ACS with that of bone graft (used for a two-stage maxillary sinus floor augmentation procedure) to induce bone that successfully supported dental implant–borne restorations after 6, 12, 18, and 24 months of functional loading.

For the intent-to-treat population, the patient success rate in the bone graft group (91% or 69 of 76 patients) was significantly higher ($P = .05$) than that of the rhBMP-2/ACS treatment group (79% or 64 of 81 patients) at 6 months of functional loading. The significant difference in patient success rates between the two groups increased

at later time points, as more patients treated with rhBMP-2/ACS than patients treated with bone graft withdrew or did not return for follow-up visits.

More patients in the rhBMP-2/ACS group were deemed failures in the time between initial surgery and dental implant placement. In the bone graft group, 95% of patients (74 of 78) received dental implants in newly induced bone, while in the rhBMP-2/ACS group, 82% of patients (67 of 82) received implants. Based on this observation, patient success rates were evaluated in the subpopulation of patients who received dental implants in newly induced bone. This analysis showed no significant differences in success rates at any time point, suggesting that the significant difference in efficacy between rhBMP-2/ACS and bone graft was the result of surgical failures that occurred before the time of dental implant placement.

The observation that bone graft patient success rates were stable while rhBMP-2/ACS rates decreased over time could be attributed to patients who were lost to follow-up or withdrew during the functional loading period rather than to documented treatment failure. Seven patients in the rhBMP-2/ACS group withdrew at various functional loading time points, compared with two patients who withdrew from the bone graft group, both before the 6-month functional loading visit. In comparison, among patients who successfully received prostheses, one patient in the rhBMP-2/ACS group was deemed a failure during the functional loading period (at the 24-month functional loading time point), while no patient in the bone graft group was deemed a failure during this period.

Dental implant success

The effectiveness of rhBMP-2/ACS and that of bone graft were also compared using the dental implant as the unit of analysis. For the purpose of this analysis, a dental implant was defined as a success after loading if the previously described criteria were met.

Dental implant success rates in each treatment group appeared to follow a similar trend to that observed at the patient level (Table 13-4). Dental implant success rates decreased from 6 months to 12 months of functional loading in both treatment groups and then stabilized. Variations in success rates from visit to visit reflect the fact that the loading status of dental implants could change over time. There was no statistically significant difference in success rate or in trend across functional loading time points between the two treatment groups when dental implants were used as the unit of analysis.

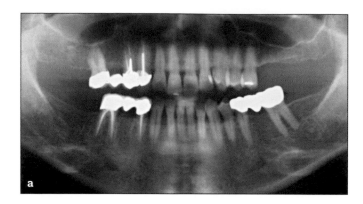

Fig 13-9a Preoperative panoramic radiograph revealing deficient alveolar bone in the posterior maxilla.

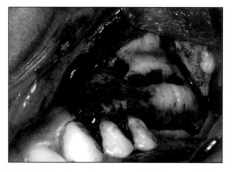

Fig 13-9b Development of a sinus window in preparation for membrane elevation.

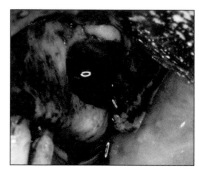

Fig 13-9c Site ready to receive augmentation material.

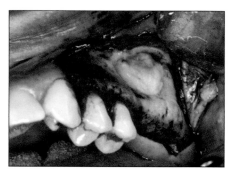

Fig 13-9d ACS loaded with rhBMP-2 (1.50mg/mL) in the maxillary sinus.

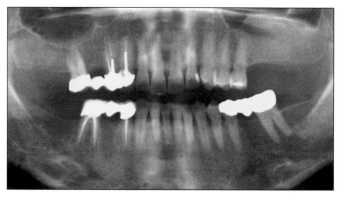

Fig 13-9e Postoperative panoramic radiograph at 6 months, revealing the de novo bone formation.

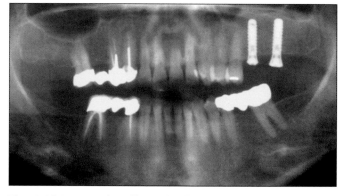

Fig 13-9f Panoramic radiograph of the dental implants in place.

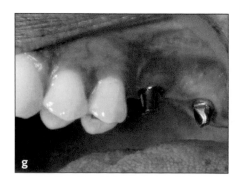

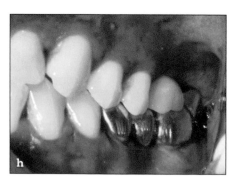

Fig 13-9g Abutments ready to receive the implant-supported prosthesis.

Fig 13-9h Implant-supported fixed partial denture 6 months after functional loading.

Table 13-4 Number (%) of dental implants that received a prosthesis and maintained functional loading (intent-to-treat population*)

Dental implants placed	Bone graft (n = 251)	rhBMP-2/ACS (n = 241)	P[†]
After 6 mo functional loading			
n[‡]	243	240	
Success[§‖]	201 (82.7)	199 (82.9)	> .99
Failure[‖]	42 (17.3)	41 (17.1)	
After 12 mo functional loading			
n[‡]	243	237	
Success[§‖]	199 (81.9)	188 (79.3)	.49
Failure[‖]	44 (18.1)	49 (20.7)	
After 18 mo functional loading			
n[‡]	243	230	
Success[§‖]	200 (82.3)	179 (77.8)	.25
Failure[‖]	43 (17.7)	51 (22.2)	
After 24 mo functional loading			
n[‡]	243	222	
Success[§‖]	204 (84.0)	173 (77.9)	.12
Failure[‖]	39 (16.0)	49 (22.1)	

*The intent-to-treat population included all enrolled patients in their respective randomized treatment group, regardless of whether they actually received their assigned treatment, provided they had at least one documented outcome.

[†]P value is from Fisher exact test.

[‡]Dental implants from patients who successfully received a prosthesis but were lost to follow-up or withdrew anytime thereafter were excluded from the intent-to-treat analysis.

[§]Success is defined as a dental implant placed in newly induced bone that received a prosthesis and maintained functional loading.

[‖]For patients who missed a functional loading visit but whose dental implant status at flanking visits was known, the known status at the last visit was used.

Because the literature often reports dental implant success rates that are independent of loading status, this same analysis was included under the term *dental implant survival*. The dental implant survival rate represents the percentage of dental implants remaining in the treated sinus, regardless of functional loading status, over the course of the study. The dental implant survival rate was the same (about 87%) in both treatment groups (219 of 251 in the bone graft group and 209 of 241 in the rhBMP-2/ACS group).

For the purpose of evaluating the number and percentage of dental implant failures in newly induced bone, the term *failure* was applied only to dental implants that had to be removed. Based on this definition, the percentage of dental implant failures in newly induced bone was comparable in the two treatment groups: 12.7% (32 of 251) and 13.3% (32 of 241) in the bone graft and rhBMP-2/ACS treatment groups, respectively.

Safety

A total of 1,884 adverse events occurred during the entire study. The number and percentage of patients with the most frequently occurring adverse events for the entire study period (occurring in at least 10% of the patients) by treatment group and body system are presented in Table 13-5. All 82 patients in the rhBMP-2/ACS

Table 13-5 Number (%) of subjects with adverse events* by treatment group/body system

	Bone graft (n = 78)	rhBMP-2/ACS 1.5 mg/mL (n = 82)	Total (n = 160)	P value†
Subjects with records	78 (100)	82 (100)	160 (100)	NA
Subjects with adverse events	77 (99)	82 (100)	159 (99)	NA
Body as a whole				
Edema	28 (36)	2 (2)	30 (19)	< .001‡
Facial edema	44 (56)	59 (72)	103 (64)	.046‡
Headache	7 (9)	11 (13)	18 (11)	.46
Infection	32 (41)	22 (27)	54 (34)	.07
Pain	40 (51)	20 (24)	60 (38)	.001‡
Digestive system				
Mouth pain	66 (85)	71 (87)	137 (86)	.82
Oral edema	50 (64)	54 (66)	104 (65)	.87
Oral erythema	50 (64)	41 (50)	91 (57)	.08
Hemic and lymphatic system				
Ecchymosis	18 (23)	14 (17)	32 (20)	.43
Metabolic and nutritional disorders				
Hyperglycemia	15 (19)	8 (10)	23 (14)	.11
Musculoskeletal system				
Arthralgia	19 (24)	9 (11)	28 (18)	.04‡
Bone disorder	9 (12)	9 (11)	18 (11)	> .99
Nervous system				
Abnormal gait	34 (44)	0 (0)	34 (21)	< .001‡
Respiratory system				
Sinusitis	10 (13)	9 (11)	19 (12)	.81
Skin and appendages				
Rash	28 (36)	8 (10)	36 (23)	< .001‡

*Only those adverse events experienced by at least 10% of subjects were included.
†P value obtained from two-sided Fisher exact test.
‡Statistically significant at P < .05.
NA = not applicable.

treatment group and 77 of 78 patients in the bone graft group experienced an adverse event. The most frequent adverse events were primarily consistent with the surgical procedures performed (maxillary sinus floor augmentation, bone graft harvest, or dental implant placement and uncovering).

Patients in the bone graft treatment group experienced a significantly greater amount of edema (P < .0001), pain (P = .001), arthralgia (P = .04), abnormal gait (P < .001), and rash (P < .001) than did those in the rhBMP-2/ACS treatment group. The increased frequency of these events reflected the morbidity associated with the bone graft harvesting procedure. Many patients complained of pain at the harvest site (eg, pain in left hip); thus the event was coded as arthralgia.

Patients in the rhBMP-2/ACS treatment group exhibited a significantly greater amount of facial edema than did those in the bone graft treatment group ($P = .046$). The facial edema observed in the rhBMP-2/ACS treatment group was consistent with the results reported in the prior phase II sinus study[15] and is thought to be secondary to the activity of the rhBMP-2, which causes an influx of fluid and cells in the treatment area.

The severity of adverse events was comparable between the treatment groups. A majority of the adverse events were mild (grade 1: 34% [55 of 159]) or moderate (grade 2: 50% [80 of 159]) in severity. In addition, 15% of the adverse events were considered severe (grade 3), but no events were life threatening (grade 4).

The immunogenicity developed with rhBMP-2/ACS was low in this study and did not represent an increased risk compared with bone graft treatment. The proportion of patients who developed treatment-emergent elevation in anti–rhBMP-2 antibodies was 0 of 78 (0%) in the bone graft treatment group and 2 of 82 (2%) in the rhBMP-2/ACS treatment group. The proportion of patients who developed treatment-emergent elevation in antibodies to bovine type I collagen was 25 of 78 (32%) in the bone graft treatment group and 24 of 82 (29%) in the rhBMP-2/ACS treatment group. No clinical manifestations of an immune response or a neutralizing effect of the biologic activity of rhBMP-2 were identified in any of the study patients.

Conclusions

Prior to initiating this study, face-to-face discussions were held with all the investigators, and training was conducted to standardize the technique and familiarize each investigator and treatment center staff with the rhBMP-2/ACS device. An end point success target of 73% for functionally loaded implant prostheses was arrived at by a literature review, individual investigator experience, and the report from the consensus conference on maxillary sinus floor grafting.[18] It was agreed that a 73% success rate was a value that was acceptable clinically to avoid an autograft and the associated morbidity.

It is not surprising that the bone density was greater in the bone graft group 6 months after grafting; however,

after functional loading, the density of the rhBMP-2/ACS surpassed that of the bone graft, indicating that formation and maturation were slightly slower in the de novo bone induced by rhBMP-2. After maturation, the bone performed as well as the bone graft. This conclusion was also supported by the histologic specimens. There was no evidence of inflammatory infiltration in de novo bone, nor was there any evidence of residual collagen from the absorbable collagen sponge.

The 6-month postoperative mean bone height was 14.98 mm for the bone graft and 13.23 mm for the rhBMP-2/ACS. Of the 82 patients randomized to the rhBMP-2/ACS groups, one patient was lost to follow-up prior to the 6-month functional loading time point. While 74 of 78 patients (95%) in the bone graft group received implants, only 67 of 82 (82%) in the rhBMP-2/ACS group did.

Several factors influenced the higher number of patients in the rhBMP-2 group who failed to continue to the 6-month functional loading period. There were five protocol violations in the rhBMP-2 group that excluded these patients, who actually grew significant amounts of bone. This was an inadvertent error by the test site. Although most of these patients formed new bone, investigators made a clinical decision to add bone allograft at the time of the dental implant placement. Furthermore, seven patients in the rhBMP-2/ACS group withdrew at various time points before 6 months of functional loading was assessed, compared with only two patients in the bone graft group. This affected the percentage of patients who continued in the study.

Among patients who successfully received a prosthesis, only one patient in the rhBMP-2/ACS group was deemed to fail at the 6-month functional loading period, and no patients in the bone graft group were failures. The dental implant success rates after 12 and 18 months of functional loading (see Table 13-4) demonstrated that the de novo bone that was induced by rhBMP-2/ACS was of excellent quality and quantity (height and density) and was capable of supporting functional loading. Additionally, the crestal bone loss exhibited from the time of dental implant placement to prosthetic delivery was comparable between groups. At 18 months of functional loading, the crestal bone loss stabilized to 0.1 mm or less per year, which further supported the results of previously reported studies[19,20] and substantiated the ability of the rhBMP-2 to support long-term functional loading.

The rhBMP-2/ACS device has previously shown an excellent record of safety,[15,21,22] which was further substantiated in this pivotal trial. The most frequent adverse event was consistent with the surgical procedure that was performed. The bone graft group had a significantly greater number of patients who experienced edema, pain, arthralgia, abnormal gait, and erythema than the rhBMP-2 group, reflecting the morbidity associated with bone graft harvest. Facial edema was more notable in the rhBMP-2 group; this has been documented in other studies and trials intraorally and in orthopedic indications.[19] This edema, although notable, did not adversely affect the outcome.

No clinical manifestation of an immune response or neutralizing effect of the biologic activity of rhBMP-2 was identified in any of the study patients. This factor has continued to be monitored in both oral and orthopedic applications.

Summary

These multicenter randomized clinical trials demonstrated the effectiveness and safety of rhBMP-2/ACS for sinus floor augmentation. The results were comparable to those achieved with conventional augmentation procedures with bone graft. Although rhBMP-2 grafting did not equal the implant placement rate achieved by conventional bone grafting, the primary efficacy goal of 73% was exceeded, and a success rate of 79% was achieved. The implants placed in both rhBMP-2/ACS and bone graft performed exactly the same after functional loading. In addition, in response to functional loading, the density of the bone in the rhBMP-2/ACS group equaled that of the bone graft.

The ability to use a recombinant product that eliminates the need for harvesting of autologous bone and the morbidity associated with the harvesting procedure strongly supports this indication and use for rhBMP-2. Investigators were unanimous in their support of the effectiveness of the rhBMP-2 in inducing a sufficient quantity of bone de novo to support functional implant-borne prostheses. This device will be an outstanding addition to the armamentarium for bone graft augmentation in the oral environment.

References

1. Boyne PJ, James RA. Grafting of the maxillary sinus floor with autogenous marrow and bone. J Oral Surg 1980;38:613–616.
2. Tatum H Jr. Maxillary sinus and implant reconstructions. Dental Clin North Am 1986;30:207–229.
3. Smiler DG, Johnson PW, Lozada JL, et al. Sinus lift grafts and endosseous implants. Treatment of the atrophic posterior maxilla. Dent Clin North Am 1992;36:151–186.
4. Kent JN, Block MS. Simultaneous maxillary sinus floor bone grafting and placement of hydroxylapatite-coated implants. J Oral Maxillofac Surg 1989;47:238–242.
5. Damien CJ, Parsons JR. Bone graft and bone graft substitutes: A review of current technology and application. J Appl Biomater 1991;2:187–208.
6. Urist MR. Bone: Formation by autoinduction. Science 1965;150:893–899.
7. Bentz H, Nathan RM, Rosen DM, et al. Purification and characterization of a unique osteoinductive factor from bovine bone. J Biol Chem 1989;264:20805–20810.
8. Wozney JM, Rosen V, Celeste AJ, et al. Novel regulators of bone formation: Molecular clones and activities. Science 1988;242:1528–1534.
9. Wozney JM. Bone morphogenetic proteins and their gene expression. In: Noda M (ed). Cellular and Molecular Biology of Bone. San Diego: Academic Press, 1993:131–167.
10. Cochran DL, Nummikoski PV, Jones AA, Makins SR, Turek TJ, Buser D. Radiographic analysis of regenerated bone around endosseous implants in the canine using recombinant human bone morphogenetic protein-2. Int J Oral Maxillofac Implants 1997;12:739–748.
11. Hanisch O, Tatakis DN, Boskovic MM, Rohrer MD, Wikesjö UM. Bone formation and reosseointegration in peri-implantitis defects following surgical implantation of rhBMP-2. Int J Oral Maxillofac Implants 1997;12:604–610.
12. Zellin G, Linde A. Importance of delivery systems for growth-stimulatory factors in combination with osteopromotive membranes. An experimental study using rhBMP-2 in rat mandibular defects. J Biomed Mater Res 1997;35:181–190.
13. Nevins M, Kirker-Head C, Nevins M, Wozney JA, Palmer R, Graham D. Bone formation in the goat maxillary sinus induced by absorbable collagen sponge implants impregnated with recombinant human bone morphogenetic protein-2. Int J Periodontics Restorative Dent 1996;16:9–19.
14. Boyne PJ, Marx RE, Nevins M, et al. A feasibility study evaluating rhBMP-2/absorbable collagen sponge for maxillary sinus floor augmentation. Int J Periodontics Restorative Dent 1997;17:11–25.
15. Boyne PJ, Lilly LC, Marx RE, et al. De novo bone induction by recombinant human bone morphogenetic protein-2 (rhBMP-2) in maxillary sinus floor augmentation. J Oral Maxillofac Surg 2005;63:1693–1707.
16. Wolff J. Das Gasetz der Transformation der Knochen. Berlin: Hirschwald, 1892.
17. Blomqvist JE, Alberius P, Isaksson S. Two-stage maxillary sinus reconstruction with endosseous implants: A prospective study. Int J Oral Maxillofac Implants 1998;13:758–766.
18. Jensen OI, Shulmann LB, Block MS, Iacono VJ. Report of the Sinus Consensus Conference of 1996. Int J Oral Maxillofac Implants 1998;13(suppl):11–45.
19. Carmichael RP, Apse P, Zarb GA, McCulloch CAG. Biological, microbiological, and clinical aspects of the peri-implant mucosa in the Brånemark osseointegrated implant. In: Albrektsson T, Zarb GA (eds). The Brånemark Osseointegrated Implant. Chicago: Quintessence, 1989:58.
20. Adell R. Long-term treatment results. In: Brånemark P-I, Zarb GA, Albrektsson T (eds). Tissue-Integrated Prostheses. Chicago: Quintessence, 1985:181.
21. Govender S, Csimma C, Genant HK, et al. Recombinant human bone morphogenetic protein-2 for treatment of open tibial fractures: A prospective, controlled, randomized study of four hundred and fifty patients. J Bone Joint Surg Am 2002;84A:2123–2134.
22. Burkus JK, Heim SE, Gornet MF, Zdeblick TA. Is INFUSE bone graft superior to autograft bone? An integrated analysis of clinical trials using the LT-CAGE lumbar tapered fusion device. J Spinal Disord Tech 2003;16:113–122.

Alveolar Distraction Osteogenesis and Tissue Engineering

Ole T. Jensen, DDS, MS

Zvi Laster, DMD

Hideharu Hibi, DDS, PhD

Yoichi Yamada, DDS, PhD

Minoru Ueda, DDS, PhD

Bone formed by distraction osteogenesis mimics developmental bone growth.[1] The mechanoadaptive capacity of bone permits formation of new bone when the existing bone is appropriately strained.[2–4] Viable cellular elements must be present for the morphogenetic signal to be propagated within the milieu of what is essentially a stretching callus.[5,6] Osteocompetent cells proliferate, differentiate, and operate, but when an inadequate number of osteogenic cells are present, the distraction wound is compromised and bone formation does not occur. The secondary application of bone-forming cells to a compromised distraction site augments the osseous wound-healing potential.

In addition to cellular competency, alveolar augmentation requires a structural strategy, or the augmentation will fail.[7] The use of distraction osteogenesis is one such structural strategy for establishing new bone, because it provides a dimensional substrate on which osteoblasts can function to enable hard tissue formation.[8]

The use of alveolar distraction osteogenesis for alveolar reconstruction is often complicated by insufficient bone mass, so that two surgical procedures for augmentation are required. A common clinical treatment challenge for surgeons is the vertically and horizontally deficient alveolar ridge. Distraction osteogenesis, as it is currently applied, will increase vertical bone mass or horizontal bone mass but not both simultaneously, necessitating a secondary bone-grafting strategy to finalize alveolar form.[9]

This chapter will discuss the current state of the art of distraction osteogenesis therapy. In addition, the discussion will include ongoing clinical research, performed at Nagano University in Japan, on autogenous ex vivo cultured bone-forming cells applied to improve the osteogenic performance of distraction osteogenesis wounds.

Vertical Alveolar Distraction Osteogenesis

The general indication for vertical alveolar distraction osteogenesis is a vertical defect greater than 5 mm.[10] Other bone augmentation strategies such as onlay (mandibular) block bone grafting and guided bone regeneration have a variable limit as to how far from basal bone functional graft incorporation will occur. Interpositional (sandwich) bone graft augmentation has a better blood supply for incorporation, but vertical gain is limited by investing soft tissues.[11]

Each of these conventional augmentation strategies becomes compromised with attempts to obtain a 10-mm vertical gain. Although gains of 10 mm have been achieved with iliac block onlay grafts, there is considerable variation in postsurgical remodeling bone loss, even when a barrier membrane is used. It is not uncommon to find 3 mm or greater vertical bone loss as a result of remodeling within the first year.[12]

A second complicating factor to consider in the use of vertical distraction osteogenesis is the bone level of adjacent teeth. Bone distracted significantly beyond the bone support of adjacent teeth will not persist. Therefore, the distraction occasionally may require the inclusion of adjacent teeth to displace the defect adequately in order to move the overall bone level crestally. Unlike conventional bone grafts, typical vertical distractions of 10 mm or more generally maintain architectural stability.[13]

The transport bone fragment being distracted should be of sufficient size to maintain blood supply and avoid sequestration or late resorption. A bone fragment that is too small, such as a one-tooth segment, or too narrow can easily be compromised by manipulation during the fixation process or by an aggressive distraction protocol.[14]

The technical procedure for device application, as well as the latency, rate, and frequency for alveolar bone manipulation has largely been extrapolated from exoskeletal or total jaw distraction studies.[2] A rate of 1.0 mm per day has been advocated, but is probably excessive for small bone fragments. Ueda et al[14] showed that a rate of 1.0 mm per day in the rat mandible resulted in less mineralized tissue in the distraction zone than was found at a slower rate of 0.5 to 0.8 mm per day. At 0.5 to 0.8 mm per day, chondroblastic bone develops, resulting in nearly twice the mineralized component in the distraction zone.[15] This suggests that use of a slower pace during the distraction treatment interval is prudent.

There is also no apparent harm done by distraction periodicity, that is, at intervals, skipping a day during the distraction phase, for example, every fourth or fifth day.[16] Patients who experience pain from distraction activation will benefit from periodicity as well as by dividing activation into intervals of two to four times per day.

The complexity of treatment of significant vertical defects cannot be overstated, because more often than not a horizontal bone deficiency must be addressed either prior to or after distraction.

Case 1

A 45-year-old patient received an implant to replace the maxillary right lateral incisor. The implant became infected and was removed. By 1 year after removal, the infection had led to the loss of several millimeters of vertical root surface bone support from the adjacent teeth (Fig 14-1a). Bone grafting with guided bone regeneration procedures was used without success to treat the defect.

A Mommaerts-Laster bi-phase distractor (Figs 14-1b and 14-1c) was used to perform an osteotomy that included the compromised adjacent teeth to mobilize the defect site (Fig 14-1d). The defect site was moved downward 10 mm and advanced 3 mm (Figs 14-1e and 14-1f).

Four months later the device was removed, and the right canine tooth was extracted. An implant was placed in the extraction site. Crown lengthening was performed on the central incisor. The defect at the site of the lateral incisor was eliminated to establish near ideal alveolar form. The treatment proceeded to a complete-crown restoration on the central incisor and a cantilevered implant restoration including the canine and lateral incisor (Figs 14-1g to 14-1i).

Horizontal Alveolar Split Distraction Osteogenesis

The indication for alveolar widening by distraction osteogenesis is an alveolus that is too narrow for implant placement, usually interpreted as less than 4 mm in crestal width, or situated too far lingually or palatally. Regenerative procedures for dehiscence and fenestration lesions around teeth or implants have been well studied, and there are numerous reports using block grafts or particulate grafts with barrier membranes.[17–19] An alveolar split bone-grafting approach is also used; this technique requires interpositioning of a structural graft or simultaneous placement of an implant to maintain width.[20,21]

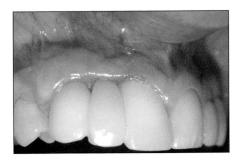

Fig 14-1a A three-unit provisional partial denture is unesthetic because of bone loss on adjacent teeth and in the pontic site following removal of a failed implant.

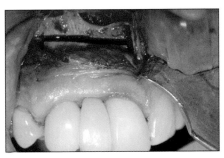

Fig 14-1b An alveolar segmental osteotomy includes the maxillary right canine and central incisor in order to move the defect of the lateral incisor site crestally.

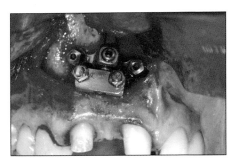

Fig 14-1c A Mommaerts-Laster bi-phase alveolar distractor (Surgi-Tec) is placed to move the segment downward and forward.

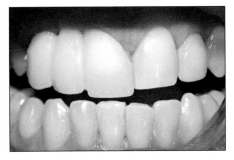

Fig 14-1d Early distraction is observed at the incisal edge of the provisional prosthesis prior to equilibration.

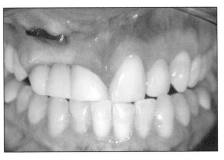

Fig 14-1e The defect site has moved downward 10 mm and has advanced 3 mm.

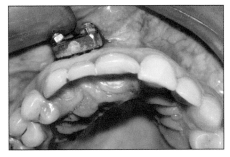

Fig 14-1f Forward projection of the canine eminence is achieved by differential tightening of the horizontal activation screws.

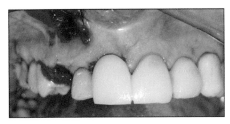

Fig 14-1g Following a crown-lengthening procedure, a provisional crown with a cantilever lateral incisor pontic is made for the right central incisor. The canine has been removed.

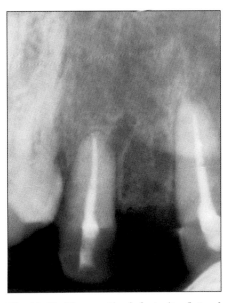

Fig 14-1h The pontic defect site (lateral incisor) is now in orthoalveolar form, but the canine root is ghost and exhibits a facial bone dehiscence.

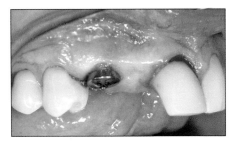

Fig 14-1i The canine is replaced with an implant.

A delayed placement approach is frequently used for all of these techniques, requiring a 4-month bone graft incorporation period prior to implant placement. Osseointegration in these settings is highly reliant on the success of the bone graft.

One of the major advantages of the split alveolar graft is the ability to obtain a mature lamellar plate of bone (both facially and lingually). This is highly desirable on the facial side, where marginal bone stability affects the cervical crown form of the final dental restoration. Alveolar distraction to increase width establishes a mature facial plate on each side of the alveolus so that dehiscence is less likely to occur following implant placement.

The use of alveolar crest widening by distraction osteogenesis not only has the advantage of avoiding a bone graft but also is favorable for early implant placement. Implants are typically placed 6 weeks after osteotomy, which is about 3 to 4 weeks after distraction, into a woven matrix that is highly conducive to osseointegration.[22] Overall treatment time is therefore significantly reduced when compared with the time involved in a bone graft.[17]

The method used for split alveolar bone exposure is important because excess periosteal reflection will lead to vascular embarrassment and subsequent plate loss from late bone resorption. Therefore, the use of minimal flap reflection and careful manipulation are of utmost importance.

Two types of narrow ridge are commonly encountered: the triangular ridge and the parallel ridge. Triangular bone plates may be split apart quite easily. The buccal plate is out-fractured to facilitate a tilting movement by distraction, thus expanding the top of the triangle. The base of the triangle is generally wide enough to host the implant. All bone cuts are performed through the mucoperiosteal incisions without periosteal stripping.

The parallel-shaped ridge has to be distracted with a bodily movement of the buccal plate. A so-called stop-cut made at the point of the desired out-fracture is often needed to allow complete mobilization of the buccal plate. However, it is difficult to make the stop-cut without detaching the blood supply to the facial plate. This problem has been solved by a two-stage surgery. In the first surgery, a stop-cut osteotomy is made through an open flap, and then the wound is sutured closed. Three weeks later, after minimal crestal reflection, the crestal and two vertical bone cuts are made, and the plate is out-fractured. The distraction device is then placed.

A second option to manage the parallel ridge is to make the stop-cut through a tunnel flap, keeping the crestal portion of the flap attached without completely reflecting the flap away from the facial plate. With this approach, the distraction device can be placed the same day.

One week after placement of the distractor, the device is activated by the patient at a very slow rate of 0.3 to 0.4 mm per day. This is done for 4 days, followed by a rest day, and then the sequence is started again. The desired expansion is achieved in about 10 days, on average. Four weeks later, the device is removed. Implants can be placed transgingivally on the day of device removal or later. The dental restoration proceeds 3 months later.

Case 2

A 39-year-old woman was referred for bone augmentation (Fig 14-2a). Examination revealed a narrow crest with sufficient vertical height (Fig 14-2b). Crest expansion by distraction osteogenesis using an alveolar crest expander was the treatment of choice.

After local anesthesia was administered to the patient, three transmucoperiosteal incisions were performed. A crestal and two vertical incisions defined the area to be distracted. The top of the crest was minimally exposed toward the lingual side (Fig 14-2c), and a microcrestal trough was made with a small round bur. A scalpel reciprocating saw was used to make a sagittal bone cut, followed by anterior and posterior transgingival bone cuts (Fig 14-2d). An osteotome was then used to split and out-fracture the facial segment (Fig 14-2e). A securing titanium wire was threaded through a hole in one of the distractor arms (Fig 14-2f), and the device was inserted in the bone (Figs 14-2g and 14-2h). After suturing of the soft tissue, the crest expander was activated one full turn (0.4 mm) to stabilize the device.

Distraction started after 1 week at a rate of a one-quarter turn three times a day (0.3 mm) for 4 days followed by a rest day. The rest day was intended to reduce the tension at the distraction callus and allow time for protein synthesis. Activation was performed by the patient.

The desired crestal width was achieved by day 20, when activation was stopped. The crest expander was removed under local anesthesia and the callus was allowed to consolidate for 1 more week. The implants were then inserted transmucosally and left with healing caps (Fig 14-2i). Final prosthetic rehabilitation was finished 3 months later (Fig 14-2j).

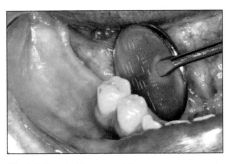

Fig 14-2a A 39-year-old woman presents with missing mandibular molars and moderate alveolar atrophy.

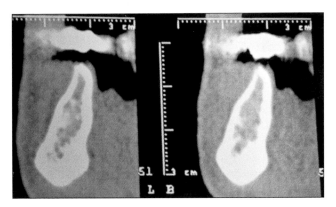

Fig 14-2b A CT reveals a 3-mm-wide (crestal) alveolar process that has sufficient vertical height.

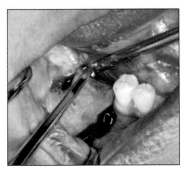

Fig 14-2c Incisions are made over the crest and at the border of the area to be distracted.

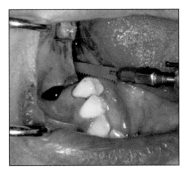

Fig 14-2d Saw cuts are made without periosteal reflection.

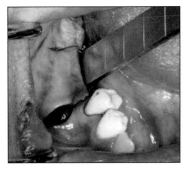

Fig 14-2e Greenstick out-fracture of the segment is achieved with an osteotome.

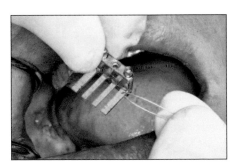

Fig 14-2f Laster horizontal distractor (Crest Expander, Surgi-Tec).

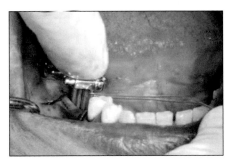

Fig 14-2g The distractor is inserted with finger pressure.

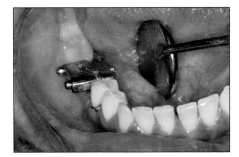

Fig 14-2h The distraction device is tapped into place and secured to an adjacent tooth with a wire ligature.

Fig 14-2i After horizontal distraction is completed (27 days after distractor placement), two implants are placed.

Fig 14-2j The final restoration has been completed 3 months after implant placement.

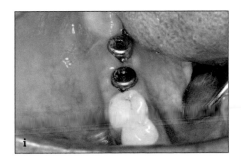

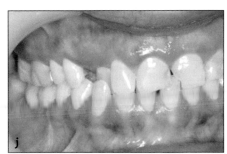

Segmental Alveolar Repositioning

Segmental alveolar distraction can be performed to advance a retrognathic maxilla. The anterior alveolar process is segmented in front of the sinuses and distracted to an advanced position. This is done in a mostly horizontal direction as an alternative to complete Le Fort I jaw advancement. When the maxilla needs to be moved downward and advanced significantly, the Le Fort I approach is preferred. If the maxilla is in a generally favorable vertical position but is retrognathic, the anterior segment can be distracted forward 10 mm or more to increase lip support and improve alveolar form.[23]

Another maxillary segmental distraction approach is performed in the posterior maxilla for the patient with an alveolar cleft. If the cleft is wide and the dental occlusion parameters are favorable, the posterior alveolar segment can be surgically advanced horizontally to reduce or even close the cleft site. A distraction approach may be more favorable than a strictly orthognathic approach, because palatal soft tissue tension is more easily overcome by gradual distraction.[24]

Palatal Distraction Osteogenesis

The modification of arch relationships by expansion of the maxilla at the palatal suture is well known in orthodontic care. The use of so-called rapid palatal expansion in the maxilla is most stable when performed by the slow method of distraction osteogenesis at a maximum rate of 1 mm or less per day for distraction. The process can be used in the growing or adult patient equally well.

One aspect that has not been adequately investigated is the use of distraction to widen the edentulous maxillary arch. The pattern of resorption commonly observed in the edentulous maxilla may leave axial arch form in relative crossbite to the mandible, or there may have been a preexisting crossbite relationship in the dentate state. If alveolar bone mass is otherwise sufficient, expansion of the maxillary arch via palatal distraction may be indicated. A partially edentulous segment can be treated in this same way.

One advantage of a palatally placed distractor is that the segments move bodily instead of tipping buccally, which favors stable buccal plate projection.

Case 3

A 17-year-old girl was referred by her orthodontist after unsuccessful treatment with a tooth-borne expander. She had hemifacial microsomia in addition to a considerable transverse arch deficiency. The tooth-borne device had caused a severe tipping of the teeth (Fig 14-3a).

A new treatment plan involved unilateral distraction osteogenesis with an osseous-based transpalatal distraction device (Surgi-Tec) (Fig 14-3b). The bone cuts and the positioning of the device with the desired vector were planned in advance through stone cast "surgery" (Fig 14-3c).

The unilateral horizontal bone cut was made in the anterior maxilla. Activation started 1 week after placement of the device; the progress was monitored with weekly follow-up and routine occlusal radiographs (Fig 14-3d).

After sufficient distraction of the left-side bone segment (Fig 14-3e), the device was locked for 2 months to allow consolidation of the callus.

The final occlusion was achieved by orthodontic treatment (Fig 14-3f). The high horizontal bone cut provided good bone-healing capacity and achieved a stable solution to the facial asymmetry (Figs 14-3g and 14-3h).

This type of device must be used in the partially or fully edentulous setting.

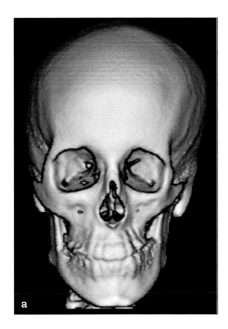

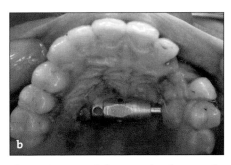

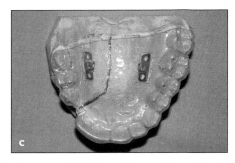

Fig 14-3a A tooth-borne palatal expansion device caused tipping of the teeth and inadequate osseous widening at the palatal suture. Note the posterior crossbite.

Fig 14-3b An osseous-based transpalatal expander is placed.

Fig 14-3c Surgery on the cast is used to establish the alveolar movement vector.

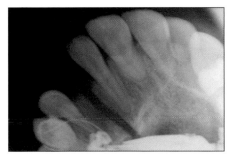

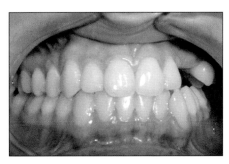

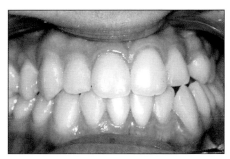

Fig 14-3d An occlusal radiograph reveals the bone cut made in the anterior maxilla.

Fig 14-3e The site exhibits sufficient expansion.

Fig 14-3f The final occlusion is established orthodontically.

Figs 14-3g and 14-3h Pretreatment (*g*) and posttreatment (*h*) facial photographs.

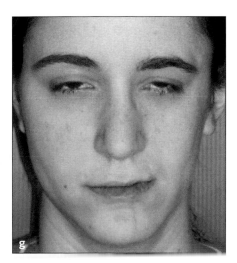

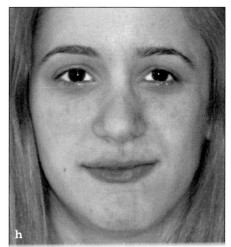

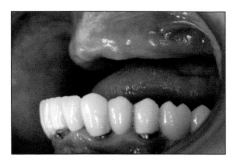

Fig 14-4a A completely edentulous 36-year-old woman exhibits maxillary retrognathic positioning.

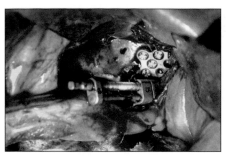

Fig 14-4b Following Le Fort I osteotomy with incomplete downfracture and sinus grafting, the maxilla is fitted with bilateral distraction devices for a downward and forward distraction vector.

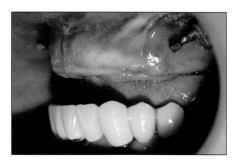

Fig 14-4c Distraction is continued until the alveolar projection is even with the mandibular incisor teeth.

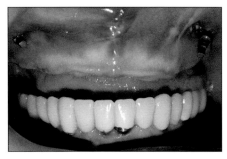

Fig 14-4d The maxilla remains tilted to the left following distraction.

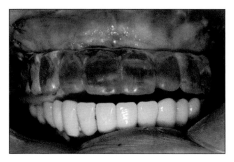

Fig 14-4e Following a 4-month consolidation period, a guide stent is used for transgingival placement of eight implants, excluding the four incisor positions.

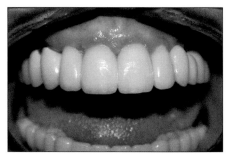

Fig 14-4f The final restoration is completed, 4 months after implant placement, with a porcelain single-unit fixed partial denture with gingival display anteriorly.

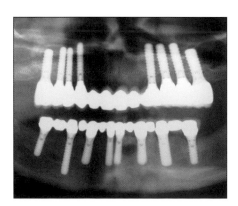

Fig 14-4g A 2-year postsurgical panoramic radiograph shows the implant-supported prosthesis.

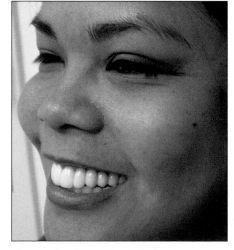

Fig 14-4h The perioral facial tissues are supported by the anteriorized maxillary complex.

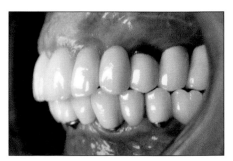

Fig 14-4i Two years posttreatment, the prosthesis and the occlusion remain stable.

Fig 14-5 A Class II maxillomandibular relationship following total joint replacement is treated by distraction osteogenesis at the body of the mandible.

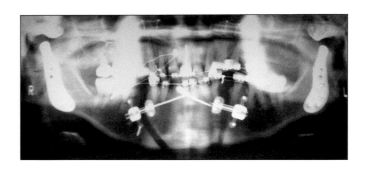

Le Fort I Distraction Osteogenesis

The indication for Le Fort I distraction osteogenesis in the reconstructive surgery setting is the need for improvement of the maxillomandibular relationship and a desire for natural gingival display. Inherent in the decision to distract an edentulous arch is the need to improve the esthetic presentation of the anterior alveolar process to be restored with an implant-supported prosthesis. The maxilla is distracted to the point where no prosthetic flange is required to support the lip, and the arches develop Class I axial alignment.

Tissue engineering with a combination of morphogens or cultured osteoblasts and a structural framework, without a change in maxillary position, seems unlikely at present to perform as well as distraction displacement in recreating an ablated or highly atrophic and retrognathic maxilla. With distraction, even if the residual maxilla is highly atrophic and needs considerable bone mass augmentation, the improvement in basal bone relationship to the opposing arch greatly reduces the amount of supplemental bone graft required and improves the stability of the graft regardless of which grafting procedure is used.

Presently, the process of distraction of a fully edentulous maxilla is typically combined with sinus bone grafts. The downfractured maxilla with elevated sinus and nasal membranes is grafted in the sinus floor with autogenous particulate bone. This site could easily be augmented with osteoblasts and alloplast as well.

Case 4

A 36-year-old completely edentulous woman had an atrophic and severely retropositioned maxilla (Fig 14-4a). Distractors were fastened bilaterally to the zygomatic buttresses (Fig 14-4b). The maxilla was advanced 12 mm and moved downward about 5 mm (Fig 14-4c). At the end of distraction, a Class I relationship had been obtained. The gingival display was visible, and the provisional denture flange had to be cut away, indicating that advancement was sufficient to allow ovate pontiform emergence of the final prosthetic restoration (Fig 14-4d).

Four months after the completion of distraction, eight implants were placed according to a prosthetic guide (Fig 14-4e). Four months after implant placement, the fixed partial denture was made (Figs 14-4f and 14-4g). The resulting orthoalveolar form allowed a biomechanically favorable and esthetically pleasing final restoration (Figs 14-4h and 14-4i).

Mandibular Body Distraction Osteogenesis

A Class II jaw relationship is most often managed by sagittal ramus osteotomy but can on occasion be managed by body osteotomy and subsequent distraction to couple the anterior occlusion. In edentulous patients, this may affect implant placement. Figure 14-5 shows a dentate patient in whom total temporomandibular joint prostheses were placed. A bilateral body distraction procedure was performed to improve the incisor relationship.

The spaces created by distraction can be treated with conventional fixed partial dentures or dental implants.

Tissue Engineering in Distraction Osteogenesis

The use of alveolar distraction osteogenesis for reconstruction of bone defects without bone grafting is now widely accepted, but a relatively long healing time is required. To shorten the consolidation period, hyperbaric oxygenation as well as electrical, ultrasonic, and chemical stimulation have been attempted with modest positive effect.[25] In contrast, cell-based therapy has been shown to significantly improve osteogenic potential in the distracted callus and to decrease healing time.[26–30] The application of tissue-engineered cells ("injectable bone") to distraction osteogenesis sites where there is a compromised host or in unfavorable situations, such as grafted bone or previous irradiation, may significantly advance therapeutic outcome.[31–33]

Injectable bone preparation

Injectable bone is prepared with autogenous stromal stem cells and platelet-rich plasma (PRP).[32] The stromal stem cells are isolated from iliac marrow aspirate, expanded in culture media for a few weeks, and then differentiated in osteogenesis induction media for another week. The PRP is isolated from autologous blood using density gradient centrifugation and a selective collection technique. The induced cells, the PRP, calcium chloride, and human thrombin are mixed for 5 seconds into an injectable mixture, which maintains as a gel for about 20 seconds.

Injection protocol

At the completion of distraction, an 18-gauge needle is percutaneously placed in the center of the distraction gap under C-arm fluoroscopy guidance. The mixture is injected over a 5-second period. The needle is left in place for an additional minute to allow the injected gel to increase in viscosity to prevent it from leaking out of the puncture site.

Case 5

A 54-year-old man was referred for rehabilitation of a previously reconstructed edentulous mandible.[31] Two years earlier, he had undergone segmental resection and immediate reconstruction of the mandible and the oral floor to treat squamous cell carcinoma. Surgery was followed by chemotherapy and irradiation of 60 Gy. The reconstruction consisted of a 9-cm vascularized fibular graft osteotomized into three segments and fixed with eight miniplates for the mandible and its cutaneous flap for the oral floor (Figs 14-6a and 14-6b). Computerized tomography (CT) demonstrated that the grafted fibula remodeled into a bi-angled body approximately 1 cm in height and width (Fig 14-6c).

A vertical distraction procedure was planned in the area between the right mental foramen and the left reconstructed segment to allow placement of dental implants. From the submandibular approach through the previous scar line, osteotomies were performed with a sagittal saw after the removal of six plates and screws, all done after administration of general anesthesia. A transport segment, which was 7 cm long and 5 mm high and attached by a pedicle to the lingual periosteum, was created from the reconstructed mandible. A distraction device (Track 1.5, Gebruder Martin) was positioned and fixed with microscrews (Fig 14-6d). The periosteum labial to the horizontal osteotomy line was disturbed because of simultaneous removal of the previously placed osteosynthesis hardware. After a latent period of 7 days, the distractor was activated at a rate of 0.5 mm, twice a day, for 15 days (Fig 14-6e).

The injectable bone was applied to the distraction callus at the end of activation. The cultured cells had been derived from 10 mL of iliac marrow aspirate expanded in culture to 5×10^7 cells, and 20 mL of PRP was isolated from 200 mL of autologous blood. The PRP contained 1.6×10^9 platelets/mL, a concentration 8.3 times greater than that of whole blood. The induced cells and PRP were used to prepare 3 mL of injectable bone, which was infiltrated for 15 seconds into the distraction gap while the patient was under intravenous sedation (Figs 14-6f and 14-6g). No complications were observed during the injection, and the subsequent course of healing was uneventful.

A series of monthly panoramic radiographs revealed that radiopacity had begun to appear in the distraction gap by 1 month. After 2 to 3 months, during which the

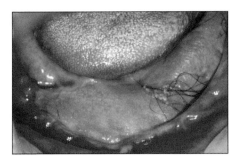

Fig 14-6a The mandible and oral floor have been reconstructed with a vascularized osteocutaneous fibular flap.

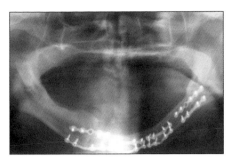

Fig 14-6b Panoramic radiograph of the reconstructed mandible.

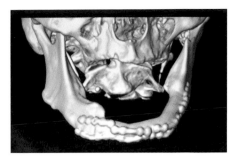

Fig 14-6c The grafted fibula has remodeled into a bi-angled body of 1 cm in height and width.

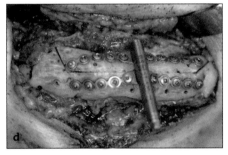

Fig 14-6d The distraction device is positioned on the reconstructed mandible.

Fig 14-6e At the end of distraction (22 days after placement of the distractor), the transported segment has been repositioned 15 mm superiorly.

Fig 14-6f Injectable bone is applied to the distracted tissue.

Fig 14-6g A fluoroscope is used to guide the application of injectable bone.

(Fig 14-6 continued on next page.)

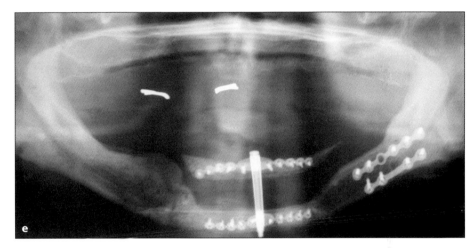

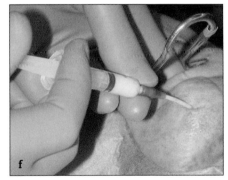

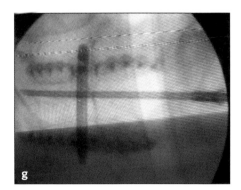

transport segment resorbed marginally (Fig 14-6h), the distraction regenerate became wholly radiopaque. CTs obtained at 3 months revealed newly formed bone in the distraction gap with a clearly delineated lingual cortical surface but an undefined labial cortex. The intercortical area was relatively evenly calcified. The bone mineral density scored higher in Hounsfield units than adjacent cancellous bone in the mandible or fibular graft (Fig 14-6i and 14-6j).

The distraction device was removed, and six titanium screw-type implants, 3.75 × 18.00 mm (Brånemark System, Nobel Biocare), were placed (Fig 14-6k). During the implant preparation, hard tissue specimens were taken with a trephine. The distalmost implant on the patient's right side was placed in native mandibular bone, while the other five implants were placed in distracted bone. All implants required a torque of 40 Ncm for placement and achieved primary stability.

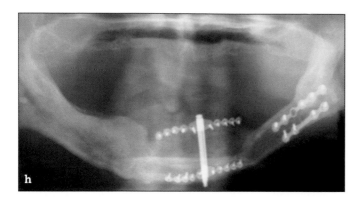

Fig 14-6h Three months after completion of distraction, the distraction gap exhibits radiopacity.

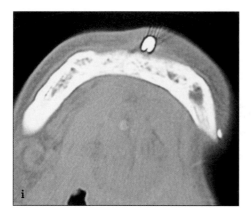

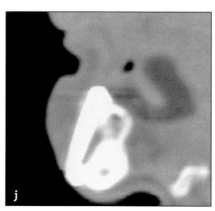

Fig 14-6i The newly formed bone in the distraction gap appears unclear at the labial aspect but clear on the lingual cortical surface.

Fig 14-6j The cortical bone, which has a relatively even density, is higher in terms of Hounsfield units than the adjacent cancellous area.

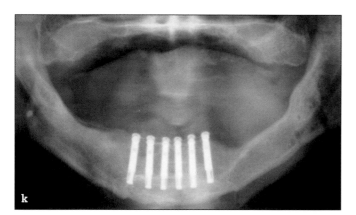

Fig 14-6k Immediately after implant placement, 3 months post-distraction.

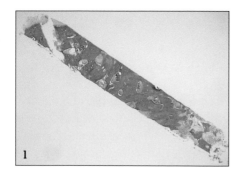

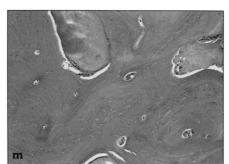

Fig 14-6l Representative decalcified histologic specimen from the bone core, harvested from the distraction zone at the time of implant placement (hematoxylin-eosin stain; original magnification ×1.25).

Fig 14-6m The specimen reveals remodeling lamellar bone and abundant osteocytes in the lacunae within the distraction zone (hematoxylin-eosin stain; original magnification ×10).

Fig 14-6n A CT taken 1 year after implant placement reveals well-mineralized bone in the distraction gap with distinct labial and lingual cortical plates.

Fig 14-6o Clinical appearance 2 years after seating of the prostheses. (Figs 14-6a to 14-6i, 14-6k to 14-6m, and 14-6o from Hibi et al.[31] Reprinted with permission.)

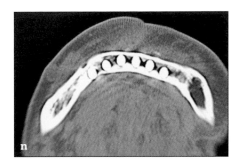
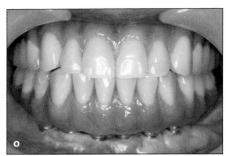

Fig 14-6p Panoramic radiograph of the fully restored site 2 years after prosthetic reconstruction.

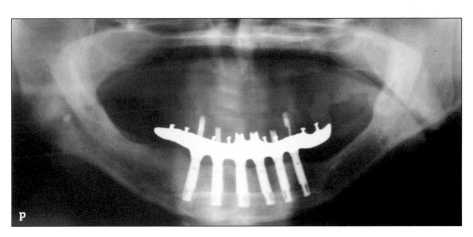

The two distalmost implants on the patient's right side had insufficient surrounding bone with a dehiscence gap in the bone between them. To augment this site, a 0.1-mm-thick titanium mesh (Micromesh, Stryker) was fixed to the platforms of all six implants using low-profile cover screws, creating additional space both marginally and labially. This space was filled with 3 mL of injectable bone prepared with 6×10^7 induced bone-forming cells and PRP containing 3.6×10^9 platelets. The postoperative course was uneventful.

A decalcified section of the histologic specimens taken at implant placement revealed remodeling lamellar bone with abundant viable osteocytes in the lacunae within the distraction zone (Figs 14-6l and 14-6m).

Three months after implant placement, the implants were uncovered, and the mesh was removed. All implants had achieved osseointegration, and healing abutments were connected. Under the mesh, a regenerated hard tissue covered with a periosteum-like membrane was observed. Palatal mucosa was transplanted over this membranous covering on the labial and lingual sides of the regenerated ridge, while the cutaneous flap was debulked, defatted, and repositioned lingually and apically to establish a vestibule.

Three weeks after the uncovering procedures, attached mucosa had formed around the implant abutments. A maxillary complete denture and a mandibular implant-supported prosthesis were placed.

CTs obtained 1 year after implant placement revealed well mineralized bone in the distraction gap with distinct labial and lingual cortical plates (Fig 14-6n). The prostheses functioned without complication (Figs 14-6o and 14-6p).

Vascularized fibular bone expansion

A vascularized fibular flap is often selected for mandibular reconstruction. However, to follow the mandibular arch, the fibula requires multiple osteotomies, which interrupt the medullary vasculature and thereby vascular supply, because the entire flap depends on the periosteum.[34] The fibular periosteum supplies the external two thirds of the cortex after revascularization, while its internal third and the medulla have a reduced vascular supply.[35] Preservation of periosteal attachment is therefore considered a

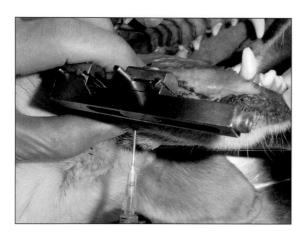

Fig 14-7 Injectable bone is applied to a distracted site in a canine mandible.

critical factor in distraction osteogenesis, even after graft-ed fibular segments have healed and united to adjacent mandibular bone.

Several authors have reported successful vertical dis-traction osteogenesis of the fibula grafted to reconstruct the mandible.[35,36] These cases were less complex than case 5 (described above), which included a patient with older age, a higher dose of irradiation, a larger transport segment, a longer distance of distraction, and damage to the labial periosteum resulting from simultaneous removal of osteosynthetic plates and screws. These conditions suggest the etiology for the partial resorption of the superior portion of the transport segment in this patient. Despite periosteal reflection, the patient demonstrated new bone formation on the labial access side of the regenerate, as well as higher-quality bone formed lingual-ly, without extension of the consolidation period.

These favorable histologic and radiographic findings may be attributed to the biomaterial injected into the dis-tracted tissue. Tissue engineering combines three key ele-ments: cells, signaling molecules, and scaffolds.[37] In this patient, for cells, autogenous osteogenic cells and PRP were applied; for signaling molecules, there were the growth and transforming factors in the PRP; and for scaf-folding, there was the isotropic fibrous tissue of the dis-traction zone.

Several animal studies have shown that the injection of cells with osteogenic potential into distraction gaps en-hances new bone formation with respect to volume and strength and shortens the consolidation period.[26–30] Sim-ilar results have also been observed in a bilateral distrac-tion osteogenesis model in the canine mandible.[22] The study used a standard protocol with a 7-day latency suc-ceeded by distraction of 1 mm per day for 10 days. After distraction was completed, 1 mL of injectable bone was

administered to the distracted tissue on one side, and the same amount of saline was administered to the opposite side (Fig 14-7). Serial occlusal radiographs of the man-dibles indicated that radiopacity of the distraction zone increased earlier in the side that received injectable bone than the side that received saline (Figs 14-8 and 14-9). The timing of cellular injections has been investigated fur-ther, but the timing of injection appears to have no effect on experimental outcome.[4]

In the patient described in case 5, the injection was administered at the end of the distraction process because that is when the distraction gap has the lowest number of cells with osteogenic potential. Injected cells function before gradual recruitment via the vasculature. Growth factors from the alpha granules of the platelets help activate cells, including stem cells and local osteo-blasts, through their membrane receptors.[38] Distraction osteogenesis appears to have few limitations regarding distraction length but can require a longer treatment time than bone grafting. These innovative methods combining distraction techniques and tissue engineering can allow more effective bone regeneration for adequate implant placement and jawbone reconstruction.

Discussion

Tissue engineering implies the extracorporeal replication or enhancement of a naturally occurring biologic process, or the production of an implantable regenerative product for modification of a deficient tissue or organ system. The growth of bone at the epiphyseal plate in long bones

Fig 14-8 Serial occlusal radiographs of a canine mandible show the injectable bone–treated experimental side *(left)* and saline-treated control side *(right)*. *(a)* Immediately after distraction. *(b)* One week after distraction. *(c)* Two weeks after distraction. *(d)* Three weeks after distraction.

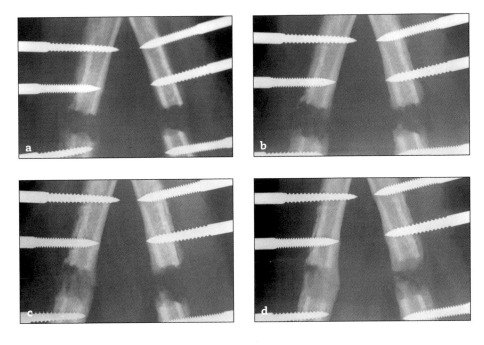

Fig 14-9 Surface plots reveal the density of the occlusal radiographs using an image processing and analyzing program. *(left)* Mandible treated with injectable bone; *(right)* control mandible. *(a)* Immediately after distraction. *(b)* One week after distraction. *(c)* Two weeks after distraction. *(d)* Three weeks after distraction.

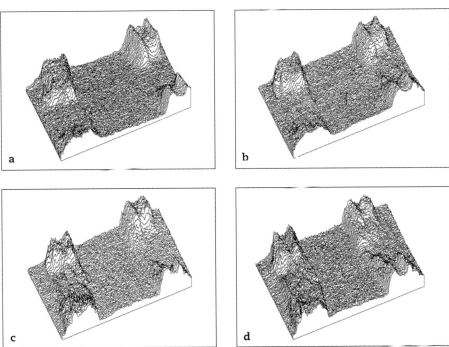

is analogous to, if not replicated by, mechanically engineered displacement resulting from distraction osteogenesis. Neurohumoral and mechanocellular signals mimic the intrinsic mechanism of primordial bone generation as bone morphogenetic protein and matrix-forming enzyme concentrations increase during both forms of osteogenesis. The use of distraction osteogenesis to regenerate bone stock in miniim clinically well founded, but technical problems persist, and improvements are still desirable.

There is a difference in bone formation on the two sides of the bone being distracted. The wound access side, which is the side on which the osteotomy and distraction plate are placed, must undergo periosteal stripping while the internal (medial side) periosteum is left largely undisturbed. The reflected periosteum is unable to function fully in callus formation; in contrast, the undisturbed side functions fully and easily expands a woven callus. The net effect is a relatively less mineralized product and sometimes defect formation on the wound side of the distraction regenerate. The use of osteoblasts injected subsequent to distraction has been shown to regain bone mass and establish a cortex.

The advantages of distraction osteogenesis over conventional bone grafting are a more predictable augmentation spatially, both hard and soft tissue histogenesis that does not require extensive creeping substitution remodeling, and greater long-term stability. In the anterior maxilla, the distraction approach can lead to more esthetic alveolar form than other approaches. One additional advantage of distraction is that it can reduce the size of a significant osseous defect and make it manageable for conventional bone grafting.

The addition of cultured osteoblasts to the protocol opens a new avenue of treatment in which the distraction approach may become even more reliable, and the bone morphology at the end of treatment may be improved.

Conclusion

The use of distraction osteogenesis in the jaws to augment alveolar bone mass or improve jaw or alveolar positioning is well founded as a biomechanical "tissue engineering" principle, but optimal technical and biologic procedures still have not been fully established. Although distraction osteogenesis is often less invasive or more dependable than bone grafting at achieving the desired bone augmentation, clinicians continue to hesitate to prescribe its use. At present, treatment plans for augmentation of deficient sites in the jaws frequently advance conventional bone-grafting strategies, and the use of distraction osteogenesis is relegated to ablated sites where bone grafts have failed or the defect is entirely unmanageable with conventional grafting.

The need for secondary augmentation with bone grafting to gain bone mass in distraction sites suggests that application of autogenous osteoblasts to the wound side or within the regenerate may be beneficial. Osteoblasts promote accelerated bone formation and reduced healing time. Indeed, the use of distraction osteogenesis and the grafting of osteoblasts are complementary procedures and may, with further research, allow the regeneration of hard tissue conformations that would not otherwise be possible.

References

1. Ilizarov G. The tension-stress effect on the genesis and growth of tissues. 2. The influence of the rate and frequency of distraction. Clin Orthop Relat Res 1989;239:263–285.

2. Ilizarov G. The tension-stress effect on the genesis and growth of tissues. 1. The influence of stability of fixation and soft-tissue preservation. Clin Orthop Relat Res 1989;238:249–281.

3. Nosaka Y, Tsumokuma M, Hayashi H, Kakudo K. Placement of implants in distraction osteogenesis; A pilot study in dogs. Int J Oral Maxillofac Implants 2000;15:185–192.

4. Gaggl A, Schultes G, Regauer S, Karcher H. Healing process after alveolar ridge distraction in sheep. Oral Surg Oral Med Oral Pathol Oral Radiol Endod 2000;90:420–429.

5. Tavakoli K, Yu Y, Shahidi S, Bonar F, Walsh WR, Poole MD. Expression of growth factors in the mandibular distraction zone: A sheep study. By J Plast Surg 1999;52:434–439.

6. Sato M, Yasui N, Nakase T, et al. Expression of bone matrix proteins mRNA during distraction osteogenesis. J Bone Miner Res 1998;13:1221–1231.

7. Jensen OT, Greer RO, Johnson L, Kassebaum D. Vertical guided bone-graft augmentation in a new canine mandibular model. Int J Oral Maxillofac Implants 1995;10:335–344.

8. Jensen OT, Kuhlke L, Reed C. Prosthetic considerations and treatment planning by classification for alveolar distraction osteogenesis. In: Jensen OT (ed). Alveolar Distraction Osteogenesis. Chicago: Quintessence, 2002:29–40.

9. Jensen OT, Cockrell R, Kuhlke L, Reed C. Anterior maxillary alveolar distraction osteogenesis: A prospective 5-year clinical study. Int J Oral Maxillofac Implants 2002;17:52–68.

10. Jensen OT, Ueda M, Laster Z, Mommaerts M, Rachmiel A. Alveolar distraction osteogenesis. Selected Readings Oral Maxillofac Surg 2002;10(4):1–48.

11. Jensen OT, Kuhlke L, Bedard JF, White D. Alveolar segmental sandwich osteotomy for anterior maxillary vertical augmentation prior to implant placement. J Oral Maxillofac Surg 2006;64:290–296 [erratum 2006;64:997].

12. Williamson RA. Rehabilitation of the resorbed maxilla and mandible using autogenous bone grafts and osseointegrated implants. Int J Oral Maxillofac Implants 1996;11:476–488.

13. Rachmiel A, Srouji S, Peled M. Alveolar ridge augmentation by distraction osteogenesis. Int J Oral Maxillofac Surg 2001;30:510–517.

14. Ueda M, Hibi H, Yamada Y. In: Diner PA, Vazquez MP (eds). 2nd International Congress on Cranial and Facial Bone Distraction Processes. Bologna: Monduzzi, 1999.

15. Rowe NM, Mehrara BJ, Dudziak ME, et al: Rat mandibular distraction osteogenesis. 1. Histologic and radiographic analysis. Plast Reconstr Surg 1998;102:2022–2032.

16. Aronson J. Experimental and clinical experience with distraction osteogenesis. Cleft Palate Craniofac J 1994;31:473–481.

17. Collins TA, Nunn W. Autogenous veneer grafting for improved esthetics with dental implants. Compend Contin Educ Dent 1994;15:370–376.

18. Misch CM. Ridge augmentation using mandibular ramus bone grafts for the placement of dental implants: Presentation of a technique. Pract Periodontics Aesthet Dent 1996;8:127–135.

19. Kuroe K, Iino S, Shomura K, Okubo A, Sugihara K, Ito G. Unilateral advancement of the maxillary minor segment by distraction osteogenesis in patients with repaired unilateral cleft lip and palate: Report of two cases. Cleft Palate Craniofac J 2003;40:317–324.

20. Dolanmaz D, Karaman AI, Ozyesil AG. Maxillary anterior segmental advancement by using distraction osteogenesis: A case report. Angle Orthod 2003;73:201–205.

21. Richardson D, Cawood JI. Anterior maxillary osteoplasty to broaden the narrow maxillary ridge. J Oral Maxillofac Surg 1991;20:342–348.

22. Oda T, Sawaki Y, Ueda M. Alveolar ridge augmentation by distraction osteogenesis using titanium implants: An experimental study. Int J Oral Maxillofac Surg 1999;28:151–156.

23. Jensen OT, Leopardi A, Gallegos L. The case for bone graft reconstruction including sinus grafting and distraction osteogenesis for the atrophic edentulous maxilla. J Oral Maxillofac Surg 2004;62:1423–1428.

24. Chin M, Toth BA. Distraction osteogenesis in maxillofacial surgery using internal devices: Review of five cases. J Oral Maxillofac Surg 1996;54:45–53.

25. Swennen G, Dempf R, Schliephake H. Cranio-facial distraction osteogenesis: A review of the literature. 2. Experimental studies. Int J Oral Maxillofac Surg 2002;31:123–135.

26. Takushima A, Kitano Y, Harii K. Osteogenic potential of cultured periosteal cells in a distracted gap in rabbits. J Surg Res 1998;78:68–77.

27. Tsubota S, Tsuchiya H, Shinokawa Y, Tomita K, Minato H. Transplantation of osteoblast-like cells to the distracted callus in rabbits. J Bone Joint Surg Br 1999;81B:125–129.

28. Richards M, Huibregtse BA, Caplan AI, Goulet JA, Goldstein SA. Marrow-derived progenitor cell injections enhance new bone formation during distraction. J Orthop Res 1999;17:900–908.

29. Takamine Y, Tsuchiya H, Kitakoji T, et al. Distraction osteogenesis enhanced by osteoblastlike cells and collagen gel. Clin Orthop Relat Res 2002;399:240–246.

30. Kitoh H, Kitakoji T, Tsuchiya H, et al. Transplantation of marrow-derived mesenchymal stem cells and platelet-rich plasma during distraction osteogenesis—A preliminary result of three cases. Bone 2004;35:892–898.

31. Hibi H, Yamada Y, Kagami H, Ueda M. Distraction osteogenesis assisted by tissue engineering in an irradiated mandible: A case report. Int J Oral Maxillofac implants 2006;21:141–147.

32. Yamada Y, Ueda M, Hibi H, Nagasaka T. Translational research for injectable tissue-engineered bone regeneration using mesenchymal stem cells and platelet-rich plasma: From basic research to clinical application. Cell Transplantation 2004;13:343–355.

33. Hibi H, Yamada Y, Ueda M, Endo Y. Alveolar cleft osteoplasty using tissue-engineered osteogenic material: Technical note. Int J Oral Maxillofac Surg 2006; 35:551–555.

34. Nocini PF, Wangerin K, Albanese M, Kretschmer W, Cortelazzi R. Vertical distraction of a free vascularized fibula flap in a reconstructed hemimandible: Case report. J Craniomaxillofac Surg 2000;28:20–24.

35. Bähr W. Blood supply of small fibula segments: An experimental study on human cadavers. J Craniomaxillofac Surg 1998;26:148–152.

36. Klesper B, Lazar F, Sießegger M, Hidding J, Zöller JE. Vertical distraction osteogenesis of fibula transplants for mandibular reconstruction—A preliminary study. J Craniomaxillofac Surg 2002;30:280–285.

37. Lynch SE, Genco RJ, Marx RE (eds). Tissue Engineering: Applications in Maxillofacial Surgery and Periodontics, ed 1. Chicago: Quintessence, 1999.

38. Marx RE. Platelet-rich plasma: Evidence to support its use. J Oral Maxillofac Surg 2004;62:489–496.

15

Dentoalveolar Modification with an Osteoperiosteal Flap and rhPDGF-BB

Ole T. Jensen, DDS, MS

The use of angiogenic growth factors such as platelet-derived growth factor BB (PDGF-BB), which upregulates vascular endothelial growth factor and therefore is favorable for early vascularization of a wound, provides an opportunity to improve wound healing of bone-grafting sites. The relatively closed flap procedure, the osteoperiosteal flap, may provide the most ideal environment for effecting angio-osteogenesis.

The osteoperiosteal flap, a relatively new approach to bone graft augmentation, has the advantage of less disturbance of osteogenic periosteum, improved continuity of crestal gingival form, and greater resistance of the augmentation to resorption remodeling. It also allows ready access to the marrow vascular space. The addition of recombinant human PDGF-BB (rhPDGF-BB) in this setting provides opportunity for an augmentation strategy that may further enhance wound healing and overall bone graft performance.

The osteoperiosteal flap, also known as the *bone flap*, is commonly used in segmental orthognathic surgery or alveolar distraction osteogenesis—a bone fragment moved in space without detachment of the investing periosteum (see chapter 14). The best example of this concept in reconstructive alveolar surgery as it relates to implant osseointegration is the interpositional osteotomy

bone graft, or sandwich graft. Other uses of the bone flap in dentoalveolar augmentation are the alveolar split graft, the edentulous alveolar repositioning osteotomy, and various alveolar distraction approaches that add width or height to an alveolar segment. This chapter describes the use of the osteoperiosteal flap to approach these bone augmentation techniques. Although the incidence of graft failure or infection with any of these techniques is low, compromised sites, such as those undergoing retreatment, those with severe ablation from trauma, those subjected to lesion removal, and those in patients with poor healing potential, may benefit from the use of rhPDGF-BB.

Interpositional Bone Graft

The interpositional bone graft can be performed anywhere in the mouth but is most indicated in the esthetic zone and the posterior mandible. A horizontal incision is made to the bone at the depth of the vestibule. The flap is reflected away from the alveolar crest and reflected minimally crestally. This not only maintains the vitality of the bone segment

Fig 15-1a The exposed mandibular gingiva with marked bone loss at the infected mandibular teeth poses a significant problem for placement of esthetic implant restorations.

Fig 15-1b A buccal incision is used to raise a small segmental osteotomy 5 or 6 mm vertically. An interpositional graft and a bone plate are placed.

Fig 15-1c Radiograph taken after grafting, showing the graft and the bone plate.

Fig 15-1d Four months later, the site is exposed for removal of the bone plate.

Fig 15-1e Implants are placed, and supplemental grafting to increase the width is performed with a nonresorbable alloplast.

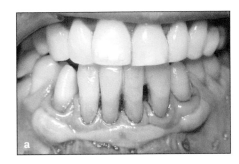

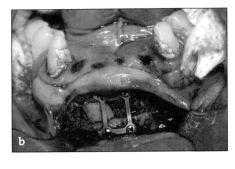

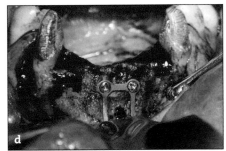

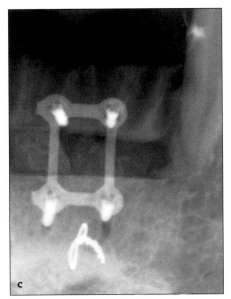

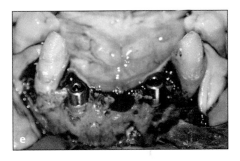

but also preserves osteogenic periosteum. Vital structures such as nerves, tooth roots, and the respiratory space are identified and avoided.

The osteotomy design in the posterior mandible is a "smile line," tapering anteriorly and posteriorly. The osteotomy segment is preferably at least 4 mm high in the middle, although it is possible to perform the procedure with less bone height. A through-and-through osteotomy is performed from the buccal plate to the lingual plate, and an osteotome is used to gently free the segment. The segment can be elevated in excess of 10 mm. Segments in the anterior maxilla, especially if they are small, can only be moved about 4 or 5 mm. Larger segments or posterior segments, however, can be moved up to 10 mm vertically despite the resistance of the palatal mucosa.

Both a bone plate and interpositional graft material, usually an autograft or alloplasts, are placed (Figs 15-1a to 15-1c). Both of these types of graft are augmented with rhPDGF-BB. The use of alloplasts next to nerve tissue should be avoided, however.

Four months after placement of the graft the plate is removed and dental implants are placed (Figs 15-1d and 15-1e). The inclusion of rhPDGF-BB may accelerate healing time, but its most significant effect is more likely to be qualitative than quantitative. Following healing of the interpositional graft, the alveolar ridge may have to be split or grafted laterally at the time of implant placement, but the vertical augmentation should be adequate.

The major advantage of using an interpositional site for bone grafting is the accessibility it provides to the endosteal surface, or marrow space, a highly vascular area conducive to graft incorporation. Very few seams, scar encleftations, bone graft exposures, bone graft resorptions, or infections occur when this approach is used. Other advantages for using the interpositional graft technique are undisturbed alveolar crestal bone, improved gingival esthetic form in anterior locations, and an overall stable postgrafting architecture. Presumably these advantages will be enhanced by the addition of growth factor.

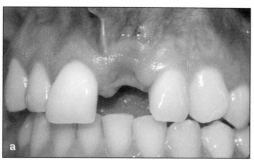
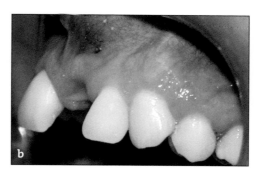
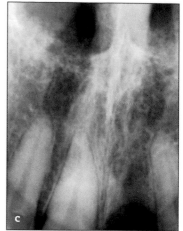

Fig 15-2a When the buccal plate is lost in a central incisor location, it becomes both a restorative and an esthetic challenge.

Fig 15-2b Loss of the buccal plate leads to a lack of alveolar projection and the apical movement of the attached gingival margin.

Fig 15-2c When adequate bone mass is present, as revealed on the radiograph and during the physical examination, a bone flap can be performed.

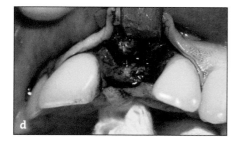
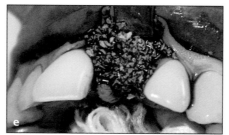
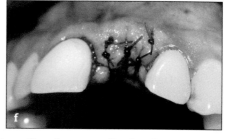

Fig 15-2d A palatocrestal incision is used to free the buccal plate without disturbing the subpapillary bone or reflecting the mucoperiosteal flap off the segment. The segment is then opened like a book.

Fig 15-2e Graft material is interposed.

Fig 15-2f The site is closed or nearly closed with sutures, and an additional gain in width is noticeable.

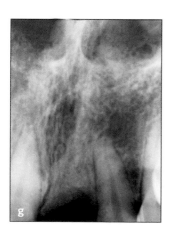
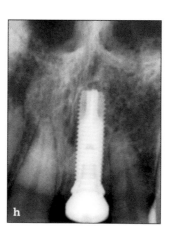
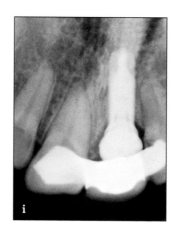

Fig 15-2g Postoperative radiographic results are shown.

Fig 15-2h Four months postsurgery, an implant is placed transgingivally.

Fig 15-2i An additional 4 months after implant placement, the tooth is restored.

Fig 15-3a An anterior alveolar crossbite is present, but there is adequate alveolar width for implants.

Fig 15-3b Following segmental osteotomy to move the alveolus forward 4 mm, the guide stent shows the improved alveolar projection.

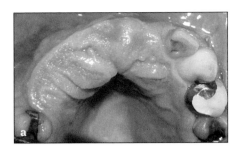
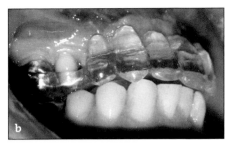

Figs 15-3c and 15-3d Transgingival implants are placed 3 mm below tissue level according to the guide stent.

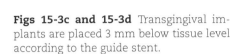
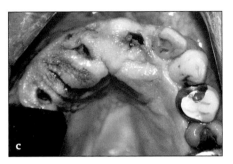
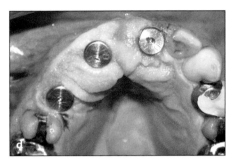

Alveolar Split Graft

The common alveolar finding in a late-healed extraction socket is a loss of alveolar width because of resorption of the buccal plate (Figs 15-2a to 15-2c). The alveolus can be widened with a crestal incision that does not reflect beyond the crest buccally but serves to identify the set point for osteotomy with an osteotome or a piezoelectric knife. This technique generally requires a minimum alveolar width of about 4 mm, but if a piezoelectric knife is used, a 3-mm width is easily managed.

Vertical cuts in the buccal plate are made blindly, without flap reflection, 1 or 2 mm away from adjacent tooth roots and connected sagittally to a depth of about 10 mm. The buccal plate is then split sagittally. Out-fracture is accomplished without detachment of the mucoperiosteum from the mobilized osseous segment, ie, the bone flap (Fig 15-2d). The mobilized segment can be moved laterally up to 5 mm.

The interosseous defect that has been created is grafted, or an implant is placed with proximate bone grafting (Fig 15-2e). Primary closure or near primary closure is obtainable if the crestal incision is placed a few millimeters palatally (Figs 15-2f and 15-2g). An implant can be placed 4 months later (Figs 15-2h and 15-2i).

The alveolar split bone flap readily augments the majority of healed maxillary dental extraction sites. It can be used in the mandible as well, although hard bone is less flexible to allow greenstick fracture, and flap detachment is a greater risk.

Alveolar Repositioning Osteotomies

Sometimes the alveolus has enough bone mass, but the alveolar crest is in a nonaxial position, such as in anterior or lateral crossbite. An alveolar segment can be freed by osteotomy, repositioned, and fixed without grafting (Fig 15-3). The use of a biomimetic can aid in the healing of this process.

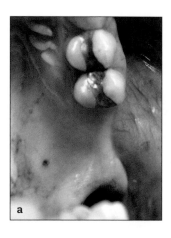

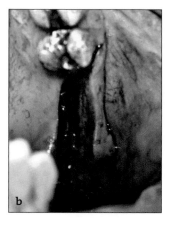

Figs 15-4a and 15-4b A narrow maxillary posterior alveolus can be split through a crestal incision without periosteal reflection.

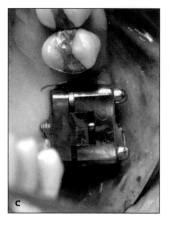

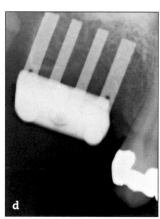

Fig 15-4c A Laster bone spreader (Surgi-Tec) is tapped into place.

Fig 15-4d The bone spreader extends 8 to 10 mm vertically into the alveolus.

Horizontal Alveolar Distraction Osteogenesis

One location in which alveolar width can be increased by distraction is the posterior mandible. This area, which is sometimes difficult to bone graft, can be split in a relatively brief operation in which no bone graft is required. The bone flap spreader is tapped into place and activated 1 week later. Adequate width is achieved in 7 to 10 days, because activation is 0.2 to 0.4 mm per day. A biomimetic can be applied either at the time of osteotomy or in the peridistraction period.

The site is left to heal for about 6 weeks after distraction is completed, and the distractor is removed. At that time, implants are placed through the distraction zone into apical bone. Compared with onlay bone grafting, the distraction approach generally results in shorter treatment time, reduced morbidity, and improved stability. An example of horizontal alveolar distraction to increase the width of the posterior maxilla is shown in Fig 15-4.

Vertical Alveolar Distraction Osteogenesis

Vertical alveolar distraction osteogenesis is now considered a well-founded technique but still is not widely used. Vertical distraction almost always requires supplemental bone grafting before or after distraction. Vertical distraction osteogenesis is technically difficult, a consideration that may discourage selection of this treatment alternative. Once again, rhPDGF-BB can be applied either at the time of osteotomy or during the distraction period.

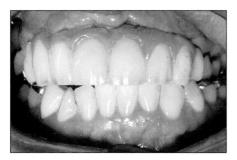

Fig 15-5a A failed anterior bone graft that had involved both block bone grafting and guided bone regeneration led to a prominent vertical defect.

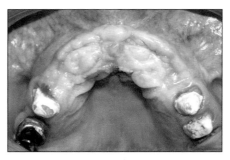

Fig 15-5b The crestal width is adequate, but the height is inadequate.

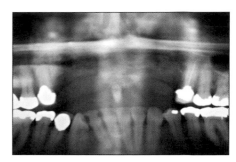

Fig 15-5c A preoperative panoramic radiograph reveals the defect.

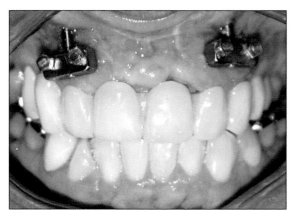

Fig 15-5d Following creation of an alveolar bone flap, two Mommaerts-Laster distractors have been placed to move an eight-tooth segment 10 mm vertically.

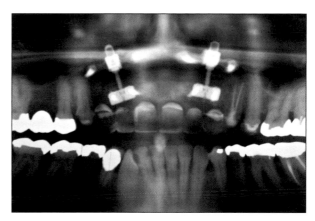

Fig 15-5e The radiographic findings following distraction are shown.

The most common indication for vertical distraction osteogenesis is the maxillary anterior alveolar ridge that has to be moved downward and, usually, forward for esthetic reasons.

Figure 15-5 shows an anterior maxillary defect treated with a bone flap translated by bilateral distraction. After it is cut and fixed with the distractor, the segment is moved downward and advanced at a rate of 0.5 to 0.8 mm per day until the segment engages the provisional or prosthetic guide. A 4-month consolidation period ensues after the distraction is complete. Implants follow with eventual prosthetic rehabilitation.

Conclusion

The use of an osteoperiosteal flap with the biomimetic rhPDGF-BB allows the surgeon to handle most dentoalveolar defects with a relatively simple surgical technique that avoids major bone grafting. It also facilitates the development of bone that is more stable, less likely to resorb, and more likely to consolidate into the graft site. The use of an interpositional bone graft engages the marrow vascular space, a place where graft material is less likely to sequester, become infected, or resorb. Application of an angiogenic material should only enhance this outcome.

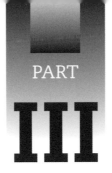

PART

III

Craniofacial Reconstruction

16

Clinical Applications of rhBMP-2

Alan S. Herford, DDS, MD
Philip J. Boyne, DMD, MS, DSc

For the last several decades, autogenous bone has been regarded as the gold standard of sources for osseous bone graft material in major oral and maxillofacial defects. Although autogenous bone has numerous advantages over allogeneic and xenogeneic sources, its use requires additional surgery to access the donor site. The recent availability of recombinant growth factors seems to offer the potential to avoid a second surgical harvest site and the morbidity associated with the procedure.

Bone morphogenetic proteins (BMPs) belong to a family of cytokines, the members of which have varying degrees of osteogenic potential. Recombinant human BMP-2 (rhBMP-2) and rhBMP-7, also known as *osteogenic protein 1*, are the BMPs most commonly used in clinical and experimental oral and maxillofacial studies. In preclinical investigations, rhBMP-2 has been shown to be effective in restoring critical-sized defects in *Macaca fascicularis*.[1] Additional animal studies on BMPs have demonstrated successful regeneration of simulated anterior maxillary cleft palate defects.[2] Toriumi et al[3] used a canine model to study BMP-2–stimulated growth in mandibular continuity defects. In the BMP-2 group, they found that 68% of the defect was replaced by mineralized bone at 6 months. Boyne[1] found that rhBMP-2 was an effective inductor of osseous regeneration in nonhuman primates in critical-sized mandibular continuity defects.

In 2004, Warnke et al[4] used BMP-7 and bone mineral blocks (xenografts) to create a custom vascularized bone graft in a human. They found bone remodeling and mineralization inside the titanium transplant.

Different approaches have been used to deliver BMP in order to produce effective reconstructive procedures without the need for bone grafting as it is currently employed. A series of three human multicenter studies have shown that rhBMP-2 successfully induces bone formation in the maxillary sinus prior to implant placement[5,6] (Boyne et al, unpublished data, 2007).

Clinical oral and maxillofacial surgical application of BMP-2 has evolved from the initial sinus studies to include defects involving the facial skeleton, such as congenital deformities (anterior maxillary clefts) as well as facial segmental defects. This chapter discusses the promising results, limitations, and future applications of rhBMP-2 in oral and maxillofacial surgery. The chapter will focus on the use of BMP-2 in the repair and reconstruction of *(1)* mandibular continuity defects following tumor resection; *(2)* preprosthetic maxillomandibular deficiencies; *(3)* traumatic facial bone loss that has produced mandibular and maxillary continuity defects; and *(4)* bony clefts of the anterior maxilla. Four cases have been selected for presentation from a series of 25 cases representing these four principal areas of major bony oral and maxillofacial reconstruction and repair.

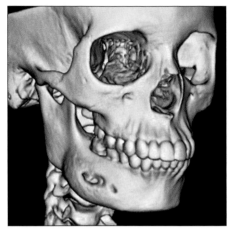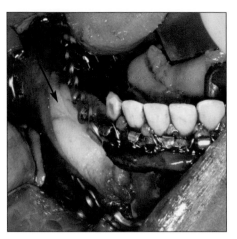

Fig 16-1a Preoperative three-dimensional computerized tomography (CT) showing the tumor with perforation of the lateral bony cortex.

Fig 16-1b Superior and inferior plates placed to bridge the defect and maintain space for bone regeneration. (*Arrow* indicates rhBMP-2/absorbable collagen sponge.)

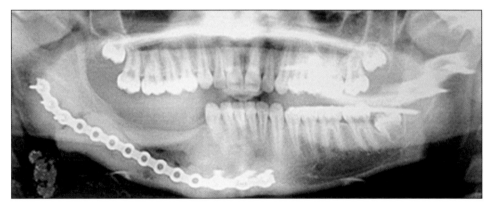

Fig 16-1c Postoperative radiograph obtained after removal of the superior plate and before removal of the inferior plate.

Mandibular Continuity Defects Secondary to Tumor Resection

Mandibular continuity defects that follow tumor resection result in significant morbidity if not appropriately reconstructed. Autogenous grafting in the form of both particulate marrow and cancellous bone (PMCB) grafts and free-tissue transfer procedures provides choices presently used to treat each defect. As an alternative to such techniques, the authors have used cytokines either alone or together with autogenous bone. Application of rhBMP-2 without harvesting of bone graft material has been used

in five patients with this category of defect; one of these cases is presented.

Case 1

A 12-year-old female patient presented for evaluation of a mandibular swelling charaterized as a soft and hard tissue mass. The tumorlike lesion was biopsied and found to be an aggressive juvenile ossifying fibroma. The patient underwent surgical resection of the tumor and primary reconstruction of the defect in one stage (Figs 16-1a and 16-1b).

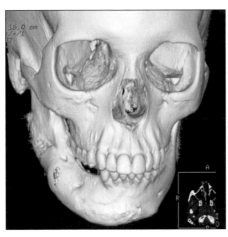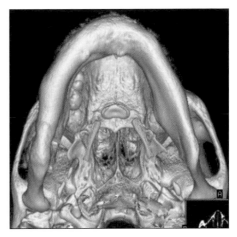

Fig 16-1d Postoperative three-dimensional CT scan showing complete mandibular reconstruction 1 year after surgery.

A 2.0-mm locking plate (Synthes) was placed inferiorly, and a similar plate was placed superiorly, to "bridge" and stabilize the defect. An absorbable collagen sponge (ACS; InFuse, Medtronic Sofamor Danek) was saturated with 8.0 mL of a 1.5-mg/mL solution of rhBMP-2. The superior plate was placed to provide tenting of the periosteum and to maintain the surgically created space for the rhBMP-2/ACS sponge. The tenting effect maintained a space for formation of an optimal amount of regenerated bone.

During the postoperative course, the patient experienced exposure of the superior plate 7 weeks after surgery. The superior plate was removed transorally in the clinic 4 months postoperatively, and the patient was noted to have excellent bone formation. There was complete reconstruction of the intraoperative bony defect, as shown by a panoramic radiograph and CT (Figs 16-1c and 16-1d). Three weeks after removal of the superior plate, the inferior plate was removed in the operating room. The patient will undergo implant placement and, subsequently, functional prosthodontic restoration.

cluding guided bone regeneration with onlay bone grafts. The more common procedures include osseous ridge augmentation and sinus floor augmentation. The choice of surgical procedure often depends on the physical characteristics of the defect.

Jovanovic et al[7] performed a histologic study using a canine ridge augmentation model.[5] They found no statistically significant difference between implants placed in rhBMP-2–induced bone and those placed in resident host bone. Boyne et al[5,6] recently reported the results of a multicenter study utilizing rhBMP/ACS in the maxillary sinus. They found that rhBMP-2 combined with the ACS carrier predictably and safely induced adequate bone for the placement and functional loading of endosseous dental implants in patients who required staged maxillary sinus floor augmentation.

In addition to being used without autogenous bone, rhBMP-2 can also be used in conjunction with a PMCB autograft. In case 2, the combination of an autograft and rhBMP-2 was used in the maxilla, and rhBMP-2 was used, without a bone graft, in the mandible.

Preprosthetic Maxillo-mandibular Deficiencies

Preprosthetic maxillomandibular ridge augmentation with autogenous grafts and bone graft substitutes is a commonly used procedure. Many techniques are available, in-

Case 2

A 45-year-old woman with a long history of smoking presented for evaluation of the possibility of bone grafting and implant placement. Her examination revealed knife-edged ridges and a lack of adequate maxillary and mandibular bone for dental implant placement (Figs 16-2a and 16-2b).

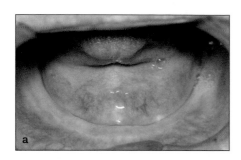

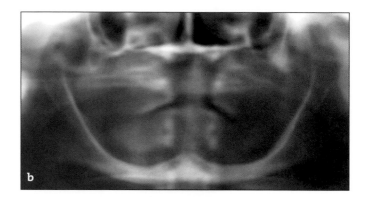

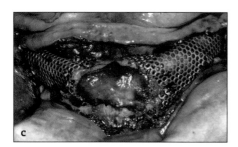

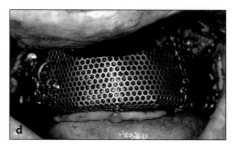

Fig 16-2a Deficient alveolar ridge.

Fig 16-2b Preoperative radiograph showing that the bone is inadequate for implant placement.

Fig 16-2c Mesh secured in place to maintain space for the rhBMP-2/ACS.

Fig 16-2d Mesh secured to the maxilla.

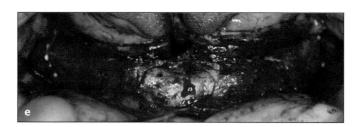

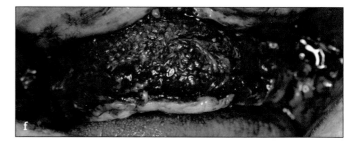

Figs 16-2e and 16-2f Regenerated mandibular (*e*) and maxillary (*f*) ridges 6 months after the initial surgery.

Fig 16-2g Six-month postoperative radiograph.

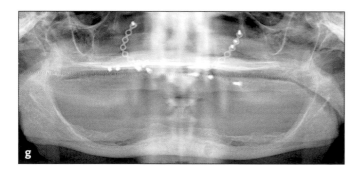

She underwent reconstruction in the maxilla with a combination of autogenous iliac crest bone graft and rhBMP-2. The reconstruction included both bilateral sinus augmentation (sinus floor) grafts and maxillomandibular ridge augmentation. Titanium mesh was used to provide stability and confinement of the rhBMP-2/ACS (Figs 16-2c and 16-2d).

The posterior mandible was reconstructed with rhBMP-2 alone. A total of 8 mL of rhBMP-2 was used (1.5 mg/mL).

Four months postoperatively, the patient underwent removal of the titanium hardware, revealing excellent bony reconstruction of the mandible (Fig 16-2e) and maxilla (Fig 16-2f). The mandible, in which rhBMP-2 was used alone, showed excellent radiographic evidence of bone regeneration (Fig 16-2g). The extent of the mandibular bone regeneration was demonstrated 6 months postoperatively, at the time of implant placement.

Fig 16-3a Avulsion of soft and hard tissues as a result of a gunshot wound to the face.

Fig 16-3b Three-dimensional CTs showing significant loss of bony tissue.

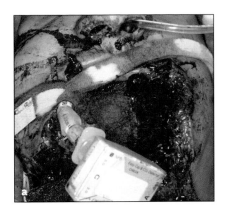
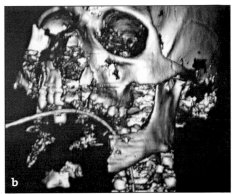

Fig 16-3c Placement of rhBMP-2/ACS adjacent to the mucoperiosteum.

Fig 16-3d Placement of rhBMP-2/ACS over particulate bone graft (beneath the periosteum).

Figs 16-3e and 16-3f Postoperative radiograph (*e*) and clinical view (*f*).

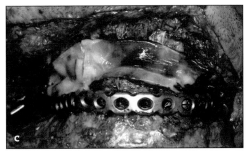
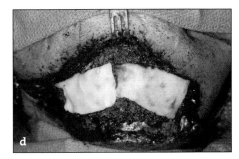

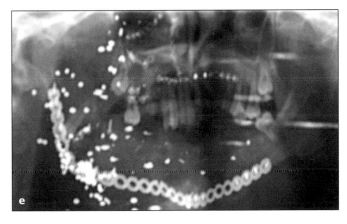
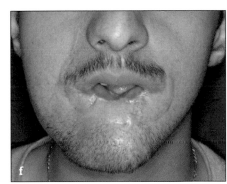

Traumatic Facial Bone Loss

Case 3

Trauma to the face can result in a wide range of defects and deformities. The extent and type of injuries are related to the mechanism of the traumatic force. Motor vehicle collisions produce characteristic injuries that are quite different from those resulting from gunshot wounds. Fractures may heal improperly, leading to the formation of fibrous tissue between the bone segments rather than a bony union. These nonunions usually require bone grafts to obtain definitive symmetric junctional healing. In the treatment of major gunshot wounds, autogenous PMCB may be used with rhBMP-2.

An 18-year-old man sustained a close-range shotgun blast to the face during a robbery (Figs 16-3a and 16-3b). Treatment included a staged secondary reconstruction using a 2.4-mm locking reconstruction plate. An iliac crest bone graft was combined with rhBMP-2 in a layered sandwich technique using a special xenograft collagen membrane (Mucograft, Geistlich; Figs 16-3c and 16-3d), which serves to protect the rhBMP-2 and the graft in areas of thin or deficient soft tissue and/or skin. Two collagen sponges were treated with 8 mL of rhBMP-2 (1.5 mg/mL). The first collagen sponge was placed directly on the residual host bone.

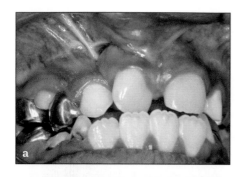

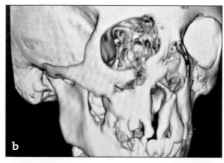

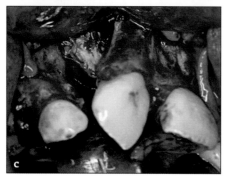

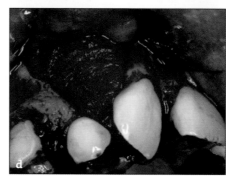

Fig 16-4a Clinical view of a right-side anterior maxillary cleft.

Fig 16-4b Three-dimensional CT showing the cleft.

Fig 16-4c Intraoperative view showing closure of the nasal floor.

Fig 16-4d Placement of the rhBMP-2/ACS in the area of the cleft defect.

This was followed by placement of a corticocancellous particulate bone graft. A second collagen sponge was placed over the graft, and the incision was closed.

The bone healing was uneventful (Fig 16-3e). The patient is awaiting final reconstruction of the dentition with root-form implants (Fig 16-3f).

Anterior Maxillary Alveolar Clefts

The standard procedure to effect bony repair of anterior maxillary clefts is to obtain particulate marrow and cancellous bone from the iliac crest, as first reported by Boyne and Sands[8] in 1976. PMCB obtained from the iliac crest has remained the ideal bone graft material and donor site for cleft repair for the past 30 years. However, Boyne et al[2] later compared rhBMP-2 with iliac crest bone grafts in simulated alveolar cleft defects in nonhuman primates. They found no statistically significant difference between the autogenous grafts and those defects reconstructed with rhBMP-2 alone.

More recently, many clinical patients (n = 16) treated by the authors have benefited from the use of rhBMP-2 to induce bone formation in clefts, thus eliminating the need for a secondary surgical site to obtain an autogenous graft.

Case 4

A 6-year-old boy presented with a unilateral premaxillary bony cleft (Figs 16-4a and 16-4b). He underwent repair with rhBMP-2 alone on the collagen sponge without a bone graft. A standard technique was used that involved careful closure of the nasal floor (Fig 16-4c) and extension of the graft material at least 1.5 cm palatal to the alveolus. An ACS with 4 mL of rhBMP-2 (1.5 mg/mL) was placed in the cleft defect (Fig 16-4d). The palatal and labial mucosal flaps were then closed.

The patient healed uneventfully. Four-month postoperative CT revealed excellent bone regeneration of the entire anterior maxillary cleft (Figs 16-4e to 16-4i). The patient is now undergoing orthodontic treatment.

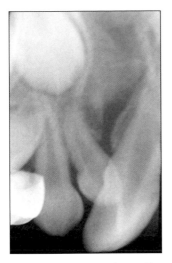

Fig 16-4e Preoperative radiograph.

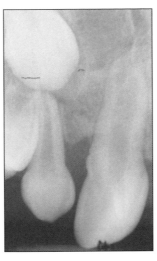

Fig 16-4f Eight-month postoperative radiograph showing complete bone regeneration of the defect.

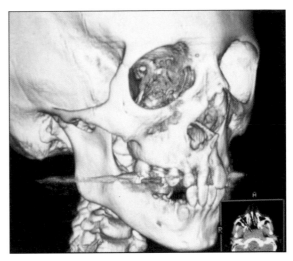

Fig 16-4g Eight-month postoperative three-dimensional CT showing bridging of the defect.

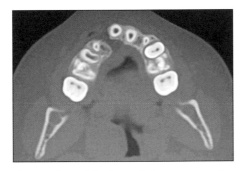

Fig 16-4h Axial view of the preoperative situation.

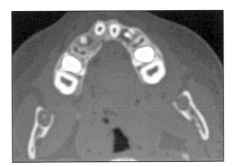

Fig 16-4i Eight-month postoperative result.

Discussion

Autogenous bone grafts in various forms have long been the gold standard for maxillofacial reconstruction. Advantages such as their high success rate, optimal availability, and biocompatibility make the use of autogenous bone grafts an excellent treatment choice in many patients. Nevertheless, autogenous grafts also may be associated with disadvantages including the cost of the procedure, the necessity for a secondary donor site, the need for hospitalization, and donor site–specific postoperative morbidity, including limitations of activity, gait disturbances,

infection, and paresthesia. Thus, a "bone in a bottle" type of osteoinductive material for reconstructing oral and maxillofacial defects would have great appeal.

The application of specific growth factors for osteoinduction without the need for autogenous bone grafting would have tremendous impact on maxillofacial reconstructive procedures. Morphogenetic factors (eg, rhBMP-2) may be used in a collagen sponge carrier or in combination with PMCB. Polypeptide growth factors influence healing by controlling migration and proliferation of adult mesenchymal stem cells. Requirements for wound healing include cellular migration and proliferation, angiogenesis, and extracellular matrix deposition. Morphogens (eg, BMP)

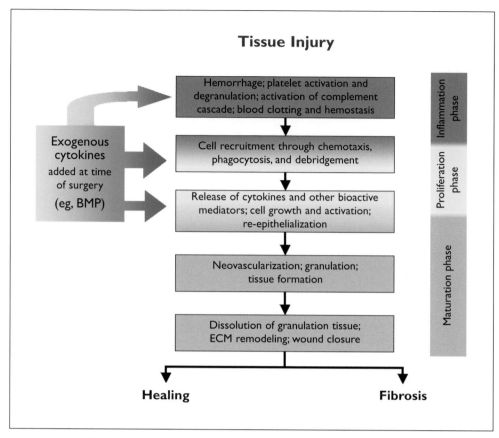

Fig 16-5 Wound-healing pathways. (ECM) extracellular matrix.

act endogenously to facilitate this pathway (Fig 16-5). As discussed earlier, morphogenetic proteins can also be introduced exogenously to the bone defect at the time of surgery, thus influencing osteoprogenitor cells to develop osteoblastic cell lines and produce bone growth.

More than 40 rhBMPs with varying abilities to enhance osteogenesis have been isolated (Fig 16-6). rhBMP-2 and rhBMP-7 seem to have the greatest ability to stimulate bone formation.

BMP-2 affects various stages of the differentiation of progenitor cells. Katagiri et al[9] reported that BMP-2 may alter the differentiation pathways of committed progenitor cells of myoblast lines and cause a differentiation of committed myoblasts to chondroblast-like cells. They also stated that BMP-2 is a potent regulator in determining osteoblastic differentiation, affecting not only pleuripotential immature mesenchymal cells (stem cells) but also committed myoblasts. This clarifies the difference between

morphogens and growth factors: Morphogens act on committed cells as well as uncommitted cells, causing differentiation or de-differentiation of cells to a specific lineage, in the case of BMPs, the osteoblastic lineage.

The optimal carrier for rhBMP-2 should slowly release the morphogen. Research is currently underway to continue development of a matrix that would fulfill these criteria.[10–12] The current carrier, ACS, is derived from highly purified bovine tendon type I collagen.[13,14] rhBMP-2, while currently approved for use with the ACS in spinal fusion procedures, has been used alone and in combination with allogeneic and xenogeneic bone grafts. Case studies will continue to provide information related to the potential synergistic effects of various carriers.

The concentration of rhBMP-2 for patients in the studies carried out by the authors was 1.5 mg/mL. Studies evaluating the cytokine (morphogen) dosage and carrier influences were evaluated to determine the optimal dose

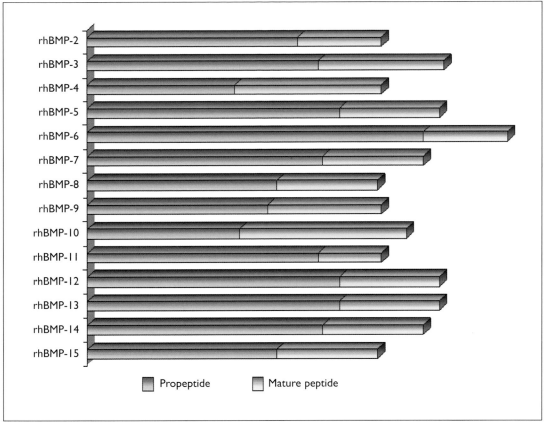

Fig 16-6 A partial list of presently available and fully characterized rhBMPs, showing the relative quantity of mature and immature peptides in each group. The mature peptides offer a stable moiety for laboratory studies.

of rhBMP-2 to stimulate bone formation. In a clinical study comparing 0.75 mg/mL and 1.50 mg/mL doses, it was found that the larger dose was more effective at inducing bone for maxillary sinus floor augmentation procedures.[7,14] However, higher doses of rhBMP-2 produce more soft tissue swelling postoperatively, including occasional facial suborbital edema (Boyne PJ, clinical data; Chin M, personal communication). It is important that the patient be aware of the possibility of this postoperative event.

A small percentage of patients (nonresponders) may not respond to BMP-2. Patients also can develop antibodies to collagen, but this does not appear to have a clinically detectable effect.

The highly osteoinductive properties of rhBMP-2, based on preclinical in vitro and in vivo results, have led to the development of a product for clinical use.[15,16] Animal studies have demonstrated its ability to successfully reconstruct a variety of defects, and successful human clinical investigations involving the maxillofacial region have been undertaken.

Conclusion

The great potential for cytokine-induced bone repair is exciting and will produce alternatives to traditional osseous grafting techniques. In the future, BMP-2 will play a significant role in the treatment of neoplastic defects, atrophic deficiencies in aging population groups, traumatic injuries, and congenital anomalies.

References

1. Boyne PJ. Animal studies of the application of rhBMP-2 in maxillofacial reconstruction. Bone 1996;19(1 suppl):83S–92S.
2. Boyne PJ, Nath R, Nakamura A. Human recombinant BMP-2 in osseous reconstruction of simulated cleft palate defects. Br J Oral Maxillofac Surg 1998; 36:84–90.
3. Toriumi DM, Kotler HS, Luxenberg DP, Holtrop ME, Wang EA. Mandibular reconstruction with a recombinant evaluation. Arch Otolaryngol Head Neck Surg 1991;117:1101–1112.
4. Warnke PH, Springer ING, Wiltfang J, et al. Growth and transplantation of a custom vascularized bone graft in a man. Lancet 2004;364:766–770.
5. Boyne PJ, Lilly LC, Marx RE, et al. De novo bone induction by recombinant human bone morphogenetic protein-2 (rhBMP-2) in maxillary sinus floor augmentation. J Oral Maxillofac Surg 2005;63:1693–1707.
6. Boyne PJ, Marx RE, Nevins M, et al. A feasibility study evaluating rhBMP-2/absorbable collagen sponge for maxillary sinus floor augmentation. Int J Periodontics Restorative Dent 1997;17:11–25.
7. Jovanovic SA, Hunt DR, Bernard GW, et al. Long-term functional loading of dental implants in rhBMP-2 induced bone. A histologic study in the canine ridge augmentation model. Clin Oral Implants Res 2003;14:793–803.
8. Boyne PJ, Sands NR. Combined orthodontic-surgical management of residual palato-alveolar cleft defects. Am J Orthod 1976;70:20–37.
9. Katagiri T, Yamaguchi A, Komaki M, et al. Bone morphogenetic protein-2 converts the differentiation pathway of C2C12 myoblasts into the osteoblast lineage. J Cell Biol 1994;127:1755–1766.
10. Johnson EE, Urist MR, Finerman GA. Resistant nonunions and partial or complete segmental defects of long bones. Treatment with implants of a composite of human bone morphogenetic protein (BMP) and autolyzed, antigen-extracted, allogeneic (AAA) bone. Clin Orthop Relat Res 1992;227:229–237.
11. Gerhart TN, Kirker-Head CA, Kriz MJ, et al. Healing of large mid-femoral segmental defects in sheep using recombinant human bone morphogenetic protein (BMP-2) [abstract]. Trans Orthop Res Soc 1991;16:172.
12. Suzuki A, Terai H, Toyda H, et al. A biodegradable delivery system for antibiotics and recombinant human bone morphogenetic protein-2: A potential treatment for infected bone defects. J Orthop Res 2006;24:327–332.
13. Zellin G, Linde A. Importance of delivery systems for growth-stimulatory factors in combination with osteopromotive membranes. An experimental study using rhBMP-2 in rat mandibular defects. J Biomed Mater Res 1997;35:181–190.
14. Nevins M, Kirker-Head C, Nevins M, et al. Bone formation in the goat maxillary sinus induced by absorbable collagen sponge implants impregnated with recombinant human bone morphogenetic protein-2. Int J Periodontics Restorative Dent 1996;16:9–19.
15. Boyne PJ. Application of bone morphogenetic proteins in the treatment of clinical oral and maxillofacial osseous defects. J Bone Joint Surg Am 2001;82A(suppl 1 pt 2):S146–S150.
16. Boyne PJ, Salina S, Nakamura A, Audia F, Shabahang S. Bone regeneration using rhBMP-2 induction in hemimandibulectomy type defects of elderly subhuman primates. Cell Tissue Bank 2006;7:1–10.

Craniofacial Osseous Reconstruction with rhBMP-2 in the Growing Patient

Ember L. Ewings, MD

Michael H. Carstens, MD

Reconstruction of craniofacial osseous abnormalities resulting from congenital disorders or traumatic destruction has traditionally relied on transplantation of autogenous bone from the calvarium, rib, iliac crest, or other donor site.[1,2] Bone grafts rely on the process of osteoconduction, whereby the grafted bone acts as a scaffold into which native cells integrate. Because the graft carries with it no blood supply, survival is based on the acquisition of nutrients from surrounding tissues until neovascularization occurs. Thus, successful grafts must be limited in size and may still resorb to some degree.[3]

Additionally, bone harvesting carries significant risk of donor site morbidity, including pain, wound dehiscence and infection, and damage to surrounding anatomy and its potential complications, such as cerebrospinal fluid leakage, pneumothorax, or paresthesias. Although autogenous bone harvesting remains a fairly reliable way to reconstruct craniofacial defects, outcomes may be compromised by tooth root resorption secondary to graft contact; poor integration of the graft; or graft resorption.

In an effort to minimize donor site morbidity and complications associated with autogenous bone grafts for craniofacial reconstruction, alternative materials have been used. These include human banked bone, anorganic bovine bone mineral, and alloplastic materials such as hydroxyapatite and carbonized apatite.[4,5] These substitutes carry their own limitations to reconstruction. Use of human banked bone and bovine-derived bone mineral requires the presence of viable bone at the periphery of the graft, because the mechanism of new bone formation is primarily osteoconductive.[6] Hydroxyapatite may interfere with orthodontic movement and tooth eruption, elicit a foreign-body reaction, or become infected, necessitating removal.

The limitations of current graft materials have prompted the continued search for reliable, safe methods to form new bone. The ideal surgical method for craniofacial reconstruction in children would overcome the challenges of large defect size, the need for functionality and durability, the potential for growth, and donor site morbidity. A technique that has been extensively studied in recent years is the application of bone morphogenetic proteins (BMPs), which have been found to induce the differentiation of host stem cells into bone-forming cells.[7,8] The proteins are placed in a soft tissue pocket in contact with muscle, periosteum, or bone marrow and incite migration and concentration of host stem cells into the area.[9,10] Recombinant human bone morphogenetic protein (rhBMP) is a commercially available agent that has been widely used in long-bone and spinal reconstruction and more recently has been studied for craniofacial applications.[11–16] This chapter will present case reports demonstrating the application of rhBMP for reconstruction of craniofacial osseous defects.

Craniofacial Reconstructive Techniques

In situ osteogenesis

In situ osteogenesis (ISO), a reconstructive technique whereby new bone is formed in a surgically created soft tissue pocket, makes use of cytokine-induced recruitment of stem cells into the pocket. These cells are then transformed into the osteoblastic cell line to facilitate new bone formation in a process known as *osteoinduction*.[3] The mechanism of rhBMP-induced osteoinduction involves six steps[17,18]:

1. Implantation: An environment containing mesenchymal stem cells (MSCs) is surgically created or modified.
2. Chemotaxis: MSCs from up to 5 cm away are attracted by rhBMP to the implantation site.
3. Proliferation: MSC multiplication is promoted in the local environment of rhBMP.
4. Differentiation: rhBMP binds to specific receptors on the MSC surface, causing transformation into osteoblasts.
5. Osteogenesis and angiogenesis: Osteoblasts respond to local mechanical forces to produce osteoid, and new blood vessel formation is observed.
6. Remodeling: Bone remodels in response to the local environment and mechanical forces.

Generation of new bone occurs in a predictable fashion based on the supraphysiologic concentration of rhBMP implanted on a collagen sponge carrier, which defines the space that the new bone will occupy. In summary, the generation of bone proceeds in a manner reminiscent of embryonic osteogenesis: growth of a cartilaginous framework with progressive replacement by bone and subsequent appearance of hematopoietic marrow.[6]

Bone formation is substantially faster in craniofacial applications than in long-bone reconstruction because craniofacial sites have an abundant blood supply and a propensity for the direct, intramembranous pathway of osteogenesis. The new bone demonstrates mechanical strength and good integration with native bone.[3] Tooth eruption and orthodontic movement may proceed normally in rhBMP-induced fields. ISO may also show promise for patients in whom autologous grafting is relatively contraindicated, such as smokers, elderly patients, and others in whom the risk of poor healing is unacceptably high.

ISO "switch"

In some patients, the use of ISO may be limited by the location or shape of the deficiency site (eg, zygomatic arch defects) if adequate soft tissue cannot be developed or maintained throughout the bone maturation process. In these cases, ISO may still be a part of the reconstructive plan when it is used to fill bony defects created by the harvesting of autogenous bone. Most notably, calvarial bone grafts can be easily cut and shaped to fit more complex craniofacial defects; the donor site is then amenable to osseous replacement by the application of rhBMP. This ISO-switch procedure extends the options for management of complicated reconstructive problems.

Distraction osteogenesis

Distraction osteogenesis is a technique whereby new bone is formed by gradual displacement of iatrogenic fracture fragments and subsequent elongation and osteoblastic development of bone in the developing periosteal interval. Use of the body's innate osteogenic abilities obviates the need for suitable graft material.[19] Distraction vectors are designed according to precise three-dimensional (3-D) cephalometric evaluation of the defect and reconstructive goals. Osteogenesis is primarily dependent on angiogenesis at the distraction site and the developing soft tissue envelope and proceeds accordingly at a rate of about 1 mm daily. Craniofacial reconstruction using distraction osteogenesis has been previously described.[20,21]

Distraction-assisted ISO

Reconstructive efforts combining the benefits of the soft tissue envelope creation inherent to distraction osteogenesis and the bone-generating properties of in situ osteogenesis have created a new pathway to craniofacial reconstruction: distraction-assisted ISO (DISO). The DISO technique uses controlled rapid tissue expansion to create a periosteal chamber between bone segments into which rhBMP can be implanted on a collagen carrier sponge.

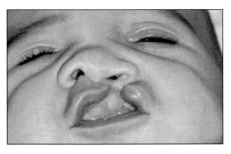

Fig 17-1a Preoperative facial view of an infant with unilateral cleft lip and palate.

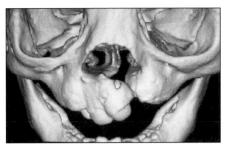

Fig 17-1b Preoperative 3-D computerized tomography (CT) demonstrating the defect.

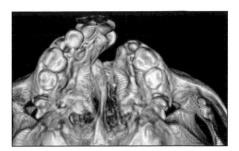

Fig 17-1c Preoperative palatal view.

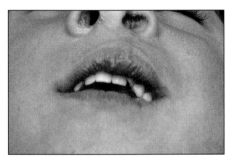

Fig 17-1d Facial view 18 months postoperative.

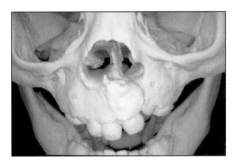

Fig 17-1e Six-month postoperative 3-D CT demonstrating restoration of the maxillary arch.

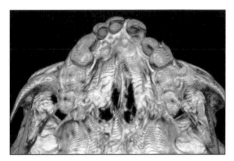

Fig 17-1f Palatal view 6 months postoperative.

This process has the advantage of eliminating the need to surgically recreate a soft tissue envelope for placement of rhBMP. Bone formation is accelerated compared with conventional distraction methods.[9] In addition, DISO allows the gradual expansion of the overlying soft tissues. DISO has been successfully applied in the clinical setting to repair congenital facial clefts and mandibular hypoplasia.[22–25]

Case 1: Unilateral Cleft Lip and Palate

The infant whose treatment is shown in Fig 17-1 had a nearly complete cleft on the left side of the lip and a wide complete palatal cleft. The scooped-out appearance of the piriform fossa reflected the absence of the frontal process zone and lateral incisor zone of the premaxilla. The nasal lining of normal developmental fields was drawn into the deficiency site, thus pulling the alar cartilage into a stretched, flattened shape. After traditional cleft repair, the surface area of the left side of the nose was reduced by approximately 30%. Nearly all patients suffer from respiratory insufficiency on the cleft side postoperatively.

Repair of this cleft with rhBMP (InFuse, Medtronic Sofamor Danek) involved the developmental field reassignment technique,[26] in which the soft tissues corresponding to the missing premaxilla are rescued from the prolabium. This zone is supplied by the anterior ethmoid arteries from the internal carotid arterial system. The nonphiltral prolabium is supplied by the nasopalatine artery from the external carotid artery.

When the nonphiltral prolabium is dissected free and brought laterally to the floor of the nose, it restores the missing lining. The nonphiltral prolabium flap is combined with periosteal flaps of the tissue lining the cleft. These are sutured together into a box that contains stem cells (periosteal mesenchymal cells). Implantation of InFuse into this site induces stem cell differentiation into the osteoblastic line, forming new bone to unify the dental arch (transversely) and provide appropriate support for the nasal floor and the canine tooth (vertically).

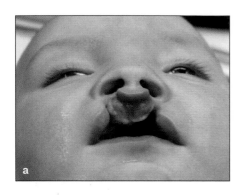

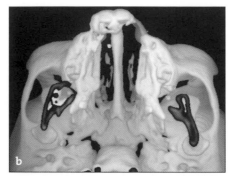

Fig 17-2a Preoperative facial view of an infant with bilateral cleft lip and palate.

Fig 17-2b Preoperative 3-D CT demonstrating palatal deficiency.

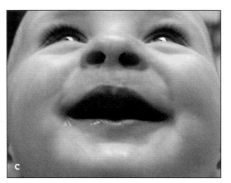

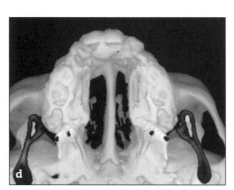

Fig 17-2c Facial view 1 year postoperative.

Fig 17-2d Six-month postoperative 3-D CT demonstrating symmetric osseous restoration of the palatal defects and stabilization of the dental arch.

Case 2: Bilateral Cleft Lip and Palate

In patients with bilateral clefts, the anterior maxilla is highly unstable. Traditional repair that incorporates only soft tissues creates forces that lead to collapse of the dental arch. Frequently, the maxillary shelves fall behind the anterior maxilla, where they remain entrapped. The only solution for these patients is jaw advancement surgery in the mid-teen years.

The patient whose treatment is shown in Fig 17-2 had symmetric bilateral alveolar bone clefts; the cleft on the right was incomplete and the one on the left was complete. For this reason, the premaxilla was rotated to the right. After developmental field reassignment repair and grafting with InFuse, soft tissue force vectors were restored. The resulting follow-up CT demonstrated rapid rotation of the premaxilla back to a normal configuration. While ISO was taking place over approximately 12 weeks, an acrylic resin splint was used for stabilization of the arch. The result was a symmetric maxilla that would not collapse and would maintain normal occlusion.

Case 3: Mandibular Atrophy

Bone grafts for large jaw defects suffer from constraints of inadequate blood supply. Critical-size defects are those with dimensions that cannot support a free graft without excessive cell death. In this instance, reconstructive surgeons may resort to vascularized bone flaps, such as the fibular flap, which are transferred to the head and neck region and connected to local blood vessels via microsurgical techniques. The operative time is long, and the donor site morbidity is considerable. In addition, the fibula does not readily accommodate the bearing of teeth.

In the absence of functional loading by teeth or dental implants, the bone flap will atrophy, as in the case of a patient with a previous fibular reconstruction of the left side of the mandibular body (Fig 17-3). Augmentation osteoplasty was performed to improve soft tissue contour and provide a potential site for future dental implants. Onlay with InFuse provided rapid and accurate correction of the irregular contour.

Figs 17-3a and 17-3b Preoperative appearance of a patient with left mandibular atrophy.

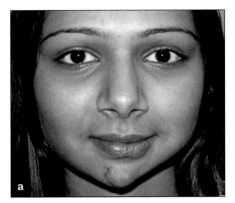

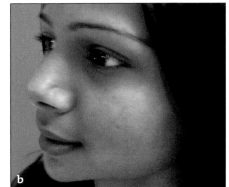

Fig 17-3c Preoperative 3-D CT.

Fig 17-3d Preoperative axial view revealing the thin, knifelike ridge of bone, which could not accommodate dental implants.

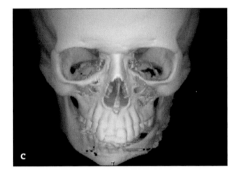

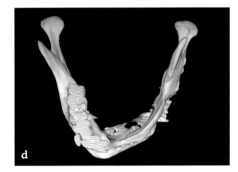

Figs 17-3e and 17-3f Facial appearance 12 months after treatment.

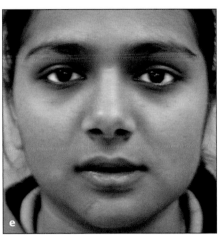

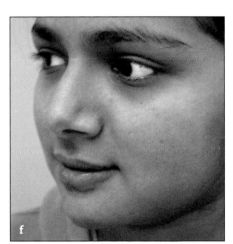

Fig 17-3g Six-month postoperative 3-D CT demonstrating new bone formation.

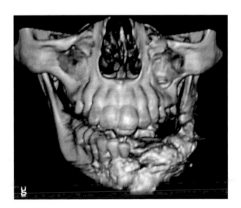

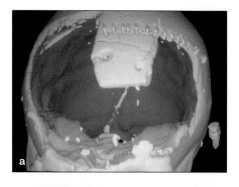

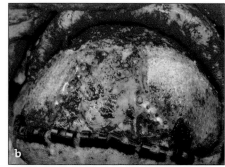

Fig 17-4a Preoperative CT demonstrating traumatic loss of the frontal calvarium bilaterally.

Fig 17-4b Intraoperative view of the frontal bone (seen from above). The BMP-2 graft has been covered by absorbable mesh to protect it from compression by the overlying soft tissues.

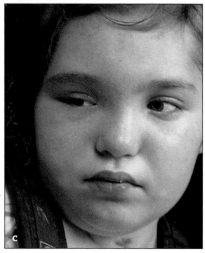

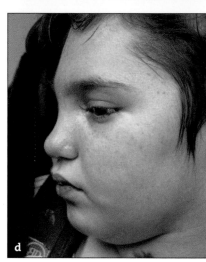

Figs 17-4c and 17-4d Facial appearance 12 months after treatment.

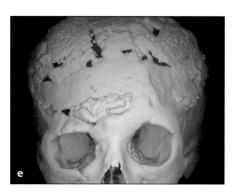

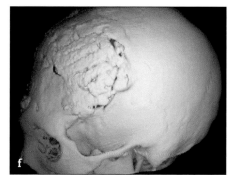

Fig 17-4e Six-month postoperative 3-D CT demonstrating calvarial ossification.

Fig 17-4f Six-month postoperative lateral 3-D CT showing healing.

Case 4: Craniofacial Trauma

A 9-year-old girl struck a pole while riding a bicycle without a helmet, sustaining a severe frontoparietal crush injury and intracranial hemorrhage. The patient underwent a bifrontal craniectomy for hematoma drainage and dural repair. In addition to bone fragment loss, the calvarial bone flap from her initial procedure was incorrectly stored and unsuitable for replantation. This resulted in a large residual defect that spanned the entire frontal bone region (Fig 17-4).

Multiple split-rib grafts would have been required to reconstruct a defect of this magnitude. An InFuse graft was instead used to close the defect. The graft was protected from overlying soft tissue compression by an absorbable mesh (KLS Martin). This reconstructive approach resulted in rapid and accurate correction of this massive defect without incurring significant instability or morbidity of the chest wall, which might have resulted from the harvesting of rib grafts.

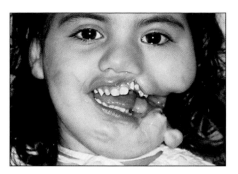

Fig 17-5a Preoperative appearance of a child with a Tessier No. 7 cleft.

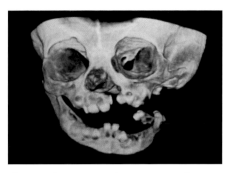

Fig 17-5b Preoperative 3-D CT demonstrating complex defects that include the left mandibular condyle, neck, and ramus.

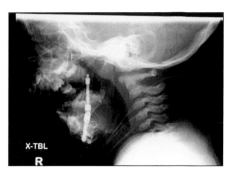

Fig 17-5c Radiographic view of the mandibular distraction device employed to lengthen the existing mandible.

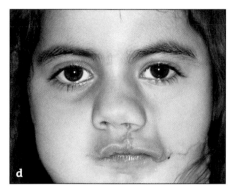

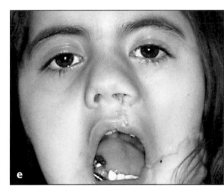

Figs 17-5d and 17-5e Photos taken 12 months after surgery show that the temporalis muscle transfer via fascia lata grafts to the neo-ramus permits control of mastication with a reasonably centric bite.

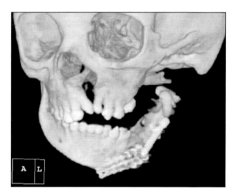

Fig 17-5f Six-month postoperative 3-D CT demonstrating biocortical neo-ramus with marrow space. (Figs 17-5b and 17-5d to 17-5f from Carstens et al.[25] Reprinted with permission.)

Case 5: Tessier No. 7 Cleft

Successful ISO is predicated on the creation of a soft tissue envelope that contains stem cells for osteoinduction, as exemplified by the neural crest mesenchymal cells present in periosteum. Creation of the periosteal chamber for placement of rhBMP by distraction allows rapid expansion and large chamber volume. The first published use of rhBMP for a craniofacial application[25] also made use of the DISO technique for reconstruction of a congenital mandibular deficiency (Fig 17-5).

The patient had a left-sided Tessier No. 7 cleft extending from the oral commissure through the horizontal embryologic axis of the ear. The mandibular defect included a foreshortened body, absent ramus, and absent masseter. Osteotomy of the proximal mandibular fragment allowed the placement of a distraction device; after 1 month, the device was adjusted to allow another sequence of distraction to establish maximal chamber length.

In a third procedure, rhBMP was applied with a Helistat collagen carrier sponge (Integra) implanted in the chamber. Eight weeks later, a procedure for muscle transfer and jaw suspension to the cranial base was performed, in addition to temporomandibular joint arthrodesis and soft tissue reconstruction. Subsequent labiomaxillary cleft reconstruction and cleft rhinoplasty were performed. An additional surgery accomplished revision of the oral commissure. The patient went on to exhibit symmetric growth and normal oral competence and dental development.

The case illustrates both the ability of rhBMP-induced bone to form rapidly when used with DISO to reconstruct deficient or absent sites (eg, the mandible) and the unique potential for growth in the growing child. The DISO technique also affords gradual expansion of overlying soft tissue as the periosteal chamber is created, reducing or eliminating the need for additional soft tissue augmentation.

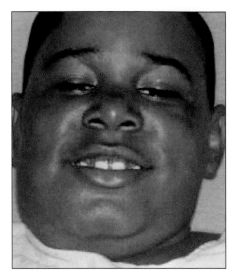

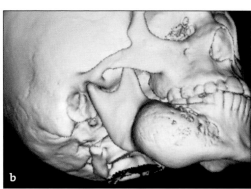

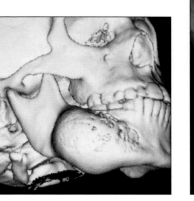

Fig 17-6a Preoperative appearance of a patient with a juvenile active ossifying fibroma on the right side of the mandible.

Figs 17-6b and 17-6c Preoperative 3-D CTs demonstrating the lesion.

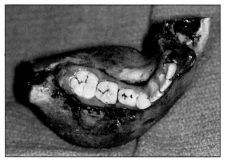

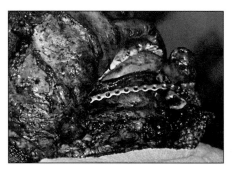

Fig 17-6d Resected mandibular segment with periosteal sleeve left in situ.

Fig 17-6e Reconstruction plate used to stabilize the mandible and support the rhBMP-2. (Figs 17-6a to 17-6e from Chao et al.[16] Reprinted with permission.)

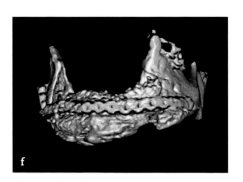

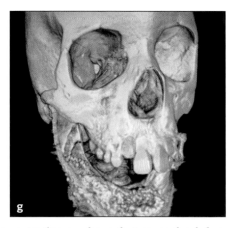

Figs 17-6f and 17-6g Postoperative 3-D CTs demonstrating new bone that spans the defect.

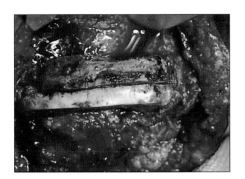

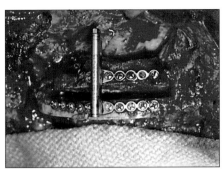

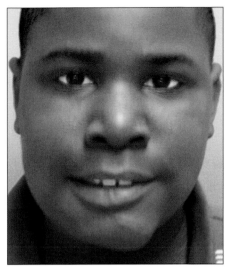

Fig 17-6h Revision osteotomy performed 24 weeks after the original surgery.

Fig 17-6i Placement of a distractor to increase the mandibular height.

Fig 17-6j Facial appearance 2 years after treatment.

Case 6: Hemimandibular Defect

The application of ISO for reconstruction of a hemimandibular defect resulting from tumor resection in a 9-year-old child demonstrates several advantages over the use of the vascularized bone flap (Fig 17-6). This case represents the first published use of rhBMP for closure of a critical-sized defect.[16] Resection of a recurrent juvenile active ossifying fibroma resulted in a 12-cm mandibular right defect. The surrounding periosteal sleeve was left intact and filled precisely with InFuse and supported by a reconstruction plate. The patient was kept in maxillomandibular fixation for stability during osteogenesis.

After 12 weeks, the entire volume of the periosteal chamber demonstrated new bone formation. The overall vertical height of the regenerated bone was appropriate, but the physical positioning of the chamber was lower than that of the contralateral side. Therefore, an osteotomy to allow placement of a vertical distractor was performed at 24 weeks. Intraoperatively, solid corticocancellous bone with bleeding marrow in the regenerated bone was noted. Further histologic examination of the osteotomy specimen demonstrated woven bone entrapped within the trabeculae of lamellar bone—characteristics of membranous bone.

The hemimandible generated by rhBMP was solid, stable, and well vascularized at 6 months and able to accommodate osteotomy and distraction without regard to vascular supply. Regenerated bone was precise in terms of periosteal chamber filling; however, establishment of accurate 3-D shape and suspension necessitates stable surrounding support of the soft tissue envelope to prevent shifting, sagging, or distortion of the bone regenerate.

Case 7: Orbital Dystopia

The challenge in some craniofacial defects is the creation of not only volumetric but also a 3-D shape, as demonstrated in this case (Fig 17-7). A 17-year-old boy had significant orbital dystopia (displacement) of the right orbit that not only was disfiguring but also affected his visual axis. Preoperative CT images showed prior reconstruction with bone graft and mesh that compressed and distorted the orbit.

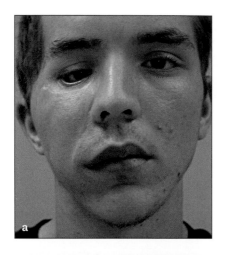

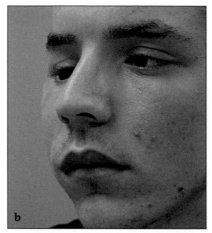

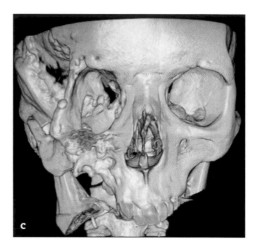

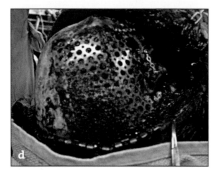

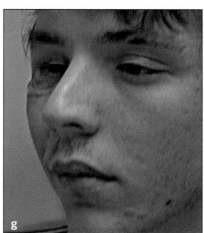

Figs 17-7a and 17-7b Preoperative appearance of a patient with a right facial neurofibroma.

Fig 17-7c Preoperative 3-D CT demonstrating right orbital and malar deformity secondary to tumor involvement.

Fig 17-7d Intraoperative view of the ISO-switch technique. Calvarial bone graft is harvested for facial reconstruction and a mesh frame placed over the harvest site.

Fig 17-7e rhBMP placed over the mesh frame to reconstitute the calvarial donor site.

Figs 17-7f and 17-7g Facial appearance 12 months after treatment.

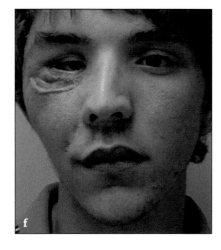

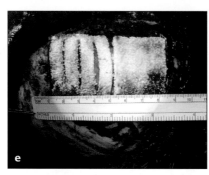

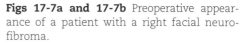

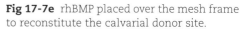

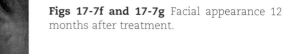

A full-thickness bone graft was harvested from the parietal skull and shaped in a jigsaw fashion to match the required dimensions. The resulting calvarial defect was replaced with InFuse. This operation is the first known example of the ISO-switch technique. The significance of this procedure is that the calvarium is especially adaptable to 3-D shaping and becomes a "never-ending bone bank" if harvesting is required for future reconstruction.

Case 8: Fronto-orbital Deformity

Another example of the ISO-switch technique demonstrates the power to produce an esthetically pleasing reconstruction (Fig 17-8). A 13-year-old boy with Saethre-Chotzen syndrome had a significant fronto-orbital deformity characterized by extreme reduction in the surface area of the orbital roof frontal bone. Prior surgery had consisted of forehead recontouring and placement of an

Figs 17-8a and 17-8b Preoperative appearance of a patient with orbital deficiency resulting from Saethre-Chotzen syndrome.

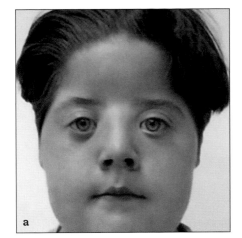
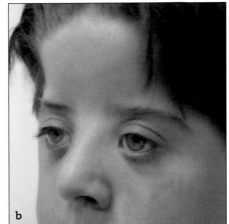

Fig 17-8c Preoperative CT revealing deficiency in the superior orbital rim.

Fig 17-8d Preoperative 3-D CT.

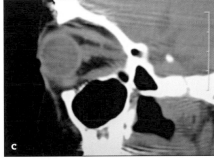
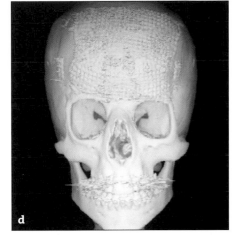

Figs 17-8e and 17-8f Facial appearance 1 year postoperative demonstrating correction of the "pinched-in" preoperative appearance.

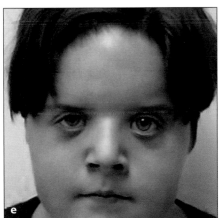
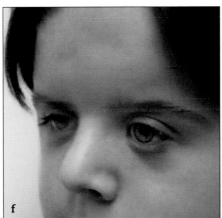

Fig 17-8g CT 6 months after ISO-switch reconstruction, demonstrating calvarial augmentation of the superior orbital rim.

Fig 17-8h Six-month postoperative 3-D CT demonstrating reconstruction of the donor site with rhBMP-2.

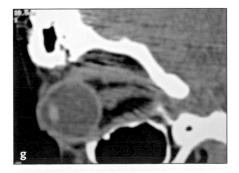
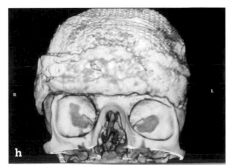

onlay graft covered with titanium mesh; the result was suboptimal projection.

The preferred method for further reconstruction would have consisted of harvesting a transverse bar of bone above the orbits and advancing it, a flap known as a *bandeau*. In similar cases, advancement of the bandeau is accompanied by removal and reshaping of the frontal bone. Unfortunately, this was prohibited by the presence of the titanium mesh. Instead, a bandeau in the form of a U-shaped bone flap was harvested from the posterior skull. The flap was then dropped forward like a visor over the existing supraorbital bone to achieve adequate supra-orbital esthetic contour and projection and associated protection of the globe. The bandeau donor site was then reconstituted with InFuse using the ISO-switch technique. Additional placement of InFuse implant at the lateral margins of the orbits was highly effective in correcting the pinched-in preoperative appearance of the face. Use of the ISO-switch technique provided an effective solution for this challenging problem, avoided entry into a postoperative site of mesh embedded into the dura, and averted significant neurosurgical morbidity.

Discussion

The induction of osseous regeneration with BMP has been well studied and widely utilized in the field of orthopedic surgery. The technique also has demonstrated great promise in the area of head and neck reconstruction. Use of rhBMP for craniofacial reconstruction circumvents several of the limitations of autogenous bone grafts, bone substitutes, and vascularized or free bone grafts. Nonbiologic implants are prone to infection, erosion, and non-incorporation and do not afford any growth potential in children. Autogenous bone must be hand shaped to accommodate the defect, may be limited in size based on the vascular supply or donor site, and may resorb to varying extents over time.

Bone formation by rhBMP is not known to be limited by defect size or volume, provided that an appropriate surrounding soft tissue envelope containing MSCs has been created. The rhBMP induces angiogenesis and essentially serves to vascularize itself. Thus, the reconstructive surgeon is freed from basing the reconstructive plan on facial blood supply as well as from laborious postoperative monitoring to prevent early flap loss arising from vas-

cular insufficiency. Furthermore, the 3-D design of the soft tissue pocket and precise filling with the collagen carrier affords relative ease and accuracy in shaping the new bony construct. Ectopic bone has not been shown to develop to any great degree beyond the confines of the sponge.

Despite these advantages, the rhBMP/absorbable collagen sponge implant must have adequate surrounding support during the period of osteogenesis to prevent malpositioning or distortion of the regenerated bone. Such support may be provided by concomitant placement of plating or mesh with muscular or fascial suspension as needed.

The ISO-switch technique may be desirable in cases where a precise shape is needed, as in midfacial or periorbital reconstruction. This provides thinner calvarial graft, which is easily cut into an exact shape to fit the defect, and uses rhBMP to fill the donor site defect. New calvarial bone formation affords an essentially endless bone bank that may be reharvested for future reconstruction, if needed.

Implantation of rhBMP is relatively rapid; single-stage operations may be possible in many cases that may have previously necessitated more arduous, multistage procedures. Bone formation is also reliably rapid; radiographic evidence of solid bone is present at 12 weeks in most cases.[12]

Autogenous bone, when placed against tooth roots, may result in tooth resorption or ankylosis. Use of nonresorbable ceramics in alveolar cleft reconstruction may interfere with the eruption and orthodontic movement of teeth. To date, no adverse effects on teeth are known to be caused by contact with rhBMP, and orthodontic movement through the regenerate has been shown to proceed normally. Additionally, the newly formed bone is solid and amenable to dental implantation in cases of absent or poor dentition.

Conclusion

Since its discovery by Urist, rhBMP has been exhaustively studied, and a number of good reviews regarding the basic science behind ISO are available.[27–34] Studies of rhBMP in the repair of alveolar clefts have demonstrated stabilization of an inherently unstable anterior maxilla. This phenomenon illustrates the advantage of ISO for cleft repair and presumably in general for pediatric craniofacial reconstruction. The pediatric face may be viewed as interlocking building blocks, all of which are growing over time. If a block (eg, the anterior maxilla) is missing, the surrounding pieces collapse into the deficient site. Reconstitution of the absent block with rhBMP allows formation of a new interlocking piece to stabilize the construct.

Perhaps the most compelling reason for considering the use of rhBMP for craniofacial reconstruction in children is the potential to accommodate growth as well as repeat operations. Early follow-up by the author (MHC) has demonstrated symmetric growth in rhBMP-created segments, which has been attributed to the principle of Wolff's law: Mechanical stress determines the architecture of bone.

Long-term observation of the growth and stability of bone formed by ISO will be essential to the establishment of rhBMP osteoconduction as a preferred technique for craniofacial reconstruction in children. Continued success of rhBMP use in the pediatric population will guide further exploration of the role for rhBMP in adult craniofacial reconstruction, as well as expanded application of the ISO technique to other anatomic sites in patients of all ages.

References

1. Boyne PJ. Use of marrow cancellous bone grafts in maxillary alveolar and palatal clefts. J Dent Res 1974;43:821–824.
2. Demas PN, Sotereanos GC. Closure of alveolar clefts with corticocancellous block grafts and marrow: A retrospective study. J Oral Maxillofac Surg 1988; 46:682–687.
3. Carstens MH, Chin M, Li XJ. In situ osteogenesis: Regeneration of 10-cm mandibular defect in porcine model using recombinant human bone morphogenetic protein-2 (rhBMP-2) and Helistat absorbable collagen sponge. J Craniofac Surg 2005;16:1033–1042.
4. Betts N, Fonseca R. Allogenic grafting of dentoalveolar clefts. Oral Maxillofac Surg Clin North Am 1991;3:617–624.
5. El Deeb M, Wolford L. Utilization of alloplastic ceramics in repair of alveolar clefts and correction of skeletofacial deformities in patients with cleft palate. Oral Maxillofac Surg Clin North Am 1991;3:625–640.
6. Wozney JM. Overview of bone morphogenetic proteins. Spine 2002;27(16 suppl 1):S2–S8.
7. Urist MR. Bone: Formation by autoinduction. Science 1965;150:893–899.
8. Urist MR, Strates BS. Bone morphogenetic protein. J Dent Res 1971;50: 1392–1406.
9. Valentin-Opran A, Wozney J, Csimma C, et al. Clinical evaluation of recombinant human bone morphogenetic protein-2. Clin Orthop Related Res 2002;395: 110–120.
10. Seeherman H, Wozney J, Li R. Bone morphogenetic protein delivery systems. Spine 2002;27(16 suppl 1):16–23.
11. Boyne PJ. Animal studies of application of rhBMP-2 in maxillofacial reconstruction. Bone 1996;19(suppl):83S–92S.
12. Boyne PJ. A feasibility study evaluating rhBMP-2/absorbable collagen sponge for maxillary sinus floor augmentation. Int J Periodontics Restorative Dent 1997; 17:11–25.
13. Boyne PJ. Application of bone morphogenetic proteins in the treatment of clinical oral and maxillofacial osseous defects. J Bone Joint Surg Am 2001;83A (suppl 1 pt 2):S146–S150.
14. Boyne PJ, Nath R, Nakamura A. Human recombinant BMP-2 in osseous reconstruction of simulated cleft palate defects. Br J Oral Maxillofac Surg 1998;36: 84–90.
15. Chin M, Ng T, Tom WK, Carstens M. Repair of alveolar clefts with recombinant human bone morphogenetic protein (rhBMP-2) in patients with clefts. J Craniofac Surg 2005;16:778–789.
16. Chao M, Donovan T, Sotelo C, Carstens MH. In situ osteogenesis of hemimandible with rhBMP-2 in a 9-year-old boy: Osteoinduction via stem cell concentration. J Craniofac Surg 2006;17:405–412.
17. zur Nieden NI, Kempka G, Rancourt DE, Ahr HJ. Induction of chondro-, osteo-, and adipogenesis in embryonic stem cells by bone morphogenetic protein-2: Effect of cofactors on differentiating lineages. BMC Dev Biol 2005;5:1–15.
18. Ebara S, Nakayama K. Mechanism for the action of bone morphogenetic proteins and regulation of their activity. Spine 2002;27(16 suppl 1):S10–S15.
19. Sato M, Yasui N, Nakase T, et al. Expression of bone morphogenetic proteins mRNA during distraction osteogenesis. J Bone Miner Res 1998;13:1221–1231.
20. Chin M. Alveolar process reconstruction using distraction osteogenesis. In: Diner PA, Vazquez MP (eds). International Congress on Cranial and Facial Bone Distraction Processes. Bologna: Monduzzi, 1997:51–54.
21. Chin M. Distraction osteogenesis in maxillofacial surgery. In: Lynch SE, Genco RJ, Marx RE (eds). Tissue Engineering: Applications in Maxillofacial Surgery and Periodontics, ed 1. Chicago: Quintessence, 1999:147–159.
22. Chin M, Boyne P, Eftimie LF. Distraction osteogenesis with bone morphogenetic protein enhancement in the extension of edentulous bone. In: Arnaud E, Diner PA (eds). 3rd International Congress on Cranial and Facial Bone Distraction Processes: 2001 Distraction Odyssey. Bologna: Monduzzi, 2001:19–22.
23. Chin M, Carstens MH. Distraction osteogenesis with bone morphogenetic protein enhancement: Facial cleft repair in humans. In: Arnaud E, Diner PA (eds). 4th International Congress of Maxillofacial and Craniofacial Distraction. Bologna: Monduzzi, 2003:197–200.
24. Chin M. Bone morphogenetic protein enhancement of alveolar distraction in humans. In: Arnaud E, Diner PA (eds). 4th International Congress of Maxillofacial and Craniofacial Distraction. Bologna: Monduzzi, 2003:49–51.
25. Carstens MH, Chin M, Ng T, Tom WK. Reconstruction of #7 facial cleft with distraction-assisted in situ osteogenesis (DISO): Role of recombinant human bone morphogenetic protein-2 with Helistat-activated collagen implant. J Craniofac Surg 2005;16:1023–1032.
26. Carstens MH. Functional matrix cleft repair: A common strategy for unilateral and bilateral clefts. J Craniofac Surg 2000;11:437–469.
27. Urist MR. Bone: Formation by autoinduction. Science 1965;150:893–899.
28. Urist MR, Strates BS. Bone morphogenic protein. J Dent Res 1971;50:1392–1406.
29. Celeste AJ, Iannazzi JA, Taylor RC, et al. Identification of transforming growth factor-β family members present in bone-inductive protein purified from bovine bone. Proc Natl Acad Sci U S A 1990;87:9843–9847.
30. Cheng H, Jiang W, Phillips FM, et al. Osteogenic activity of the fourteen types of human bone morphogenetic proteins (BMPs). J Bone Joint Surg Am 2003; 85A:1544–1552.
31. Urist MR, Huo YK, Brownell AG, et al. Purification of bovine bone morphogenic protein by hydroxyapetite chromatography. Proc Natl Acad Sci U S A 1984; 81:371–375.
32. Wozney JM, Rosen V, Celeste AJ, et al. Novel regulators of bone formation: Molecular clones and activities. Science 1988;242:1528–1534.
33. Valentin-Opran A, Wozney J, Csimma C, Lilly L, Riedel GE. Clinical evaluation of recombinant human bone morphogenetic protein-2. Clin Orthop Relat Res 2002;395:110–120.
34. Seeherman H, Wozney J, Li R. Bone morphogenetic protein delivery systems. Spine 2002;27(16 suppl 1):16–23.

18

Tissue Engineering Strategies in the Treatment of TMDs

Mary Beth Schmidt, PhD

Leslie Robin Halpern, DDS, MD, PhD, MPH

The term *temporomandibular disorders (TMDs)* describes a broad category of diseases involving both the temporomandibular joint (TMJ) and related musculoskeletal structures of the head and neck.[1-3] The origin of TMDs may be macrotraumatic or microtraumatic. Macrotrauma can result from facial injury (facial fractures or blunt injury), neck injury, or chronic dental therapy for recurrent occlusal dysfunction. Microtrauma is often the direct result of parafunctional habits with exacerbation of clenching, headaches, and grinding or bruxism. Additionally, molecular mechanisms and sexual dimorphisms, such as hormonal and inflammatory mediators, have been explored in an attempt to determine the pathophysiologic basis of TMDs.[4-6] The possible causal factors of TMDs may therefore include biologic and physiologic mechanisms as well as behavioral factors and genetic predisposition to disease based on selective expression of cellular mediators.[7,8]

TMDs affect 25% to 40% of the general population. Epidemiologic studies indicate that up to 70% of patients who exhibit some form of TMD are suffering from TMJ dysfunction. Dodson[9] reviewed the epidemiology of TMDs with respect to prevalence and treatment needs over the last 50 years. He concluded that a potential group of 7.5 to 15 million patients within the United States may have symptoms that are not being diagnosed.[9]

Significantly more females are affected than males (by ratios of 7:1 to 10:1).[9,10] Hormones and acute-phase reactants may play significant roles in the pathophysiology and sex predilection of TMDs.[7,8,11] Studies have shown that, in both animals and humans, estrogen receptors can be localized in the TMJs of females and not males.[5] While the relationship between these receptors and TMDs in humans is not clear, studies do suggest that female sex hormones play a role in pain transmission.[8]

Significant numbers of TMD patients complain of headaches, neck pain, clicking, and popping of their jaws during speech, eating, and sleeping, all of which interfere with their daily function and health-related quality of life. Many TMD patients also exhibit disc displacement that is irreversible, leading to permanent physical changes in the disc.[12-14] The number of patients who seek active treatment varies depending on the severity of their symptoms. With such a vast array of symptoms and the large number of patients with some form of TMD, dental and surgical practitioners have faced a significant dilemma with respect to treatment strategies.

Over the past 20 years, the improved ability to image the internal structures of the TMJ encouraged the use of open joint surgery to repair damaged tissue or replace it with synthetic substitutes.[12,14] Conditions requiring surgi-

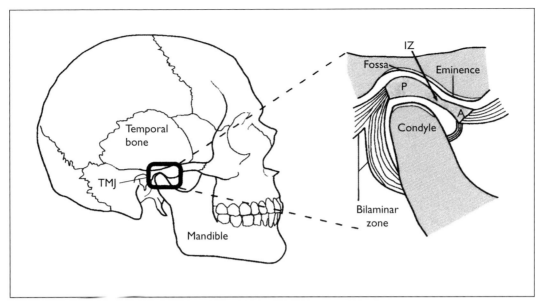

Fig 18-1 Side view of the human skull, including the bony structures forming the TMJ and an enlarged sagittal section of the TMJ. (P) Posterior band; (IZ) intermediate zone; (A) anterior band. (From Detamore and Athanasiou.[16] Reprinted with permission.)

cal intervention include internal joint derangement, ankylosis, traumatic injuries, recurrent dislocation, arthritic conditions, and tumor ablation. Many of these procedures have resulted in either equivocal success or, in some cases, irreversible sequelae that affect long-term function and health-related quality of life for the patients.

More recently, the approach to TMJ surgery has focused on less invasive techniques, such as arthroscopy and arthrocentesis. The latter technique has provided a means to characterize possible biomarkers or inflammatory mediators that may aid in determining possible success or failure for various therapeutic options.[15]

Advances in both open surgery and minimally invasive approaches, however, have failed to mitigate serious postoperative complications, including nerve damage, scarring, infection, degenerative joint disease, ankylosis, malocclusions, and implant failure.[12] The relatively high complication rate, regardless of treatment approach, poses a significant dilemma to the surgeon who must develop a treatment plan. Patients are often disappointed with interventional strategies, because full and unrestricted joint function may never return.

Researchers are beginning to apply tissue engineering strategies for reconstruction and rejuvenation of the temporomandibular joint and associated structures. Recent advances in biomaterials research and molecular biology at the genetic level may provide the key connection between joint structure and function at the biologic and molecular levels. This chapter reviews the application of tissue engineering strategies in the surgical management of TMJ disease with respect to TMJ pathophysiology. The normal anatomy of the TMJ and the possible physical and molecular mechanisms responsible for pathophysiologic changes in TMJ tissues are discussed. Experimental and preclinical studies in mammalian models and suggestions for future research design strategies are addressed.

Anatomy of the TMJ

The TMJ is a diarthrodial, ginglymoid synovial joint formed by the articulation of the mandibular condyle with the glenoid fossa and the articular eminence of the temporal bone (Fig 18-1). It is diarthrodial because it has two articulating surfaces and ginglymoid because it moves in a hingelike fashion. The TMJ is covered by a bilayered capsule with an outer fibrous layer and an inner synovial layer. The capsule is further divided into a lateral portion and an anterior portion. The anterior portion is further subdivided into three segments that are often visualized with arthroscopy. The inner synovial layer contains synovial cells (A, B, and C cells), which play an active role in secretion, debris removal, and production of inflammatory mediators that are moderators of repair.

Most synovial joints are composed of hyaline cartilage at their articular surfaces. The TMJ, however, has an articular surface that is better characterized as fibrocartilage. This fibrocartilage has a multilayered structure; the most proximal layer is characterized as the articular zone. This zone is composed of collagen fibers that are oriented parallel to the surface of the condyle and articular eminence to resist biomechanical wear during joint function. Within the layer of fibrocartilage there are scattered groups of chondrocytes that have been shown to contain active protein-synthesizing machinery (ie, Golgi complexes and endoplasmic reticulum) that secretes type II collagen, proteoglycans, and glycoproteins. Glycosaminoglycans (GAGs) are negatively charged, highly hydrophilic polysaccharides found within the extracellular matrix of the cartilage. GAGs aggregate with proteins to form large proteoglycan molecules that are entrapped within the collagen network, contributing to the compressive stiffness of cartilage.

A fibrocartilaginous disc is situated between the condyle and fossa eminence. This disc divides the joint into superior and inferior joint spaces. The function of the TMJ disc is to improve the congruity of the mating joint surfaces, reduce contact pressure, act as a shock absorber, and aid in joint lubrication. Medially and laterally, the disc is attached to the joint capsule on the head of the condyle. The disc attaches anteriorly to the eminence and condyle and posteriorly to the retrodiscal tissue and posterior condylar neck. These attachments separate the joint space into superior and inferior compartments.

The TMJ disc is biconcave and nonuniform in thickness. It is thinner in the center and thicker at the periphery, where it is connected to retrodiscal tissue that is vascularized and innervated. This variation in thickness provides the disc with sufficient flexibility during rotation and translation of the joint.

The cells found within the TMJ disc are of a heterogenous origin, consisting of a mixture of chondrocytes, fibrochondrocytes, fibroblasts, and smooth muscle cells.[17] The predominant cell type in the human TMJ disc has not yet been conclusively established; it may vary by species in animals due to differences in diet and chewing patterns.[17] Much of the research examining cell types of the TMJ disc has been based on the use of the porcine model.[18,19] The porcine disc is composed of cells that are similar to those found in the human TMJ disc; therefore, this model has been frequently used for tissue engineering studies. A recent study has isolated cell type and distribution in the porcine TMJ disc.[19]

The collagen produced in the TMJ disc is predominantly type I, but traces of type II are sometimes reported.[20,21] The fibers are arranged in a circumferential or ringlike pattern, with some branching at the peripheral attachment boundaries. This structural arrangement allows the disc to withstand the tensile stresses that are generated in the TMJ.[22] Proteoglycans have been identified throughout the body of the disc, with a slightly higher concentration toward the periphery. However, the total GAG content of the TMJ disc is about an order of magnitude lower than that of hyaline cartilage, leading to a lower compressive stiffness.

Despite the existence of established surgical techniques to repair the injured or malaligned temporomandibular joint, true regeneration of functional intra-articular tissues has been difficult to achieve. The capacity of these tissues to regenerate is limited by their low vascularity and relatively sparse cellularity. Without access to chondrogenic cells, growth factors, or other cytokines that drive these cells to migrate to a joint surface defect, proliferate, and form new fibrocartilage, a traumatic injury or accumulated microdamage is incapable of healing. Although surgical intervention may restore alignment and disc position and provide pain relief, untreated cartilage damage eventually leads to arthritic lesions on the joint surface and loss of normal joint function.

Pathophysiology of TMJ Dysfunction

Mechanical mechanisms

TMJ pain and dysfunction as a result of displacement of the intra-articular disc have been recognized as significant clinical problems for more than a century.[23] The most common causes of internal derangement are traumatic injury to the TMJ and osteoarthritis.[12,14] Human cadaver studies have indicated that disc displacement may affect as much as 67% of the population.[24] The root cause of this pathologic disease state is an acute or chronic mechanical interference of smooth joint movement secondary to an abnormal relationship between the articular disc and the condyle and fossa eminence. Wilkes[25] has described internal derangement as a series of five stages based on radiographic, clinical, and surgical criteria. Once this cascade of derangement has begun, the disc seldom returns to a complete resolution of structural and functional integrity.[25]

Chronic wear of the deranged TMJ leads to a metaplastic metamorphosis of viable joint tissues. Studies have shown that patients with internal derangement have an abundance of vascularized hyaline-like tissue with a reduced ability to conform under functional loading.[26] Histologic analyses suggest that the biologic machinery necessary to regenerate the cell population and extracellular matrix is absent.[26] In addition, it has been suggested that bony changes to the condyle and temporal bone precede or follow disc dislocation, resulting in degenerative joint disease and osteoarthritis.[27] Other mechanical causes of TMJ derangement and degeneration include an imbalance of pressure and loading during chewing and asymmetric remodeling of the articular surfaces of the condyle and articular eminence.[27]

Molecular mechanisms

The molecular mechanisms hypothesized to contribute to TMJ dysfunction have their origins within the building blocks of the discal tissue. Studies have shown that the composition of the extracellular matrix, specifically collagen, proteoglycans, GAGs, and water content, significantly contributes to the biomechanical properties of the articular surface. Tissues containing proteoglycans are resilient to compressive forces mainly because of their high water content. The destruction of the extracellular matrix and the concomitant loss of water lead to failure of TMJ tissues to resist normal joint-loading forces.

The collagen network may be initially altered by either enzymatic or nonenzymatic cascades, resulting in degradation products that are removed as debris.[28,29] The enzymatic pathway includes metalloproteinases, which are produced by chondrocytes and synoviocytes, and gelatinase, cathepsin, and elastase synthesized by polymorphonuclear lymphocytes. These biologic markers have been isolated from synovial fluid during arthrocentesis and arthroscopy, although their role in degenerative joint disease is still largely unclear. Nonenzymatic degradation mechanisms include free radicals that can generate a series of reactions that either stimulate or inhibit molecular mechanisms for repair.[27]

Inflammatory mediators

Inflammatory cytokines are small peptides that are potent at very low concentrations (10^{-9} to 10^{-12} M). These peptides can exert significant effects in response to physiologic insults to the TMJ, initiating a cascade of events that leads to the pathogenesis of degenerative joint disease. Among the many well-established cytokines isolated, interleukin 1 (IL-1), IL-6, IL-8, and tumor necrosis factor (TNF) have been most strongly associated with degenerative joint disease. IL-1 has been studied extensively using lavage fluid collections as well as in vitro tissue culture with chondrocytes that are exposed to IL-1.[30,31] Research is still underway to determine the cause-and-effect relationship between inflammatory cytokines and degeneration of the TMJ.

Another group of neuropeptides (substance P, calcitonin gene–related peptide, and bradykinin) has been implicated in the inflammatory cascade of IL-1 and TNF. This process has been referred to as *neurogenic inflammation*.[32] Substance P and calcitonin gene–related peptide have been localized with immunocytochemistry in the retrodiscal tissue and have been implicated to increase IL-1 and TNF synthesis. Studies have shown an increase of substance P in the synovial fluid with injections of IL-1.[32]

Although a cause-and-effect relationship is not clear, the cytokines and neuropeptides act in concert to affect the molecular events of TMJ disc degeneration.[27] It is suggested that three factors contribute to degeneration and inability to repair: direct mechanical trauma, hypoxiareperfusion, and neurogenic inflammation.[5]

Regardless of the cause of a TMD, once the joint tissues are damaged, they are no longer able to withstand the biomechanical stresses experienced in the temporomandibular joint during normal daily activities. The capacity for articular cartilage or the TMJ disc to undergo repair is limited, particularly after physical and morphologic degradative changes occur within these joint components. The integration of tissue engineering approaches into clinical treatment options may lead to successful regeneration of the TMJ articular surface and the fibrocartilage disc by overriding the physiologic obstacles faced by the native tissues. As such, tissue engineering could revolutionize treatment modalities for the surgical management of patients with diseases of the TMJ.

Fundamentals of Cartilage Tissue Engineering

Tissue engineering offers the means to regenerate or replace tissues that are normally incapable of intrinsic repair. The tissue engineering approach to cartilage or discal repair requires three basic elements to ensure that the morphology and mechanical properties of the repair tissue adequately resemble those of native tissue: cells, a scaffold, and biologic factors. A source of chondrogenic and/or fibroblastic cells is needed, because of the relatively small number of cells contained in healthy or degenerated cartilage in the TMJ or disc and the lack of access to a pool of potentially reparative progenitor cells. Attempts at cartilage repair using acellular approaches have often produced results inferior to those achieved with cell-based cartilage repair. Scaffolds provide a way to deliver the cells to the site of injury and ensure that they stay in place long enough to effect the desired repair. Growth factors and other anabolic cytokines stimulate migration of native cells to the wound site, differentiation of precursor cells along the proper pathway, proliferation of cells, and production of neocartilage matrix.

Most of the pioneering work in the development of tissue engineering techniques for cartilage repair has been done on the knee joint, which has a thick layer of hyaline cartilage that covers a significantly greater surface area than the TMJ. The knee joint also represents an extremely challenging mechanical environment, because it experiences very high contact stresses in the weight-bearing areas and large, complex rolling and sliding motions. Repair tissue must be robust enough to withstand these demanding conditions during long-term use. Transfer of these techniques to smaller joints such as the TMJ may present obstacles to the clinician, such as limited access, a smaller joint surface area, and a thinner fibrocartilage layer.

Scaffolds

A cartilage repair scaffold must provide a hospitable environment for cellular attachment and growth as it resorbs or remodels and is eventually replaced by a neocartilage matrix. The scaffold must have sufficient porosity to allow cellular colonization and tissue ingrowth as well as good integration with the host cartilage at the margins of the defect. The scaffold must have sufficient mechanical strength to withstand the implantation procedure and the forces generated at the joint surface during healing. A careful balance must be maintained between the rate of scaffold resorption and the rate of neocartilage formation, or the quality of the repair tissue can be adversely affected. Additional scaffold design requirements include good handling properties, ease of shaping to conform to the defect's size and shape, and retention in the defect site.

Autologous tissues such as the perichondrium and periosteum may be used as scaffolds for cartilage repair. Progenitor cartilage cells have been identified in the cambium layer of these tissues, which allows them to serve both as scaffolds and a source of cells. The clinical outcomes of this approach have been mixed, however; incomplete defect fill, detachment, and graft ossification have been noted.[33–35]

Periosteal flaps have also been used to contain cells delivered to a cartilage defect site without a scaffold. In this procedure, the periosteal flap is shaped to conform to the geometry of the defect and sutured in place. Fibrin glue is applied to ensure that a good peripheral seal is formed. The patient's own cartilage cells, obtained at biopsy and expanded in vitro, are then injected under the flap into the defect site. Histologic examination of repaired knee joint cartilage indicates that the mean fill area is 71% at 8 weeks and that the repair tissue mainly consists of hyaline-like cartilage.[36,37] Osteochondral autografting, termed *mosaicplasty*, offers another method to fill a defect with cartilage cells in their native scaffold. In this treatment, cylindrical osteochondral plugs are cored from peripheral or low weight–bearing areas of the joint surface. These plugs are subsequently implanted in damaged or diseased areas of the joint, providing a source of cells and an autologous scaffold. Although pain relief and recovery of joint function have been reported following this procedure, there is evidence to suggest that the implanted cartilage does not always survive over the long term.[38]

Other biologic materials, such as fibrin, hyaluronan, and collagen, have been used as scaffolds and cell delivery vehicles for cartilage repair. Fibrin has been used to contain and deliver chondrocytes and growth factors to a cartilage defect site.[39–41] Although fibrin is a natural part of the wound-healing cascade, it does not have the inherent mechanical strength to withstand the high forces of joint surfaces. It is also rapidly resorbed, so it is unlikely to provide an adequate foundation for new cartilage formation.

Hyaluronan (hyaluronic acid) is a linear, unbranched polysaccharide that serves as the backbone for proteoglycan aggregates within articular cartilage. Fibrous hyaluronan derivatives have been used as three-dimensional porous scaffolds for cartilage cell culture and implantation. Cell binding is reported to be significantly greater with hyaluronan scaffolds than with porous ceramic scaffolds, resulting in a greater relative amount of cartilage per unit area.[42,43] The 3-year results of a recent multicenter clinical study indicate a 76% reduction in pain and an 88% reduction in mobility problems in patients with focal knee joint cartilage lesions that were treated with hyaluronan implants seeded with autologous chondrocytes.[44]

Collagen-based scaffolds are among the most widely used biologic materials for cartilage tissue engineering. Collagen gels have been used to suspend cells in a three-dimensional matrix for in vitro culture expansion and as a delivery method for repair of a localized defect. Mesenchymal stem cells suspended in a collagen gel and placed in full-thickness defects in rabbits have resulted in formation of hyaline-like cartilage in the defect, although marginal integration was incomplete and the stiffness of the repair tissue was lower than that of the surrounding articular cartilage.[45] Collagen fiber sponges appear to favor migration, attachment, and proliferation of cartilage and progenitor cells.

In vitro studies of chondrocyte behavior suggest that type II collagen, the predominant collagen phenotype in hyaline articular cartilage, is superior for cartilage tissue engineering scaffolds. Chondrocyte morphology more closely resembles that of in situ cells, and the rate of cellular proliferation is greater on type II collagen scaffolds than on type I and type III scaffolds.[46]

Recent work using electrospinning techniques has shown that collagen fibers as small as 100 nm in diameter can be deposited in an oriented or random fashion to produce tissue engineering scaffolds that closely resemble the fiber size found in the native extracellular matrix of healthy articular cartilage.[47,48] Chondrocytes infiltrate and adhere to these fine scaffold fibrils, indicating that electrospun collagen scaffolds provide a suitable environment for cartilage tissue engineering.[46]

Fiber architecture may also play an important role in scaffold design. A cell-seeded two-layer collagen fiber scaffold was used for repair of osteochondral defects in rabbits.[49,50] This scaffold consisted of a dense layer that was in contact with the subchondral bone and a more porous layer to support the attachment and growth of the seeded cells. Better defect fill was observed after 6 months in the defects treated with the cell-seeded bilay-

er scaffold than in defects treated with scaffolds alone or no implant. The permeability and GAG content were reported to be near normal levels, and the type II collagen content was equivalent to normal.

Synthetic scaffold materials offer the opportunity to engineer the mechanical properties, porosity, and resorption rate of the scaffold to suit the conditions required for optimal neocartilage formation. Polymer materials such as polyglycolic acid (PGA), polylactic acid (PLA), and their copolymers have been used extensively for cartilage repair scaffolds. PLA/PGA copolymers provide more control of the degradation rate of the scaffold, mitigating possible release of acidic by-products into the local tissue environment. Woven meshes or porous foams can be manufactured with well-defined, uniform physical characteristics such as porosity and pore size. Additionally, microspheres of a PLA/PGA copolymer have been used to create an injectable cell-seeded scaffold for minimally invasive cartilage cell delivery. Chondrocytes coinjected with microspheres demonstrated greater cellular retention in the implant site than did chondrocytes injected without microspheres.[51]

Cells

Autologous chondrocyte transplantation to enhance hyaline cartilage repair was pioneered by the work of Grande and coworkers.[52] Since then, adult chondrocyte expansion and transplantation techniques have been developed and refined to optimize cell number and maintain phenotypic characteristics. Chondrocytes are usually isolated and expanded in culture, although the expansion potential for adult chondrocytes is limited. Cells may be derived from normal healthy cartilage that is harvested from a low weight–bearing area of the joint. Alternatively, other cell sources, such as marrow-derived progenitor cells, adipocytes, or skin fibroblasts, have been stimulated to produce cartilage in vitro.[53-56] The differentiated and expanded cells may subsequently be seeded on a scaffold and implanted, or the construct may be further cultured to initiate neocartilage formation prior to implantation.

Environmental conditions significantly influence in vitro chondrogenesis. Three-dimensional culture systems have proven to be superior to monolayer culture.[57-60] Supplementation with biologic factors that stimulate chondrocyte growth and differentiation is also beneficial, as discussed in the next section. Mechanical loading may be used to further drive pluripotent precursor cells to differentiate along the chondrogenic pathway and enhance neocartilage formation.[61–64] Chondrogenesis may also be enhanced by using low oxygen concentrations in vitro to mimic the in vivo cellular environment.[65,66]

Growth factors

The metabolism of mature hyaline articular cartilage is regulated by peptide growth factors such as insulin-like growth factor 1 (IGF-1), platelet-derived growth factor (PDGF), transforming growth factor β (TGF-β), and fibroblast growth factor (FGF), which originate from cellular production within cartilage as well as from the synovial fluid and surrounding tissues. As the mechanisms of action for these growth factors are established through well-defined in vitro studies, it is becoming clear that growth factors may eventually serve to augment current cartilage repair techniques. Chemotactic growth factors may be used to encourage migration of host cells to an injury site. Cell numbers can also be increased and matrix production upregulated by the presence of appropriate mitogenic and chondrogenic growth factors during in vitro culture expansion, controlled release of growth factors from scaffold materials, or other methods of intra-articular delivery.

IGF is the dominant anabolic growth factor for hyaline articular cartilage. It plays a key role in cartilage homeostasis, balancing proteoglycan synthesis and breakdown by the chondrocytes. In vitro studies demonstrate that IGF-1 stimulates proteoglycan production in a dose-dependent manner, as evidenced by increased ^{35}S-sulfate incorporation.[67] Similarly, IGF-1 has been shown to slow proteoglycan catabolism in a dose-dependent fashion.[68] Collagen production may also be regulated by IGF-1, although reports in the literature offer conflicting findings that may be dose-related. Blunk et al[69] showed that in vitro culture with IGF-1 (50 to 100 ng/mL) substantially increased the wet weight of tissue-engineered bovine cartilage constructs and increased the total proteoglycan and collagen contents. In contrast, no effect was observed in a similar study at lower doses of 1.25 and 2.50 ng/mL.[70]

IGF-1 treatment has been shown to improve the quantity and quality of cartilage repair tissue in several animal models. Critical-sized full-thickness defects in equine knee joint cartilage treated with IGF-1, loaded on either cell-seeded or acellular fibrin clots, were filled with more organized repair tissue, consisting predominantly of type II collagen, than were untreated controls.[39,40] In the acellular approach, it appeared that IGF-1 had a chemotactic effect, stimulating cellular migration from the surrounding tissues. Hunziker and Rosenberg[71] demonstrated that IGF-1 treatment results in an increased number of mesenchymal cells in the defect site. These cells are presumed to originate from the host synovial membrane and its underlying tissues.

PDGF plays a fundamental role in the wound-healing cascade. It is present in high concentrations in platelets and in the fluids generated during the early stages of wound healing.[72] PDGF is a potent mitogenic and chemotactic factor for cells of mesenchymal origin, including fibroblasts, osteoblasts, and chondrocytes, and is thus believed to be capable of enhancing tissue regeneration and repair. PDGF receptors have been identified on a variety of cell types, including chondrocytes, and the number of receptors is upregulated by the presence of inflammatory cytokines such as IL-1.[73]

The effect of the homodimer PDGF-BB on in vitro chondrocyte proliferation and extracellular matrix formation has been studied over a wide range of growth factor concentrations. Cell numbers were greater with all PGDF-BB concentrations of 4.7 ng/mL or more than they were in untreated controls.[74] Treatment with PDGF-BB also resulted in significantly more heterotopic cartilage formation following intramuscular implantation of chondrocyte-seeded scaffolds in rats.[75]

Indirect evidence for the role of PDGF and other growth factors active in the wound-healing process can be seen in the healing response in hyaline cartilage defects treated with microfracture. This procedure involves creating microperforations with an arthroscopic awl in the subchondral bone in and around a chondral lesion.[76] The mechanical integrity of the bone is maintained through careful placement of the holes. The awl is driven to a depth sufficient to ensure that the marrow space is accessed and bleeding is observed. A clot forms in the defect, which is anchored to the bone by the increased surface roughness produced by the microperforations. Wound-healing growth factors such as PDGF are released in the defect site, exerting chemotactic and mitogenic effects on cells in the surrounding cartilage and infiltrating mesenchymal stem cells. This provides an enriched environment for new tissue formation, which may be augmented by placement of a scaffold seeded with autologous cells.[77,78]

The TGF family includes TGF-β1, TGF-β2, and TGF-β3 and a variety of bone morphogenetic proteins (BMPs).

These growth factors regulate embryonic tissue development and also appear to play a major role in repair reactions following cartilage injury.[79] TGF-β growth factors are produced by hyaline cartilage chondrocytes and are present in the extracellular matrix of normal cartilage.

The primary effect of TGF-β appears to be matrix synthesis and inhibition of matrix breakdown. Addition of TGF-β to culture medium increases the total number of cells in tissue-engineered cartilage constructs by 1.4-fold at 4 weeks and increases the total GAG and collagen contents of the repair tissue.[69] Prolonged exposure to TGF-β through multiple intra-articular injections results in a marked increase in proteoglycan synthesis in a mouse model.[79] In response to injury or degradation, chondrocytes seem to become more sensitive to TGF-β, suggesting that it exists in the cartilage matrix in a latent form that is capable of being activated when repair is needed.[67]

Basic FGF (bFGF) is produced locally by the chondrocytes as well as systemically by the pituitary gland. This growth factor has been shown to be a powerful in vitro mitogen and thus may be a useful tool to accelerate cellular expansion for autologous transplantation.[67,79] In vitro studies suggest that bFGF can stimulate matrix synthesis, although this effect may be age dependent. In bovine cartilage explants from young animals, low doses of bFGF stimulated anabolic processes, while higher doses stimulated catabolism. In contrast, adult explants showed accelerated proteoglycan release at low bFGF concentrations but increased matrix synthesis at higher concentrations.[80]

Application of Tissue Engineering in the TMJ

Cartilage repair

TMJ cartilage is capable of limited intrinsic remodeling and repair following acute or chronic trauma. Using an adult sheep model for traumatic TMJ injury, Guven et al[81] created 0.5 × 0.5–cm experimental defects in mandibular condyle cartilage. The defects were created with a surgical bur and were observed to extend to the subchondral bone. Histologic analysis indicated that, 3 months postoperatively, the defects were filled with connective tissue and blood vessels. By 6 months fibrocartilaginous tissue was observed at the base of the defect, and by 9

months, most of the defect was filled with fibrocartilage. Small islands of loose connective tissue were observed to persist in the center of the defect. Increased cellularity was noted in the repair tissue, and immature cells resembling chondrocytes were observed parallel to the joint surface. It is likely that these cells originated from the marrow rather than the surrounding cartilage.

Similar repair tissue morphology and composition have been reported in untreated or experimental knee joint cartilage defects. Localized indentation testing has been used to demonstrate that the repair tissue is often mechanically inferior and unable to adequately withstand long-term joint loading.[82,83] Eventually, the repair tissue degrades, leading to joint pain and loss of function. Filling such defects with autologous cartilage cells or precursors, delivered on a bioresorbable scaffold, provides a promising new clinical treatment method for more successful cartilage repair outcomes.

Dysfunction of the TMJ may be related to congenital, traumatic, or chronic changes in the anatomy of the joint structures. As a result, the loading patterns across the articulating surfaces may be altered, leading to high focal stresses and gradual breakdown of the cartilage surfaces. Recent work shows that it may be possible to reconstruct the degenerated condyle with a tissue-engineered analog. Several investigators have attempted to form anatomically correct mandibular condyles by encapsulating cells and scaffold material within a mold.[84–86] This approach can be used to provide a source of autogenous bone for grafting procedures, thereby eliminating issues of limited bone availability and donor site morbidity.

Advancing the concept further, Alhadlaq et al[87–89] used predifferentiated rat mesenchymal stem cells in a bilayer mold to form a condyle analog with a cartilage-covered articulating surface (Fig 18-2). Marrow-derived precursor cells were differentiated in vitro into bone- and cartilage-forming cell populations using osteogenic and chondrogenic culture media supplements. The osteogenic medium contained 100 nM of dexamethasone, 10 mM of β-glycerophosphate, and 0.05 mM of ascorbic acid, while the chondrogenic medium was supplemented with 10 ng/mL of TGF-β1. The differentiated cells were loaded in a bilayer anatomically shaped mold and implanted in subcutaneous pockets in immunodeficient mice.

Histologic evaluation at 8 weeks indicated that a layer of neocartilaginous tissue was successfully formed over the bony construct. Positive safranin O staining was observed in the cartilage, indicating synthesis of cartilage-specific GAGs in the extracellular matrix. No mineralization was observed within the cartilage layer.[87–89] While

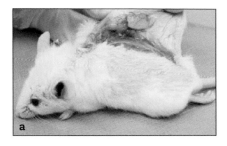

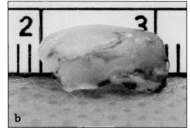

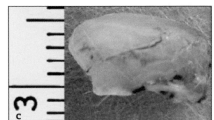

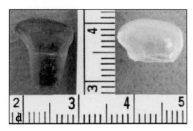

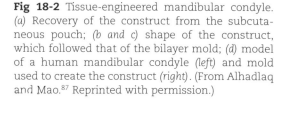

Fig 18-2 Tissue-engineered mandibular condyle. *(a)* Recovery of the construct from the subcutaneous pouch; *(b and c)* shape of the construct, which followed that of the bilayer mold; *(d)* model of a human mandibular condyle *(left)* and mold used to create the construct *(right)*. (From Alhadlaq and Mao.[87] Reprinted with permission.)

significant additional work is required before tissue-engineered TMJ condyle analogs are ready for therapeutic use, this approach offers promise for patients with anatomy-based TMJ dysfunction.

Because of the small size of the TMJ and limited surgical access to the joint surface, injectable or arthroscopic treatment modalities may offer the most practical approach to cartilage repair in symptomatic joints. Growth factors may be injected intra-articularly to promote repair and regeneration of cartilage tissue. BMP-2, a member of the TGF family, has been injected into internally deranged TMJ in a rabbit model.[90] Circular osteochondral defects, 2 mm in diameter and 2 mm deep, were created in the surface of the condylar head. A type I collagen solution containing 0.6, 3.0, or 15.0 μg of BMP-2 was injected into the defects, while controls were left unfilled or were filled with the collagen solution alone.

Three weeks postoperatively, neocartilage was observed in the defects treated with 3.0- and 15.0-μg doses of BMP-2 (Fig 18-3), while fibrous tissue filled most of the defects treated with a 0.6-μg dose. Several treated defects contained little repair tissue, suggesting that the growth factor–laden collagen may have migrated out of the defect. Unfilled control defects showed no evidence of tissue repair, and the collagen-filled defects contained only loosely organized connective tissue.[90]

Injection of TGF-β and IGF-1 in mice with osteoarthritic lesions in the TMJ cartilage has been studied by Sviri et al.[91] Repeated injections of IGF-1 (25 ng/60 μL), TGF-β (10 ng/60 μL), or IGF-1 (25 ng/30 μL) + TGF-β (10 ng/30 μL) were given at 3-day intervals over the course of 9 days. Cartilage was subsequently explanted and cultured

for 2 additional days without the presence of additional growth factors.

Histologic and immunohistochemical analyses indicated that IGF-1 alone and TGF-β alone increased protein and DNA synthesis in osteoarthritic cartilage, and a small additive effect on DNA synthesis was observed with the combined treatment. Hypertrophic cells and increased proteoglycan production were observed near the articulating surface (Fig 18-4), which may be related to the use of intra-articular injections. The results of this study further indicate that an accumulation of proteoglycans occurs during the injection period, as evidenced by increased ^{35}S-sulfate incorporation, but on termination of the growth factor injections, ^{35}S-sulfate incorporation was reduced. This finding suggests that the overall tissue responsiveness only occurs during the treatment period.

Disc repair

The TMJ disc is integral to the motion and function of the TMJ. The disc is situated between the mandibular condyle and the fossa eminence, increasing the congruity between the joint surfaces, increasing the contact area and thus distributing loads, providing shock absorption, and aiding in joint lubrication.[16,92] Disc repair is of particular interest, because the majority of patients with TMDs present with varying degrees of disc displacement or degeneration. When the TMJ disc is chronically displaced, it undergoes morphologic changes that eventually prevent normal joint function.

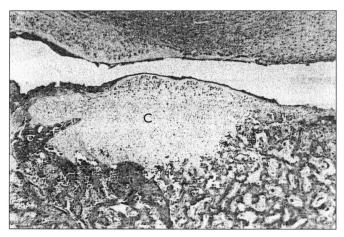

Fig 18-3a Histologic appearance of a rabbit TMJ cartilage defect treated with 15 µg of BMP-2. Cartilage (C) is observed to fill the defect (hematoxylin-eosin stain; original magnification ×6.5).

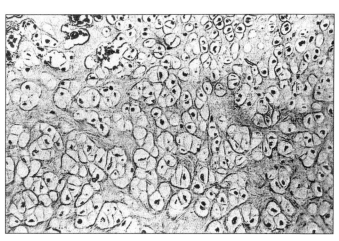

Fig 18-3b Higher magnification view of the repair tissue shown in Fig 18-3a (hematoxylin-eosin stain; original magnification ×16). (Figs 18-3a and 18-3b from Suzuki et al.[90] Reprinted with permission.)

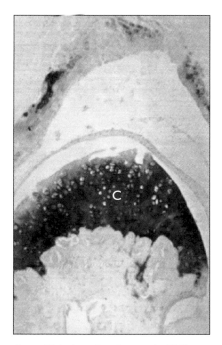

Fig 18-4 Intense staining for sulfated proteoglycans in TMJ cartilage (C) from an 18-month-old mouse following three intra-articular injections of 10 ng/mL of TGF-β plus 25 ng/mL of IGF-1 (0.1% toluidine blue stain; original magnification ×190). (From Sviri et al.[91] Reprinted with permission.)

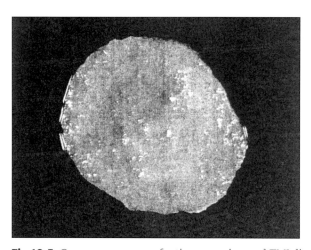

Fig 18-5 Gross appearance of a tissue-engineered TMJ disc analog (12.0 × 10.0 mm). (From Thomas et al.[94] Reprinted with permission.)

Early efforts to repair the TMJ disc include the use of autogenous dermal grafts to resurface or replace damaged discs. This approach met with marginal clinical success; few surgically treated joints returned to long-term unrestricted normal function.[93]

More recently, attempts have been made to develop an in vitro tissue-engineered disc analog.[94] Explants from rabbit TMJ discs were fragmented, and the cells were collected and expanded in culture. The cells were then seeded on a porous collagen scaffold and maintained in a static tissue culture environment for 14 days. A solid, fibrocartilaginous tissue analog resulted (Fig 18-5), with cells that resembled native disc cells. The matrix of the tissue analogs stained positively for the presence of proteoglycans, while control monolayer cell cultures differentiated into fibroblastic cells that did not synthesize proteoglycans.

Using a similar approach, Puelacher et al[95] examined TMJ disc replacements generated in vitro from three-dimensional bioresorbable porous polymer scaffolds seeded with articular cartilage chondrocytes. Following static culture for 1 week to allow cellular attachment, the constructs were implanted subcutaneously for 12 weeks. Histologic analysis showed the resulting tissues to be composed of avascular hyaline-like cartilage. Biomechanical testing of tissue samples in compression indicated that the neocartilage had a compressive stiffness that was similar to that of articular cartilage.

To successfully replicate the TMJ disc, however, tissue engineering studies must be designed with the fundamental characteristics of the specific tissue in mind. Significant differences exist in the cells, composition, and structure of the native TMJ disc and hyaline cartilage. Fibrocartilaginous tissues such as the TMJ disc and the knee meniscus consist primarily of type I collagen organized in a circumferential pattern, whereas hyaline cartilage is primarily composed of type II collagen organized in a layered structure. The cell population in fibrocartilage is mixed, containing fibroblasts as well as chondrocyte-like cells. In addition, fibrocartilage has a lower GAG content, lower compressive modulus, and higher tensile modulus than does healthy adult hyaline cartilage.[16,17,22]

Growth factors may play an important role in accurately regenerating tissues for TMJ disc replacement. Detamore and Athanasiou[22] isolated porcine TMJ disc cells from healthy young adult animals and expanded them in culture. The cells were subsequently seeded onto a three-dimensional porous PGA mesh and cultured in the presence of TGF-β (5 or 30 ng/mL), FGF (10 or 100 ng/mL), or IGF (10 or 100 ng/mL) for 6 weeks. Controls received no growth factor. Constructs were analyzed for cellular proliferation and biosynthesis at 0, 3, and 6 weeks.

In all growth factor groups, newly formed extracellular matrix was deposited uniformly throughout the scaffold, unlike control scaffolds, which exhibited complete degradation in the center. This result may be related to differences in cellular migration in the absence of growth factors. IGF and TGF-β were most effective at promoting collagen synthesis, and all three growth factors increased GAG synthesis. Cell numbers were also greater in all growth factor groups than in the control group. No significant differences in collagen and GAG synthesis or cell number were detected for any of the dose levels studied. The compressive mechanical properties of constructs exposed to growth factors were also improved over those of the untreated controls, although none of the engineered tissues in this short-term study was equivalent to native disc tissue.

Conclusion

Surgical management of TMJ dysfunction by conventional therapies continues to present significant challenges to the dental clinician. New tissue engineering approaches to cartilage and disc repair and regeneration appear to be promising future treatment strategies. An increased understanding of the cellular and mechanical mechanisms of tissue repair is being developed through the use of relevant animal models to approximate the physiology of everyday homeostasis. A key unanswered question is whether engineered cellular implants and tissue constructs possess the ability to successfully integrate with the surrounding native tissues and remain throughout the life of the individual.

Other important research hurdles still to be addressed include:

- Revascularization of the construct, which could be assisted through the use of scaffolds that contain angiogenic signals for neovascularization in areas of tissue function
- Characterization of the cell populations within the TMJ disc with respect to cell phenotype, the proportion and spatial distribution of each cell population, and the temporal response of these cells to relevant growth factors and cytokines
- Identification and validation of better animal models that incorporate joint loads and motions that are more similar to the human TMJ
- Adaptation of existing cartilage repair procedures, such as autologous cell transplantation coupled with various scaffold materials, to the significantly smaller TMJ without compromising the mechanical integrity or clinical efficacy of the repair procedure
- Examination of the role of genetics and genetic mutations as risk factors for TMJ disease, potentially using genetic markers such as human lymphocytic antigens along with clinical and serologic data to identify patients who may be better candidates for surgical treatment of TMD

As tissue engineering approaches to TMJ cartilage and disc repair and regeneration are refined and current shortcomings are addressed, they have the potential to become the new standard of care for the treatment of TMJ dysfunction. In addition, the development of these repair procedures will provide clinical practitioners with a greater scientific understanding of the structure-function relationships within the TMJ. From the patient's perspective, tissue engineering constructs offer the prospect of fully rejuvenating the functional capacity of the TMJ and improving health-related quality of life.

References

1. August M, Glowacki J. Temporomandibular joint syndrome. In: Carlson KJ, Eisenstat SA (eds). Primary Care of Women, ed 2. Philadelphia: Mosby, 2002:66–70.
2. Chase DC, Hudson JW, Gerard DA, et al. The Christensen prosthesis. A retrospective clinical study. Oral Surg Oral Med Oral Pathol Oral Radiol Endod 1995;80:273–278.
3. McNeill C. History and evolution of TMD concepts. Oral Surg Oral Med Oral Pathol Oral Radiol Endod 1997;83:51–60.
4. Christensen D. Joint and muscle dysfunction of the temporomandibular joint. TMJ Science 2003;2(1):5–15.
5. Milam SB, Schmitz JP. Molecular biology of temporomandibular disorders: Proposed mechanisms of disease. J Oral Maxillofac Surg 1995;53:1448–1454.
6. Milam SB. Failed implants and multiple operations. Oral Surg Oral Med Oral Pathol Oral Radiol Endod 1997;83:156–162.
7. Warren MP, Fried JL. Temporomandibular disorders and hormones in women. Cells Tissues Organs 2001;169:187–192.
8. Zuniga JR. Current pain research: The genetics of pain. Oral Maxillofac Clin North Am 2000;12:335–342.
9. Dodson TB. Epidemiology of temporomandibular disorders. In: Bays RA, Quinn PD (eds). Oral and Maxillofacial Surgery, vol 4. Temporomandibular Disorders. Philadelphia: Saunders, 2000:93–107.
10. LeResche L. Epidemiology of temporomandibular disorders: Implications for the investigation of etiologic factors. Crit Rev Oral Biol Med 1997;8:291–305.
11. Halpern LR, Chase DC, Gerard DA, Behr MM, Jacobs W. Temporomandibular disorders: Clinical and laboratory analyses for risk assessment of criteria for surgical therapy, a pilot study. J Craniomandib Pract 1998;16:35–43.
12. Dolwick MF. The role of temporomandibular joint surgery in the treatment of patients with internal derangement. Oral Surg Oral Med Oral Pathol Oral Radiol Endod 1997;83:150–155.
13. Mitchell RJ. Etiology of temporomandibular disorders. Curr Opin Dent 1991;1:471–475.
14. Keith DA. Complications of temporomandibular joint surgery. Oral Maxillofac Clin North Am 2003;15:187–194.
15. Holmlund A, Eckblom A, Hansson P, Lind J, Lundberg T, Theodorsson E. Concentrations of neuropeptides Substance P, neurokinin A, calcitonin gene-related peptide, neuropeptide Y and vasoactive intestinal polypeptide in synovial fluid of the human temporomandibular joint: A correlation with symptoms, signs and arthroscopic findings. Int J Oral Maxillofac Surg 1991;20:228–231.
16. Detamore MS, Athanasiou KA. Motivation, characterization, and strategy for tissue engineering the temporomandibular joint disc. Tissue Eng 2003;9:1065–1087.
17. Almarza AJ, Athanasiou KA. Design characteristics for the tissue engineering of cartilaginous tissues. Ann Biomed Eng 2004;32:2–17.
18. May B, Saha S. Animal models for TMJ studies. A review of the literature. TMJournal 2001;1:20–27.
19. Detamore MS, Hegde JN, Wagle RR, et al. Cell type and distribution in the porcine temporomandibular joint disc. J Oral Maxillofac Surg 2006;64:243–248.
20. Milam SB, Klebe RJ, Triplett RG, Herbert D. Characterization of the extracellular matrix of the primate temporomandibular joint. J Oral Maxillofac Surg 1991;49:381–391.
21. Mills DK, Fiandaca DJ, Scapino RP. Morphologic, microscopic, and immunohistochemical investigations into the function of the primate TMJ disc. J Orofac Pain 1994;8:136–154.
22. Detamore MS, Athanasiou KA. Tensile properties of the porcine temporomandibular joint disc. J Biomech Eng 2003;125:558–565.
23. Annandale T. On displacement of the interarticular cartilage of the lower jaw and its treatment by operation. Lancet 1887;1:411–412.
24. Solberg WK, Hansson TL, Nordstrom B. The temporomandibular joint in young adults at autopsy: A morphological classification and evaluation. J Oral Rehabil 1985;303–321.
25. Wilkes CH. Internal derangements of the temporomandibular joint: Pathological variations. Arch Otolaryngol Head Neck Surg 1989;115:469–477.
26. Isacsson G, Isberg A, Johansson AS, Larson O. Internal derangement of the temporomandibular joint: Radiographic and histologic changes associated with severe pain. J Oral Maxillofac Surg 1986;44:771–778.
27. Westesson PL, Rohlin M. Internal derangement related to osteoarthrosis in temporomandibular joint autopsy specimens. Oral Surg Oral Med Oral Pathol 1984;57:17–22.
28. Hamerman D. The biology of osteoarthritis. New Engl J Med 1989;320:1322–1330.
29. Milam S. Pathophysiology of articular disc displacements of the temporomandibular joint. In: Bays RA, Quinn PD (eds). Oral and Maxillofacial Surgery, vol 4. Temporomandibular Disorders. Philadelphia: Saunders, 2000:46–72.
30. Vilamitjana-Amedee J, Harmand MF. Biochemical analysis of normal and osteoarthritic human cartilage. Clin Physiol Biochem 1990;8:221–230.
31. Milam SB. Cell-Extracellular Matrix Interactions With Special Emphasis on the Primate Temporomandibular Joint [thesis]. San Antonio: University of Texas, 1990.
32. Lotz M, Vaughan JH, Carson DA. Effect of neuropeptides on production of inflammatory cytokines in human monocytes. Science 1988;241:1218–1221.
33. Nehrer S, Spector M, Minas T. Histologic analysis of tissue after failed cartilage repair procedures. Clin Orthop Relat Res 1999;365:149–162.
34. Bouwmeester SJ, Beckers JM, Kuijer R, van der Linden AJ, Bulstra SK. Long-term results of rib perichondral grafts for repair of cartilage defects in the human knee. Int Orthop 1997;21:313–317.
35. Bouwmeester P, Kuijer R, Terwindt-Rouwenhorst E, van der Linden T, Bulstra S. Histological and biochemical evaluation of perichondral transplants in human articular cartilage defects. J Orthop Res 1999;17:843–849.
36. Brittberg M, Lindahl A, Nilsson A, Ohlsson C, Isaksson O, Peterson L. Treatment of deep cartilage defects in the knee with autologous chondrocyte transplantation. New Engl J Med 1994;331:890–904.
37. Brittberg M, Nilsson A, Lindahl A, Ohlsson C, Peterson L. Rabbit articular cartilage defects treated with autologous cultured chondrocytes. Clin Orthop Relat Res 1996;326:270–283.
38. Huntley JS, Bush PG, McBirnie JM, Simpson AH, Hall AC. Chondrocyte death associated with human femoral osteochondral harvest as performed for mosaicplasty. J Bone Joint Surg Am 2005;87:351–360.
39. Fortier LA, Mohammed HO, Lust G, Nixon AJ. Insulin-like growth factor-I enhances cell-based repair of articular cartilage. J Bone Joint Surg Br 2002;84:276–288.
40. Nixon AJ, Fortier LA, Williams J, Mohammed H. Enhanced repair of extensive articular defects by insulin-like growth factor-I-laden fibrin composites. J Orthop Res 1999;17:475–487.
41. Hendrickson DA, Nixon AJ, Grande DA, et al. Chondrocyte-fibrin matrix transplants for resurfacing extensive articular cartilage defects. J Orthop Res 1994;12:485–496.
42. Solchaga LA, Yoo JU, Lundberg M, et al. Hyaluronan-based polymers in the treatment of osteochondral defects. J Orthop Res 2005;18:773–780.
43. Solchaga LA, Dennis JE, Goldberg VM, Caplan AI. Hyaluronic acid-based polymers as cell carriers for tissue-engineered repair of bone and cartilage. J Orthop Res 1999;17:205–213.
44. Marccaci M, Berruto M, Brocchetta D, et al. Articular cartilage engineering with Hyalograft C: 3-year clinical results. Clin Orthop Relat Res 2005;435:96–105.
45. Wakitani S, Goto T, Pineda S, et al. Mesenchymal cell-based repair of large, full thickness defects in articular cartilage. J Bone Joint Surg Am 1994;76A:579–592.
46. Gigante A, Bevilacqua C, Cappella M, Manzotti S, Greco F. Engineered articular cartilage: influence of the scaffold on cell phenotype and proliferation. J Mater Sci Med 2003;14:713–716.
47. Shields KJ, Beckman MJ, Bowlin GL, Wayne JS. Mechanical properties and cellular proliferation of electrospun collagen type II. Tissue Eng 2004;10:1510–1517.

48. Matthews JA, Wnek GE, Simpson DG, Bowlin GL. Electrospinning of collagen nanofibers. Biomacromolecules 2002;3:232–238.

49. Frenkel SA, Di Cesare PE. Scaffolds for articular cartilage repair. Ann Biomed Eng 2004;32:26–34.

50. Frenkel SR, Toolan B, Menche D, Pitman MI, Pachence JM. Chondrocyte transplantation using a collagen bilayer matrix for cartilage repair. J Bone Joint Surg Br 1997;79B:831–836.

51. Kang SW, Jeon O, Kim BS. Poly(lactic-co-glycolic acid) microspheres as an injectable scaffold for cartilage tissue engineering. Tissue Eng 2005;11:438–447.

52. Grande DM, Pitman M, Peterson L, Menche D, Klein M. The repair of experimentally produced defects in rabbit articular cartilage by autologous chondrocyte transplantation. J Orthop Res 1989;7:208–219.

53. Sakaguchi Y, Sekiya I, Yagishita K, Muneta T. Comparison of human stem cells derived from various mesenchymal tissues: superiority of synovium as a cell source. Arthritis Rheum 2005;52:2521–2529.

54. Bosnakovski D, Mizuno M, Kim G, Takagi S, Okumura M, Fujinaga T. Isolation and multilineage differentiation of bovine bone marrow mesenchymal stem cells. Cell Tissue Res 2005;319:243–253.

55. Guilak F, Awad HA, Fermor B, Leddy HA, Gimble JM. Adipose-derived adult stem cells for cartilage tissue engineering. Biorheology 2004;41:389–399.

56. Wickham MQ, Erickson GR, Gimble JM, Vail TP, Guilak F. Multipotent stromal cells derived from the infrapatellar fat pad of the knee. Clin Orthop Relat Res 2003; 412:196–212.

57. Manjubala I, Woesz A, Pilz C, et al. Biomimetic mineral-organic composite scaffolds with controlled internal architecture. J Mater Sci Mater Med 2005;16: 1111–1119.

58. Terada S, Yoshimoto H, Fuchs JR, et al. Hydrogel optimization for cultured elastic chondrocytes seeded onto a polyglycolic acid scaffold. J Biomed Mater Res A 2005;75:907–916.

59. Mukaida T, Urabe K, Naruse K, et al. Influence of three-dimensional culture in a type II collagen sponge on primary cultured and dedifferentiated chondrocytes. J Orthop Sci 2005;10:521–528.

60. Woodfield TB, Van Blitterswijk CA, De Wijn J, Sims TJ, Hollander AP, Riesle J. Polymer scaffolds fabricated with pore-size gradients as a model for studying the zonal organization within tissue-engineered cartilage constructs. Tissue Eng 2005; 11:1297–1311.

61. Seidel JO, Pei M, Gray ML, Langer R, Freed LE, Vunjak-Novakovic G. Long-term culture of tissue engineered cartilage in a perfused chamber with mechanical stimulation. Biorheology 2004;41:445–458.

62. Waldman SD, Spiteri CG, Grynpas MD, Pilliar RM, Hong J, Kandel RA. Effect of biomechanical conditioning on cartilaginous tissue formation in vitro. J Bone Joint Surg Am 2003;85A(suppl 2):101–105.

63. Freyria AM, Yang Y, Chajra H, et al. Optimization of dynamic culture conditions: Effects on biosynthetic activities of chondrocytes grown in collagen sponges. Tissue Eng 2005;11:674–684.

64. Waldman SD, Spiteri CG, Grynpas MD, Pilliar RM, Kandel RA. Long-term intermittent compressive stimulation improves the composition and mechanical properties of tissue-engineered cartilage. Tissue Eng 2004;10:1323–1331.

65. Nagel-Heyer S, Goepfert C, Adamietz P, Meenen NM, Portner R. Cultivation of three-dimensional cartilage carrier constructs under reduced oxygen tension. J Biotechnol 2006;121:486–497.

66. Mizuno S, Glowacki J. Low oxygen tension enhances chondroinduction by demineralized bone matrix in human dermal fibroblasts in vitro. Cells Tissues Organs 2005;180:151–158.

67. Coutts RD, Sah RL, Amiel D. Effects of growth factors on cartilage repair. Instr Course Lect 1997;46:487–494.

68. Hickey DG, Frenkel SR, Di Cesare PE. Clinical applications of growth factors for articular cartilage repair. Am J Orthop 2003;32:70–76.

69. Blunk T, Sieminski AL, Gooch KJ, et al. Differential effects of growth factors on tissue-engineered cartilage. Tissue Eng 2002;8:73–84.

70. Barone-Varelas J, Schnitzer TJ, Meng Q, Otten L, Thonar EJM. Age-related difference in the metabolism of proteoglycans in bovine articular cartilage explants maintained in the presence of insulin-like growth factor 1. Connect Tissue Res 1991;26:101–120.

71. Hunziker EB, Rosenberg LC. Repair of partial-thickness defects in articular cartilage: Cell recruitment from the synovial membrane. J Bone Joint Surg Am 1996; 78:721–733.

72. Spindler KP, Mayes CE, Miller RR, Imro AK, Davidson JM. Regional mitogenic response of the meniscus to platelet-derived growth factor (PDGF-AB). J Orthop Res 1995;13:201–207.

73. Smith RJ, Justen JM, Sam LM, et al. Platelet-derived growth factor potentiates cellular responses of articular chondrocytes to interleukin-1. Arthritis Rheum 1991;34:697–706.

74. Kieswetter K, Schwartz A, Alderete M, Dean DD, Boyan BD. Platelet derived growth factor stimulates chondrocyte proliferation but prevents endochondral maturation. Endocrine 1997;6:257–264.

75. Lohmann CH, Schwartz Z, Niederauer GG, Carnes DL Jr, Dean DD, Boyan BD. Pretreatment with platelet derived growth factor-BB modulates the ability of costochondral resting zone chondrocytes incorporated into PLA/PGA scaffolds to form new cartilage in vivo. Biomaterials 2000;21:49–61.

76. Steadman JR, Rodkey WG, Rodrigo JJ. Microfracture: Surgical technique and rehabilitation to treat chondral defects. Clin Orthop Relat Res 2001;391(suppl): S362–S369.

77. Breinan HA, Martin SD, Hsu HP, Spector M. Healing of canine articular cartilage defects treated with microfracture, a type-II collagen matrix, or cultured autologous chondrocytes. J Orthop Res 2000;18:781–789.

78. Dorotka R, Windberger U, Macfelda K, Bindreiter U, Toma C, Nehrer S. Repair of articular cartilage defects treated by microfracture and a three-dimensional collagen matrix. Biomaterials 2005;26:3617–3629.

79. van den Berg WB, van der Kraan PM, Scharstuhl A, van Beuningen HM. Growth factors and cartilage repair. Clin Orthop Relat Res 2001;391S:S244–S250.

80. Sah RL, Chen AC, Grodzinsky AJ, Trippel SB. Differential effects of bFGF and IGF-I on matrix metabolism in calf and adult bovine cartilage explants. Arch Biochem Biophys 1994;308:137–147.

81. Guven O, Metin M, Keskin A. Remodelling in young sheep: A histological study of experimentally produced defects of the TMJ. Swiss Med Weekly 2003;133: 423–426.

82. Vasara AI, Nieminen MT, Jurvelin JS, Peterson L, Lindahl A, Kiviranta I. Indentation stiffness of repair tissue after autologous chondrocyte transplantation. Clin Orthop Relat Res 2005;433:233–242.

83. Hale JE, Rudert MJ, Brown TD. Indentation assessment of biphasic mechanical property deficits in size-dependent osteochondral defect repair. J Biomech 1993; 26:1319–1325.

84. Weng Y, Cao Y, Silva CA, Vacanti MP, Vacanti CA. Tissue-engineered composites of bone and cartilage for mandible condylar reconstruction. J Oral Maxillofac Surg 2001;59:185–190.

85. Chen F, Mao T, Tao K, Chen S, Ding G, Gu X. Bone graft in the shape of human mandibular condyle reconstruction via seeding marrow-derived osteoblasts into porous coral in a nude mice model. J Oral Maxillofac Surg 2002;60:1155–1159.

86. Abukawa H, Terai H, Hannouche D, Vacanti JP, Kaban LB, Troulis MJ. Formation of a mandibular condyle in vitro by tissue engineering. J Oral Maxillofac Surg 2003;61:94–100.

87. Alhadlaq A, Mao JJ. Tissue-engineered neogenesis of human-shaped mandibular condyle from rat mesenchymal stem cells. J Dent Res 2003;82:951–956.

88. Alhadlaq A, Elisseeff JH, Hong L, et al. Adult stem cell driven genesis of human-shaped articular condyle. Ann Biomed Eng 2004;32:911–923.

89. Alhadlaq A, Mao JJ. Tissue-engineered osteochondral constructs in the shape of an articular condyle. J Bone Joint Surg Am 2005;87:936–944.

90. Suzuki T, Bessho K, Fujimura K, Okubo Y, Segami N, Iizuka T. Regeneration of defects in the articular cartilage in rabbit temporomandibular joints by bone morphogenetic protein-2. Br J Oral Maxillofac Surg 2002;40:201–206.

91. Sviri GE, Blumenfeld I, Livne E. Differential metabolic responses to local administration of TGF-β and IGF-1 in temporomandibular joint cartilage of aged mice. Arch Gerontol Geriatr 2000;31:159–176.

92. Detamore MS, Athanasiou KA. Structure and function of the temporomandibular joint disc: implications for tissue engineering. J Oral Maxillofac Surg 2003;61: 494–506.

93. Meyer RA. The autogenous dermal graft in temporomandibular joint disc surgery. J Oral Maxilliofac Surg 1988;46:948–954.

94. Thomas M, Grande D, Haug RH. Development of an in vitro temporomandibular joint cartilage analog. J Oral Maxillofac Surg 1991;49:854–856.

95. Puelacher WC, Wisser J, Vacanti CA, Ferraro NF, Jaramillo D, Vacanti JP. Temporomandibular joint disc replacement made by tissue-engineered growth of cartilage. J Oral Maxillofac Surg 1994;52:1172–1177.

PART

IV

Orthopedic Indications

19

Application of rhPDGF-BB in Foot and Ankle Fusion Procedures

Tim R. Daniels, MD

Jeffrey O. Hollinger, DDS, PhD

Cross-fertilization of ideas from multiple medical disciplines plays an important role in translating best practices. Much of this book is devoted to the biologic principles and surgical techniques of tissue repair and regeneration in the orofacial region; however, increasing attention is being devoted to tissue engineering in the field of orthopedics, where surgeons are looking to combine tissue-specific scaffolds with growth factors to facilitate faster, more predictable bone healing with less morbidity for patients.

Although craniomaxillofacial bones and bones of the axial and appendicular skeleton differ in their developmental pathways, it is well known that the compositional elements of each (cells, matrix, and signaling molecules) are virtually identical, and each is capable of healing without a scar. The concept of regional anatomic domains (integrating anatomic, embryologic, biomechanical, and physiologic properties in the anatomic areas of the craniofacial, axial, and appendicular skeletons) and the similarities between these domains were discussed extensively in chapter 1. As a consequence of these similarities, bone at various skeletal sites can be expected to respond in a very similar manner to different treatment modalities. The autograft, which has a remarkable history of efficacy across skeletal sites, is a key example of this effect.

Expanding the use of effective treatment modalities across skeletal sites will broaden clinical opportunities throughout musculoskeletal medicine, with a profound beneficial effect on patient care. One new therapeutic modality that has shown great promise in orofacial applications is the use of recombinant growth factors to enhance wound healing and bone regeneration. Recombinant human platelet-derived growth factor BB (rhPDGF-BB) is the first recombinant protein therapeutic cleared for treatment of periodontal defects. Because the elements and properties of bone healing are similar throughout the body, it is likely that the success of this material in orofacial sites will translate to orthopedic indications. This chapter describes an evolving clinical treatment in orthopedics that combines rhPDGF-BB with a tissue-specific matrix to enhance bone regeneration in foot and ankle fusion procedures.

Development of rhPDGF-BB

Although grafting alone has been useful in the treatment of a variety of bone defects, this passive treatment modality dependent on the healing capacity of the individual patient and the inherent osteoconductive properties of the grafting material, has resulted in variable, unpredictable regenerative outcomes. This fact has led clinical researchers to develop new therapies that combine bioactive proteins with conductive matrices to enhance regenerative outcomes.

In 2003, pilot human histologic studies found that rhPDGF-BB in combination with demineralized freeze-dried bone allograft resulted in periodontal regeneration in both class II furcations and interproximal intrabony defects.[1,2] This was the first report of periodontal regeneration demonstrated histologically in human class II furcation defects.

Subsequently, the effectiveness of a purified rhPDGF-BB product (Gem 21S, BioMimetic Therapeutics) was demonstrated by the results of a pivotal clinical trial required for clearance by the US Food and Drug Administration (FDA).[3] Moderate to severe periodontal intrabony defects treated with 0.3 mg/mL of rhPDGF-BB plus β-tricalcium phosphate (β-TCP) had significantly greater gains in clinical attachment level and less gingival recession at 3 months and significantly greater radiographic linear bone growth and percentage bone fill at 6 months than did sites treated with the active control (β-TCP plus buffer).

GEM 21S, combining rhPDGF-BB (0.3 mg/mL) and β-TCP, is now commercially available for the treatment of periodontal defects, including intrabony and furcal periodontal defects and gingival recession associated with periodontal defects. The highly concentrated rhPDGF-BB provided in this product contains approximately 1,000 times greater concentration of rhPDGF-BB than that which is commonly obtained through platelet concentration.[4–7]

Foot and Ankle Fusion

From an evolutionary perspective, the foot is what separates *Homo sapiens* from other species. Its unique design allows enough flexibility to function as a shock absorber yet provides adequate stability to become an effective lever arm during the midportion of the gait cycle. A 150-lb person walking a mile places 62 tons of accumulative force through the feet, yet the surface area of the hindfoot joints is one third that of the hip or knee.[8–10] If the joint complex of the hindfoot or midfoot begins to malfunction, it often is the result of joint arthritis and/or deformity.

When arthritis develops in the knee, hip, shoulder, or elbow, it is often surgically managed by joint replacement. This is an anatomic replication of the joint made of plastic and steel that allows the restoration of pain-free motion. In the foot and ankle, the development of durable joint replacements has been a challenge because of the small surface area of the joints, the excessive forces, and the complex biomechanics involved. Consequently, joint fusion (arthrodesis) has remained the mainstay for management of foot and ankle pain caused by arthritis or deformity.[11–13]

In the United States, an estimated 1 million surgeries are performed annually on the foot and ankle, including fracture fixation, joint fusions, and corrective osteotomies. Many of these procedures incorporate bone grafts to encourage the bone-healing process. Foot and ankle fusion is primarily performed in patients with severe osteoarthritis who do not respond to more conservative treatments. In a fusion procedure, the joint space between adjacent bones is surgically prepared and treated with a graft material to stimulate a fusion, or permanent connection of the two bone ends. This connection eliminates the pain associated with the movement of the joint.

Clinical indications

The two primary indications for fusion of joints in the foot and ankle are arthritis and deformity. Arthritis is a condition in which the cartilage of the joint has eroded and there is bone-on-bone articulation (Fig 19-1). Despite the excessive forces and small surface area, the hindfoot joints are extremely resilient to the detrimental effects of aging; consequently, most arthritis of the hindfoot or midfoot is caused by trauma or inflammatory arthropathies (ie, rheumatoid arthritis and psoriatic arthritis).

The morbidity associated with end-stage arthritis of the hindfoot is substantial. A recent multicentered Canadian study assessing the disability associated with end-stage ankle arthritis in patients who had not yet undergone surgery demonstrated that most of the validated outcomes with regard to physical disability and pain were 2 to 3 SDs below those of healthy control subjects.[13,14]

Fig 19-1a Radiographic appearance of a normal ankle (L) and an ankle with end-stage arthritis (R). The normal joint space appears radiolucent on the radiograph. In the arthritic joint, the joint space is collapsed, with bone-on-bone articulation.

Fig 19-1b Lateral view of the arthritic joint.

Fig 19-1c Lateral view of the normal joint.

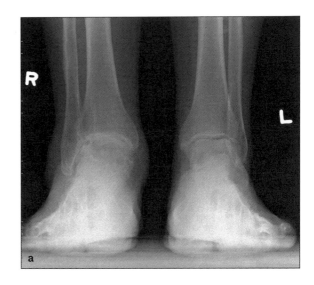

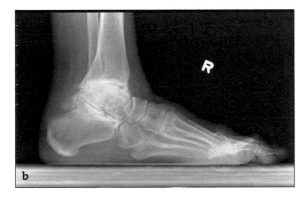

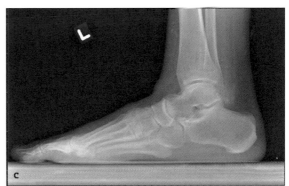

Clinical considerations

Once the patient has decided to proceed with surgical management of foot or ankle arthritis, much of the success and the patient's satisfaction with the outcome is in the hands of the treating surgeon. It is imperative that the surgeon pay particular attention to details such as proper preparation of the joint, adequate positioning of the fusion site, rigid internal fixation with compression, bone grafting to augment fusion, and careful management of the soft tissues. Any significant complication such as infection or nonunion at the fusion site can create a situation whereby the patient would have been better served without surgical management.

Complications

The most common complications following fusion of foot and ankle joints are malpositioning and nonunion at the fusion site.[15,16] Nonunion occurs when bone growth is delayed or halted at the fusion site. Several factors can increase the risk of nonunion: smoking; noncompliance by the patient (eg, weight bearing before the healing process is properly advanced); medical comorbidities such as diabetes; medications; poor surgical technique; and inadequate blood supply to the extremity. Some of these factors are beyond the control of the treating surgeon; in these cases, the patient can only be advised that the risk of nonunion is greater than average.

The primary determinants of fusion that are within the surgeon's control are correct surgical technique and interventions at the time of surgery that help to augment bony healing (union). Therefore, many surgeons choose to use autografts at the fusion site to decrease the risk of nonunion and in some cases accelerate healing.

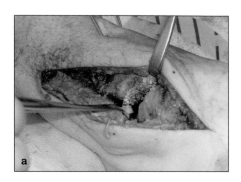

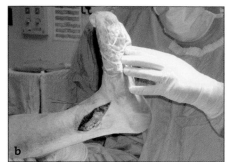

Fig 19-2a Foot and ankle fusion treatment with rhPDGF-BB–enhanced β-TCP. After the opposing surfaces of the joints are prepared, and immediately prior to rigid fixation, the PDGF-enhanced graft is placed in the fusion site. The joint space should not be overpacked. This method allows for maximum new bone ingrowth, leading to successful fusion of the joint.

Fig 19-2b The talus has been positioned on the tibia and held temporarily with two K-wires from the anterior aspect of the tibia into the talus. Foot position is being assessed prior to screw insertion.

Bone grafting

Historically, autogenous bone has been the type of bone most commonly used to graft a fracture or fusion site in orthopedic indications. The autogenous bone graft offers several key benefits, including freedom from disease transmission from donor to recipient, the absence of immunologic disparities and consequences, and, in general, desirable biomechanical properties.

However, the autogenous bone graft has a number of disadvantages. These liabilities include limitations in the amount, configuration, and quality of donor bone. In addition, depending on graft volume, type of graft format (ie, cortical or cancellous), and location, resorption and replacement with host bone may take months or years to occur, especially with block cortical bone grafts.[17,18]

Serious concerns related to autografting also include increased pain and time in the hospital. It is not uncommon for patients to report that the pain associated with harvesting of an iliac bone graft is greater than the pain they are experiencing in the surgically treated foot or ankle. Management of the pain increases the length of time the patient stays in the hospital and further delays rehabilitation. For example, learning how to walk with crutches can be delayed for several days because the patient is in too much pain to get out of bed or cannot tolerate walking with crutches because of the pain at the donor site. In addition, scarring following harvesting of iliac crest or proximal tibia bone grafts can be an esthetic concern.

Nerve damage and/or hypersensitive wounds from peripheral sensory nerve damage may lead to hyperesthesia, numbness, or dysthesia at the donor site. When an iliac crest bone graft is obtained, the lateral femoral cutaneous nerve is at particular risk of injury. Damage to this nerve can cause chronic pain and a large area of decreased sensation on the anterolateral aspect of the patient's thigh. When a proximal tibial graft is obtained, sensory branches of the saphenous and lateral sural cutaneous nerve are at risk of injury.

After autografting, recovery is subject to donor site morbidity, including significant and prolonged pain in more than 30% of cases, decreases in biomechanics leading to fracture, additional operative time, and blood loss and possible infection at the donor site.[19] Infection can lead to catastrophic outcomes, including septic shock and early renal failure. As a consequence of the well-known deficiencies of the autograft in general and in foot and ankle fusions more specifically (nonunions), there is a compelling requirement for an alternative to improve clinical outcome and diminish the problematic postoperative sequelae.

rhPDGF-BB grafting: An alternative to autograft

rhPDGF has been cleared by the FDA for dermal wound-healing procedures and represents, along with recombinant human bone morphogenetic protein 2 (rhBMP-2), one of the two recombinant protein therapeutics that have been approved for bone regenerative treatments. In animals, rhPDGF-BB has been shown to accelerate fracture repair and increase bone density.[20–22] Moreover, rhPDGF-BB has been successful in regenerating both hard and soft tissues in periodontal defects[1,2,23] and has received FDA clearance for use in the treatment of intrabony and furcation periodontal defects and recession defects associated with periodontal bone loss.[3] Because of the regenerative results demonstrated in a variety of sites in preclinical and clinical studies, rhPDGF-BB is a logical alternative to autogenous and allogeneic bone in arthrodesis of joints in the foot and ankle.

Clinical trial

Recently, a Canadian multicenter pivotal clinical trial was initiated to evaluate the safety and effectiveness of rhPDGF- BB in a β-TCP delivery system as a bone regeneration device in foot and ankle fusions.[24]

The primary inclusion criteria for the clinical study were male and female patients older than 18 years who required a hindfoot fusion procedure using a bone graft. Patient populations were stratified to ensure adequate sample sizes in representative fusion applications according to the statistical analysis plan.

Briefly, the surgical protocol provided for the interposition of the 0.3 mg/mL rhPDGF-BB particulate matrix to the site of fusion at the time of rigid fixation. The opposing surfaces of the joints were prepared in standard fashion. They were coapted and fused with compression screws to ensure rigid compressive fixation. Approximately 3 to 9 mL of graft material was inserted in the fusion site, depending on the surface area. In an effort to maintain space for new bone ingrowth, the fusion site was not overpacked with the growth factor–enhanced matrix preparation (Fig 19-2). Following final fixation of the deformity, additional graft material was placed around the fusion site to maximize exposure of the site to the graft material, thereby facilitating osseointegration across the fusion space. Careful closure of the joint capsule and surrounding subcutaneous tissue helped to contain the graft material within the fusion space.

The foot was immobilized in a below-knee cast for 1 to 2 weeks; after this time, the sutures were removed and a short leg cast was applied. The below-knee cast was changed as necessary for proper fit and integrity. Patients were instructed not to bear weight on the foot for the first 6 weeks postoperatively. Physical therapy was then initiated. At 12 weeks, the cast was replaced with a walking shoe. Follow-up included the completion of foot and ankle outcome scores, radiographic assessment, and a computerized tomographic (CT) scan to assess fusion 6 and 12 weeks following surgery.

Sixty patients from three separate centers in Canada underwent hindfoot fusion procedures using rhPDGF/

Box 19-1 Results of rhPDGF-BB/β-TCP treatment for foot and ankle arthrodesis

Patient demographics

Mean patient age (y)	53.4
Obese patients (BMI ≥ 30)	38%
Smokers/patients with a history of smoking	60%
Patients with previous failed fusion at affected site	33%

Device-related adverse events	0

*Fusion assessed by CT (osseous bridging > 50%)**

Week 6	42%
Week 12	70%

Fusion rates reported with autogenous bone graft[25]

Week 6	23%
Week 12	48%

*Data based on 56 patients.

β-TCP. The procedures were separated into ankle, subtalar, and triple fusions. The studies were performed in academic tertiary care centers and consisted of a high-risk population in which well over half of the patients presented with at least one of the following risk factors: *(1)* obesity [body mass index ≥ 30], *(2)* previous failed fusion surgery at the affected site, or *(3)* a history of smoking. In the patient population, 60% reported a positive smoking history, 38% were obese, and 33% had a failed fusion procedure (Box 19-1).

The patients have been followed from 12 to 24 weeks; to date none have experienced an adverse event caused by the product. None of the patients developed heterotopic bone formation at the fusion site or excessive callus formation, and all of the calcium phosphate particles in the soft tissues resorbed or were resorbing. Interim (6- and 12-week) results are shown in Box 19-1. Fusion, as assessed on CT scans, occurred in 42% of patients at 6 weeks and 70% of patients by 12 weeks. The data from this study for the growth factor–enhanced matrix appeared at least comparable with recently published data in studies using autogenous bone graft, which showed 23% mean fusion at 6 weeks and 48% mean fusion at 12 weeks.[25] Current orthopedic literature suggests overall rates of nonunions of up to 41% in smokers, diabetic patients, obese individuals, and patients undergoing revision

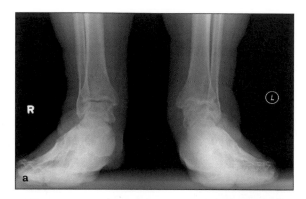

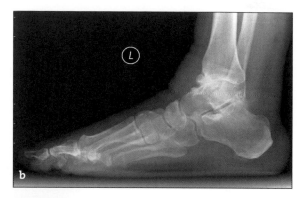

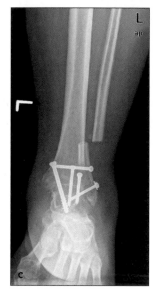

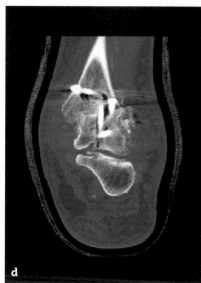

Fig 19-3a Pretreatment radiograph in which the left ankle exhibits arthritis with valgus deformity.

Fig 19-3b Lateral pretreatment view of the arthritic ankle.

Fig 19-3c Radiograph taken 6 weeks after ankle fusion using rhPDGF-BB–enhanced β-TCP. The appearance of the treated site suggests early bony union.

Fig 19-3d CT scan performed 6 weeks posttreatment. The image reveals bony cross-trabeculation, confirming bone union.

surgeries.[26,27] For the total group, the results were comparable with those achieved with autogenous bone grafting; when subtalar and ankle fusions were isolated, however, the outcomes were better than those of fusion procedures using autogenous grafting.[28]

Case 1

A 57-year-old man presented with left ankle pain and deformity. He had a history of numerous ankle sprains since he was 20 years of age. Over the past several years, he had been experiencing increasing pain. His walking and standing capacity was approximately 15 minutes. Ten years previously he had been diagnosed as having non–insulin-dependent diabetes. His blood glucose levels were being controlled with diet and oral hypoglycemics.

On examination, his peripheral pulses were palpable. On the left side, he had a slight valgus deformity with increased swelling. The range of motion of the left ankle was restricted, and there was bony crepitus at the extremes of dorsiflexion and plantar flexion. Radiographs revealed end-stage left ankle arthritis with valgus deformity (Figs 19-3a and 19-3b).

The patient underwent a left ankle fusion. The ankle fusion was performed via a medial and lateral incision, combined with a fibular osteotomy. A percutaneous tendo-achilles lengthening was performed. The ankle was positioned in neutral dorsiflexion and then stabilized with three 4.5-mm cannulated screws using the three-column technique. GEM OS1 (6 mL) was inserted in the fusion site prior to positioning and stabilization with the cannulated screws. Postoperatively the patient wore a below-knee, non–weight-bearing fiberglass cast for 6 weeks.

Radiographs at 6 weeks suggested early bony union despite the diabetes (Fig 19-3c). Bony cross-trabeculation was confirmed by a CT scan 6 weeks postoperatively (Fig 19-3d).

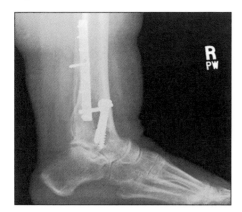

Fig 19-4a Radiograph taken at initial presentation of the patient. Hardware from a previous ankle fracture and fusion can be seen. The radiograph reveals mild arthritis of the subtalar joint and more significant arthritis of the talonavicular joint.

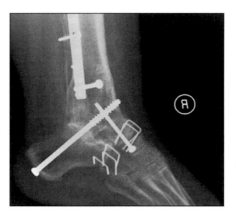

Fig 19-4b Radiograph taken 6 weeks following foot and ankle fusion treatment using rhPDGF-BB–enhanced β-TCP. The appearance suggests early bony union.

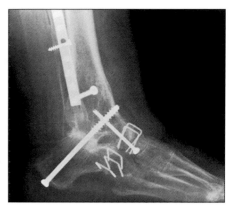

Fig 19-4c Radiograph taken 12 weeks posttreatment.

Case 2

A 63-year-old overweight woman presented with severe, chronic pain in the right foot and ankle. A previous foot and ankle fusion procedure performed on the right side had failed, resulting in persistent, chronic pain. The patient required the assistance of a walker for mobility. Her medical history was significant for morbid obesity and previous fracture of the right ankle.

Radiographs revealed hardware from her previous ankle fracture and ankle fusion. Mild arthritis of the subtalar joint was present, and there was more significant arthritis of the talonavicular joint (Fig 19-4a).

The patient underwent treatment to remove existing hardware and receive a triple fusion procedure (talonavicular, calcaneocuboid, and subtalar joints) using rhPDGF-BB and β-TCP. Postoperatively, the patient was placed in a below-knee, non– weight-bearing fiberglass cast for 6 weeks.

Radiographs at 6 weeks suggested early bony union (Fig 19-4b). By 12 weeks postoperatively, complete bone fusion across the fusion site was observed (Fig 19-4c), and the patient was free of pain and able to ambulate without the aid of a walker. Bony cross-trabeculation was confirmed by CT scans 6 and 12 weeks postoperatively.

Case 3

A 65-year-old woman presented with persistent, increasing pain in the left foot and ankle. The medical history revealed that a previous fracture at this site, 30 years earlier, had healed with a delayed union. Subsequently, an open reduction procedure was performed at the fracture site. Increasing pain had persisted at the treatment site for 2 years.

The clinical examination revealed anterior translation of the hindfoot, restricted ankle motion, and pain with activity at the ankle. Radiographs showed anterior angulation of the tibia and fibula, end-stage ankle arthritis, and maximum joint space loss in the anterior half of the ankle joint (Fig 19-5a).

The patient was managed surgically with a fibular osteotomy, posterior translation of the talus on the tibia, insertion of 6 mL of GEM-OS1, and fusion of the ankle joint with cannulated screws. The 6- and 12-week postoperative radiographs revealed bony union at the fusion site (Figs 19-5b and 19-5c).

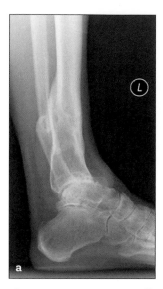
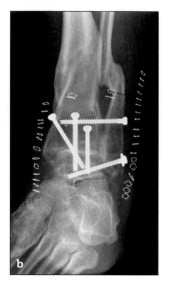
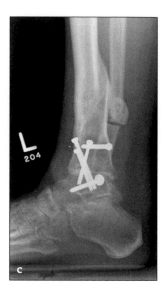

Fig 19-5a Pretreatment radiograph of a patient with evidence of anterior angulation of the tibia and fibula, end-stage ankle arthritis, and maximum joint space loss in the anterior half of the ankle joint.

Fig 19-5b Radiograph taken 6 weeks posttreatment. The pathologic conditions have been managed surgically with a fibular osteotomy, posterior translation of the talus on the tibia, and rigid fixation incorporating rhPDGF-BB. The radiograph reveals bony union at the fusion site.

Fig 19-5c Radiograph taken 12 weeks postoperatively.

Conclusion

Intramembranous and endochondral bone will heal without scar formation and will regenerate. Regardless of the developmental or healing pathway, bone has the universal capacity to regenerate. Moreover, the compositional elements (cells, matrix, and signaling molecules) of all bones are virtually identical. As a consequence of these similarities, bone at various skeletal sites may be expected to respond in a very similar manner to different treatment modalities. Extrapolation of the results of effective treatment modalities across skeletal sites has led to expanded clinical opportunities throughout areas of musculoskeletal medicine, with a profound beneficial effect on patient care.

A highly successful periodontal regenerative therapy, implantation of rhPDGF-BB in combination with an appropriate tissue matrix, was showcased in a compelling clinical study of foot and ankle arthrodesis. The outcomes achieved with rhPDGF-BB in foot and ankle arthrodesis were clinically equivalent to those achieved with the standard of care, the autograft, even in compromised patients who were recognized as being at risk for poor bone healing. These results confirm that the anatomic location of a bone site does not limit therapeutic opportunities.

References

1. Camelo M, Nevins ML, Schenk RK, Lynch SE, Nevins M. Periodontal regeneration in human Class II furcations using purified recombinant human platelet-derived growth factor-BB (rhPDGF-BB) with bone allograft. Int J Periodontics Restorative Dent 2003;23:213–225.

2. Nevins M, Camelo M, Nevins ML, Schenk RK, Lynch SE. Periodontal regeneration in humans using recombinant human platelet-derived growth factor-BB (rhPDGF-BB) and allogenic bone. J Periodontol 2003;74:1282–1292.

3. Nevins M, Giannobile WV, McGuire MH, et al. Platelet-derived growth factor stimulates bone fill and rate of attachment level gain: Results of a large multicenter randomized controlled trial. J Periodontol 2005;76:2205–2215.

4. Bowen-Pope DF, Malpass TW, Foster DM, Ross R. Platet-derived growth factor in vivo: Levels, activity, and rate of clearance. Blood 1984:64:458–469.

5. Huang JS, Huang SS, Deuel TF. Human platelet-derived growth factor. Radioimmunoassay and discovery of a specific plasma-binding protein. J Cell Biol 1983; 97:383–388.

6. Singh JP, Chalkin MA, Stiles CD. Phylogenetic analysis of platelet-derived growth factor by radio-receptor assay. J Cell Biol 1982;95:667–671.

7. Harvest Technologies Corporation. SmartPrep 2. Available at: http://www.harvesttech.com/education/prp-brochures.html. Accessed 17 Oct 2007.

8. Kimizuka M, Kurosawa H, Fukubayashi T. Load bearing pattern of the ankle joint: Contact area and pressure distribution. Arch Orthop Trauma Surg 1980;96:45–49.

9. Brown TD, Shaw DT. In vitro contact stress distributions in the natural human hip. J Biomech 1983;16:373–384.

10. Ihn JC, Kim SJ, Park IH. In vitro study of contact area and pressure distribution in the human knee after partial and total meniscectomy. Int Orthop 1993;17(4): 214–218.

11. Greisberg J, Hansen S, DiGiovanni C. Alignment and technique in total ankle arthroplasty. Oper Tech Orthop 2004;14:21–30.

12. Greisberg J, Assal M, Hansen S. Takedown of ankle fusion and conversion to total ankle arthroplasty. Clin Orthop Relat Res 2004;434:80–88.

13. Coester L, Saltzman C, Leupold J, Pontarelli W. Long-term results following ankle arthrodesis for post-traumatic arthritis. J Bone Joint Surg Am 2001;83:219–227.

14. Thomas R, Daniels TR, Parker K. Gait analysis and functional outcomes following ankle arthrodesis for isolated ankle arthritis. J Bone Joint Surg Am 2006;88: 526–535.

15. Chao W, Mizel MS. What's new in foot and ankle surgery? J Bone Joint Surg Am 2006;88:909–922.

16. Abidi N, Gruen G, Conti S. Ankle arthrodesis: Indications and techniques. Am Acad Orthop Surg 2000;8:200–209.

17. Goldberg VM, Akhavan S. Biology of bone grafts. In: Lieberman J, Friedlaender G (eds). Bone Regeneration and Repair: Biology and Clinical Applications. Totawa, NJ: Humana Press, 2005:57–65.

18. Hollinger JO. Bone dynamics: Morphogenesis, growth modeling, and remodeling. In: Lieberman J, Friedlaender G (eds). Bone Regeneration and Repair: Biology and Clinical Applications. Totawa, NJ: Humana Press, 2005:1–20.

19. Younger EM, Chapman MW. Morbidity of bone graft donor sites. J Orthop Trauma 1989;3:192–195.

20. Howes R, Bowness J, Grotendorst G, Martin G, Reddi A. Platet-derived growth factor enhances demineralized bone matrix-induced cartilage and bone formation. Calcif Tissue Int 1988;42:34–38.

21. Nash TJ, Howlett CR, Martin C, Steele J, Johnson KA, Hicklin DJ. Effect of platelet-derived growth factor on tibial osteotomies in rabbits. Bone 1994;15:203–208.

22. Mitlak B, Finkelman R, Hill EL, et al. The effect of systemically administered PDGF-BB on the rodent skeleton. J Bone Miner Res 1996;11:238–247.

23 Lynch SE, Williams RC, Polson AM, et al. A combination of platelet-derived growth factor enhances periodontal regeneration. J Clin Periodontol 1989;16: 545–548.

24. Daniels TR. rhPDGF-BB: A novel tissue engineering system for the future? Presented at the 47th Annual Denver Orthopaedic Society Meeting, Toronto, 4 Nov 2006.

25. Coughlin MJ, Grimes JS, Traughber PD, Jones CP. Comparison of radiographs and CT scans in the prospective evaluation of the fusion of hindfoot arthrodesis. Foot Ankle Int 2006;27:780–787.

26. Easley ME, Trnka HJ, Schon LC, Myerson MS. Isolated subtalar arthrodesis. J Bone Joint Surg Am 2000;82:613–624.

27. Frey C, Halikus N, Vu-Rose T, Ebramzadeh E. A review of ankle arthrodesis: Predisposing factors to nonunion. Foot Ankle Int 1994;15:581–514.

28. Valderrabano V, Pagenstert G, Horisberger M, Knupp M, Hintermann B. Sports and recreation activity of ankle arthritis patients before and after total ankle replacement. Am J Sports Med 2006;34:993–999.

The Role of Growth Factors in Tendon Healing

Joshua C. Nickols, PhD
Joshua Dines, MD

Injured tendons heal through an elaborate process involving recruitment of cells, regeneration of connective tissue, and reassembly of the tendon macrostructure. Growth factors and cytokines are of primary importance, driving cell division, inducing secretion of proteoglycans, glycosaminoglycans, and collagen and further synthesis of growth factors.

Among the growth factors expressed by injured tissues is platelet-derived growth factor (PDGF). PDGF is a soluble protein homodimer composed of the ligands PDGF-A, PDGF-B, PDGF-C, PDGF-D, or the heterodimer PDGF-AB. The molecule binds to PDGF receptor α and PDGF receptor β, which can elicit a variety of responses, notably healing in the musculoskeletal system.

Interruption of the healing events, such as that arising from infection or keloid formation, predisposes the tendon to reinjury. In addition, certain patient characteristics, such as age and smoking habits, influence the degree of tendon healing. The purpose of this chapter is to describe the natural role of PDGF in tendon healing and to examine the use of the recombinant form to improve tendon healing in patients who might otherwise experience compromised outcomes.

Anatomy of the Tendon

The tendon is a complex organization of connective fibers, cells, and extracellular matrix. The primary constituent of the tendon is type I collagen, but there are smaller quantities of other collagen isoforms, such as types III and X. The remaining structural components of the tendon are proteoglycans, glycosaminoglycans, and structural glycoproteins that support the organization of the tendon and hold water. Water imparts resilience and elasticity to the tissue. Specialized, elongated fibroblasts called *tenocytes* also reside within the tendon and secrete structural components of the tendon.

A hierarchy of fascicles and subfascicles organizes the tendon into discrete units, the smallest of which is the fibril. Interwoven collagen fibrils are clustered to form fibers. These fibers are then organized into primary, secondary, and tertiary fiber bundles. Each of these bundles is invested with and held together by a network of connective tissue called the *endotenon*. Within the endotenon are blood vessels, lymphatics, and nerves that supply the tendon. Finally, several of the tertiary fiber bundles are

Fig 20-1 Macrostructure of the tendon. (Modified from Kannus.[1] Reprinted with permission.)

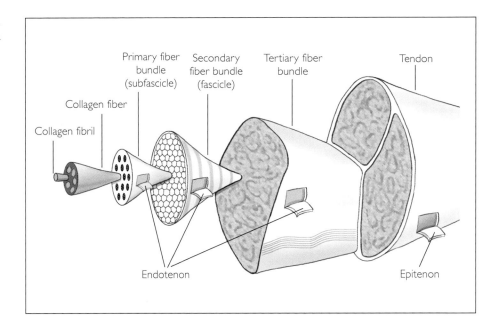

Fig 20-2 Tissue types of the tendon insertion. Tendon (T), fibrocartilage (FC), and bone (B) compose the enthesis (immunohistochemical labeling for type II collagen; bar = 100 µm). (From Benjamin.[2] Reprinted with permission.)

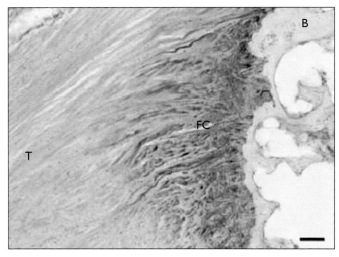

clustered into the tendon proper and wrapped by the *epitenon*[1] (Fig 20-1).

Forces generated by the muscle are transferred through the myotendinous junction to the tendon proper. The tendon is protected from friction by sheaths and synovial membranes that contain a thick synovial fluid. These membranes, especially in the hands and feet, become pulleys and points of attachment to bone. These forces are transmitted to bone by the terminal attachment of the distal tendon, called the *enthesis*. At the enthesis, the tendon transitions to fibrocartilage, first unmineralized, and then mineralized fibers called *Sharpey fibers*, which penetrate periosteum and cortical bone and anchor in lamellar bone[2] (Fig 20-2).

Healing of the Tendon

Normal healing

Tendon healing can be generalized to comprise four phases: clot formation, inflammation, proliferation, and regeneration. At avulsion or rupture, blood vessels in the tendon tear, releasing blood, platelets, and clotting factors. Macrophage, neutrophils, and leukocytes then rapidly invade the clot, secreting growth factors and cytokines and leading to inflammation. By 4 days, the tendon parenchyma is punctuated by neutrophils and ED1+ macrophage[3]

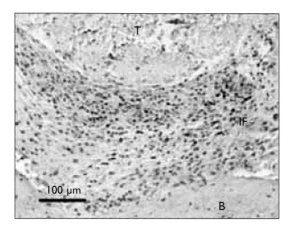

Fig 20-3a Four days postinjury, the tendon (T) to bone (B) junction (IF) is punctuated by polymorphonuclear neutrophil leukocytes.

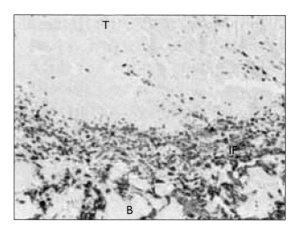

Fig 20-3b Four days postinjury, the tendon (T) to bone (B) junction (IF) also contains ED1+ macrophages (immunohistochemical staining for ED1+ macrophage; original magnification ×80). (Figs 20-3a and 20-3b from Kawamura et al.[3] Reprinted with permission.)

(Fig 20-3). Neighboring tissue also contributes to the release of growth factors, marking the onset of neovascularization and replacement of the fibrin clot by granulation tissue.

Gradually, the normal short, crimped collagen bundles within tendon are replaced with long, crimped, and disorganized strands of collagen and extracellular matrix molecules. Later in the process, growth factors promote the removal of tissue debris, chemotaxis, and proliferation of mesenchymal stem cells and fibroblasts. Eventually specialized fibroblasts establish a network of collagens, proteoglycans, glycoproteins, and hyaluronic acid. As the tendon matures, the cellularity of the tissue decreases, and a network of highly cross-linked collagen replaces scar tissue. The repair, however, is never histologically or biomechanically normal, and the result is a weaker tendon or ligament prone to tearing.

Compromised healing

Many factors can have a negative effect on the healing process. Among the common causes of incomplete healing are infection, keloid formation, bleeding, and blood clots. Age is also a significant factor in the outcome of injury of the supraspinatus tendon of the shoulder. A multivariate analysis of shoulder function demonstrated that these tendons heal only 43% of the time in patients older than 65 years.[4]

Other tendons, irrespective of the patient's age, have a weak intrinsic ability to heal. The Achilles tendon has a poor blood supply along its length and few blood vessels in its cross-sectional area. Subclinical injuries of the tendon set the stage for ischemia, degenerative changes, and incomplete scarring.[5]

Repair technique is also a major determinant of success or reinjury. Supraspinatus tendons under tension or secured to bone by a single point fail more frequently. These findings have influenced sports surgeons to reduce forces placed on the tendon and to employ techniques aimed to better approximate tendon to bone.[6,7]

In addition to intrinsic and technical properties that compromise the healing of tendons following injury, many pharmacologic causes of tendon repair failure have been reported. In rats, the antimicrobial agent doxycycline decreases the biomechanical force to failure in the Achilles tendon. Doxycycline inhibits the activity of matrix metalloproteases believed necessary to remodeling damaged tendons.[8]

Corticosteroid injections, a common treatment for tendon injuries, may actually initiate prolonged degenerative changes in the tendon. Treatment of tenosynovitis with triamcinolone caused a delayed rupture of the flexor digitorum superficialis and profundus tendons, possibly by slowing cellular proliferation and migration in the tendon.[9,10]

Fig 20-4a Expression of VEGF 10 days after laceration of the canine flexor tendon (immunohistochemical staining for VEGF; original magnification ×200). *(circle)* Blood vessel.

Fig 20-4b Expression of PDGF-BB 10 days after laceration of the canine flexor tendon. Expression of PDGF-BB and VEGF overlaps at this time point (immunohistochemical staining for PDGF-BB; original magnification ×400).

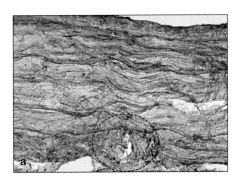
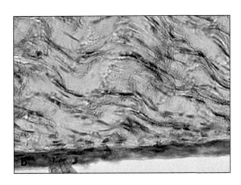

Fig 20-4c Control for VEGF immunostaining in Fig 20-4a (no stain; original magnification ×100).

Fig 20-4d Control for PDGF-BB immunostaining in Fig 20-4b (no stain; original magnification ×400). (Figs 20-4a to 20-4d from Tsubone et al.[13] Reprinted with permission.)

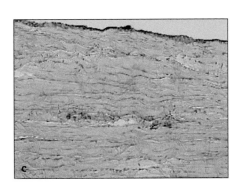
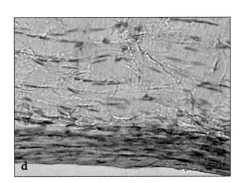

Of greater consequence to the broader population may be the effect that smoking has on tendon healing. A recent study demonstrated that the chronic administration of nicotine to an animal model of rotator cuff repair reduced collagen production, cellular proliferation, and tendon mechanical force.[11]

Postinjury Growth Factor Expression

Shortly after the onset of an inflammatory reaction in the tendon, injured tissues express PDGF, insulin-like growth factor 1 (IGF-1), basic fibroblast growth factor (bFGF), and transforming growth factor β (TGF-β). The rise of these factors is partly responsible for the early influx of inflammatory cells that generate other cytokines and clear tissue debris.

In a rabbit model of supraspinatus injury, the expression of IGF-1 and TGF-β begins almost immediately, followed by the appearance of bFGF at 3 days, and synthesis of PDGF by 7 days. Immunostaining of the tissue neighboring the full thickness transection reveals PDGF expression localized to cells of the tendon midsubstance and blood vessels.[12] In a similar study of acute flexor tendon injury and repair, robust staining for PDGF-AA and PDGF-BB is detected adjacent to the repair site by 10 days.[13] In both studies, vascular endothelial growth factor (VEGF), a potent angiogenic factor, overlapped PDGF expression in the endotenon and epitenon (Fig 20-4).

Expression of these two factors may be causal and not coincidental. In cardiac or vascular smooth muscle, the injection of PDGF promotes an upregulation of VEGF and growth of blood vessels in ischemic tissue.[14] Antagonists of PDGF show an ability to stall the formation and maturation of blood vessels in ischemic cardiac tissue.[15]

Within the field of tendon repair, much attention has been directed to the induction of mitogenesis, chemotaxis, and matrix in cells of the tendon by PDGF-BB. In particular, PDGF exerts chemotactic and proliferative effects on tenocytes, fibroblasts, and multipotent mesenchymal stem cells (MSCs). MSCs that migrate to the tendon injury become a source of future myoblasts, chondrocytes, fibroblasts, and other cell types. A recent study by Chong and colleagues[16] reported that injection of a fibrin glue and MSC solution in the Achilles tendon transection increased the modulus or tendon stiffness at 3 weeks. Furthermore, MSCs serve as a rich source of bioactive factors that in the context of the microenvironment stimulate regeneration, turnover, and hematopoiesis.[17]

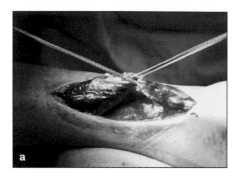

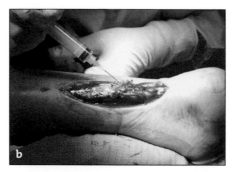

Fig 20-5a In the treatment group, which is to receive PRP, ruptured Achilles tendons are first reattached with suture.

Fig 20-5b The tendons are injected with an unclotted platelet-rich solution.

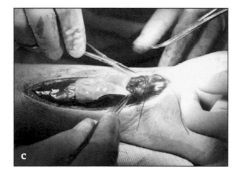

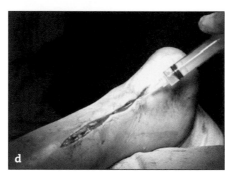

Fig 20-5c The wound is covered with a PRP/fibrin matrix.

Fig 20-5d Before closure, the wound is infiltrated with additional unclotted PRP.

Application of Growth Factors to Injured Tendons

Achilles tendon

Achilles tendon rupture often occurs traumatically during athletics with a sudden pop and pain, and many athletes report feeling as though they were kicked in the back of the leg. The most frequent site of the rupture is within the tendon midsubstance, but avulsions from the tendon's calcaneal insertion are common as well. Midsubstance tears are treated by resuturing the proximal and distal ends of the ruptured tendon and protecting the surrounding sheath. Tendon avulsions are repaired with bone anchors used to reinsert the Achilles tendon in the calcaneus. Physicians may also elect to cast the leg, but nonsurgical treatment tends to have a higher rate of rerupture.[18]

An approved recombinant human PDGF-BB (rhPDGF-BB) treatment for tendon injury does not yet exist; however, two products based on rhPDGF-BB are currently marketed. Regranex (becaplermin, Ethicon) and GEM 21S (BioMimetic Therapeutics) are cleared by the US Food and Drug Administration for the treatment of deep neuropathic diabetic foot ulcers and periodontally related bone defects, respectively.

As a surrogate to rhPDGF-BB, several orthopedic clinical and preclinical studies have used a concentrated blood fraction, platelet-rich plasma (PRP). In a study by Sanchez and colleagues,[19] PRP was applied to the repair of Achilles tendon ruptures in a small number of athletes. During surgery, the tendons of six patients were repaired using standard techniques plus a platelet-rich fibrin matrix overlay and subcutaneous injection of PRP adjacent to the tendon (Fig 20-5). Another six matched patients treated with the standard of care served as controls. Postoperatively, all patients were treated according to a standard clinical protocol, and the treated leg was immobilized with a cast for 2 or 3 weeks; this was followed by physical rehabilitation.

Over time, each patient was evaluated for functional outcomes, including a full range of ankle motion, capacity for gentle running, and resumption of athletic training. Patients who received PRP demonstrated a statistically faster improvement in all three outcome measures by at least 3 weeks[19] (Fig 20-6).

The finding that PRP provides a detectable healing difference as long as 14 weeks after surgical repair is a bit of a paradox, given the short half-life of both growth factors and the fibrin matrix. It appears that physical rehabilitation in conjunction with growth factor injection is fundamental to the healing of tendons. In one study, the injection of botulinum toxin A into the calf muscle after repair of the

Fig 20-6 The functional outcomes of motion, running, and training occurred earlier in patients who underwent Achilles tendon repair with a preparation rich in growth factors (PRGF) than in control patients who received treatment consistent with the standard of care. *P < .05. (From Sanchez et al.[19] Reprinted with permission.)

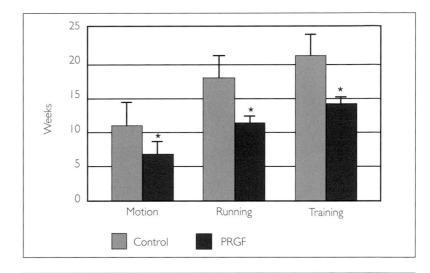

Fig 20-7 Achilles tendon fibroblasts respond to PDGF-BB by increased secretion of VEGF under hypoxic (5% O$_2$) and normoxic (20% O$_2$) conditions. (From Petersen et al.[24] Reprinted with permission.)

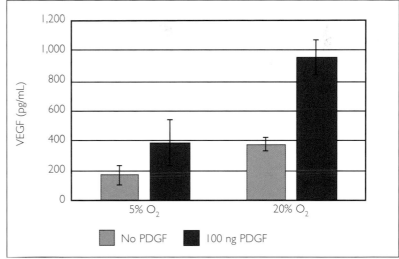

transected Achilles tendon in a rat eliminated the benefit of PRP injection.[20,21] Thus it appears that the addition of PDGF creates an initial pro-healing environment that is extended by movement of the tendon well after the added growth factor is cleared.

The trauma of an Achilles tendon tear destroys both collagen fibers and the supporting vasculature. The blood-deprived tissue thus becomes ischemic and potentially necrotic. Under ideal conditions, this environment stimulates angiogenesis; however, failures in the synthesis of new vessels are common and often cited as the cause of rerupture.[22] Principally responsible for new blood vessel formation is VEGF, a soluble, glyscosylated homodimer. When deprived of oxygen, healthy tissue and cells secrete hypoxia-inducible factor, which in turn stimulates release of VEGF. Free VEGF, bound to its cognate receptors (VEGF receptor 1 and receptor 2), results in the proliferation of vascular smooth muscles and sprouting and maturation of blood vessels.

The injection of VEGF into the rat Achilles tendon following transection and repair yields higher tensile strength of the healing tendon at early time points (1 and 2 weeks) than does control treatment.[23] Under the hypoxic conditions of tendon rupture (5% oxygen), Achilles tenocytes jumpstart angiogenesis by expressing twofold greater amounts of VEGF than they do under normoxic (20% oxygen) conditions. This endogenous response to ischemia was found to increase in vitro after the application of PDGF. Treatment of cultured tendon fibroblasts with 100 ng/mL of PDGF raised VEGF secretion to five times that of normoxic conditions.[24] In conjunction with the ability of PDGF to induce proliferation of smooth muscle cells, this effect on VEGF expression creates a rich environment for new vessel sprouting in the tendon and potentially more rapid tendon healing[24–26] (Fig 20-7).

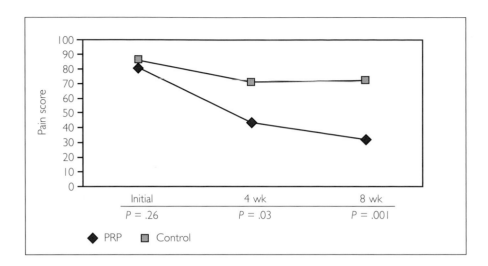

Fig 20-8 A single injection of PRP resulted in a statistically significant improvement in visual analog pain scores 4 and 8 weeks posttreatment (From Mishra and Pavelko.[32] Reprinted with permission.)

Patellar tendon

Patellar tendinitis ("jumper's knee") is a condition brought on by repetitive overloading of the patellar tendon during sports such as tennis, football, baseball, and volleyball. Although the patellar tendon can withstand large forces of 12 to 15 times body weight, repetitive strain causes microtearing of fibers. Early tendinitis is treated conservatively with rest, ice, compression, and elevation. Without adequate time to heal, these weak points predispose the tendon to rupture, particularly with the high linear stresses generated during sports.

In response to tendon damage, epitendinous cells proliferate and form a callus of collagen around the injury. Remodeling of the scar is carried out by two sources of tenocytes: those that multiply within the endotenon and bundles and those that invade the callus and lay down new collagen fibrils.[27] The result is hypercellularity, observed in biopsy specimens from patients with subclinical patellar tendinitis. These patients show a nearly fivefold greater immunoreactivity for the mitosis marker, proliferating cell nuclear antigen, than normal. This response, in part, is grounded in PDGF signaling.

Within the same tissues, approximately three times more tenocytes express the PDGF-BB receptor (PDGF receptor β).[28] Upregulation of the receptor amplifies the proliferative response of patellar tenocytes in the proximity of the injury. As has been reported, treatment of sheep patellar tendon explants with 50 ng/mL of PDGF-AB induces a fourfold rise in new DNA synthesis and results in a larger pool of cells to regenerate the tendon.[29] Also, studies of mouse embryonic fibroblasts demonstrated that a gradient of PDGF stimulates migration to the source of the growth factor.[30]

The intracellular messengers that cause PDGF signaling to instruct proliferation versus chemotaxis are not entirely understood. However, elevated intracellular calcium appears to cause motility, whereas mitogen-activated protein kinase signaling appears to induce DNA synthesis.[31] Although these in vitro findings require in vivo validation, the observations imply that PDGF may arrest or reverse tendinitis in the patellar tendon. PRP has been used successfully to treat patients with another type of tendinitis, tennis elbow. Following a single injection of PRP, significant decreases in pain were measured with a visual analog pain scale[32] (Fig 20-8).

Anterior cruciate ligament

The patellar tendon serves the additional purpose of providing bone-tendon-bone grafts to reconstruct the anterior cruciate ligament (ACL). The harvest of these tissues involves removing a central third band of patellar tendon and a small block of bone at its attachments to the patella and tibia. As a consequence of the harvest, the tendon is weakened, and, although rare, there are reports of patellar tendon rupture at the harvest site.[33]

Fig 20-9 Tendinous ACL grafts are affixed with PDGF-coated sutures. (From Weiler et al.[35] Reprinted with permission.)

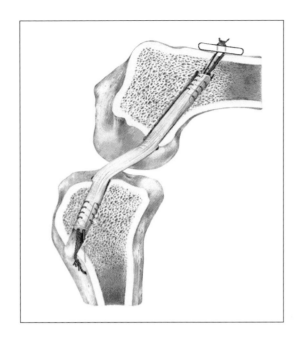

A more frequent problem is the failure of the patellar tendon that serves as an ACL graft. Approximately 8% of ACL procedures require revision because of graft elongation, failure of fixation, or intrinsic failure.[34]

PDGF applied to the living graft at implantation may improve the long-term outcome of ACL reconstruction. Weiler and colleagues[35] tested this hypothesis on tendinous ACL grafts by affixing the tendon with PDGF-coated sutures. The study employed a sheep model of ACL reconstruction, and the intact knees were evaluated at 3, 6, and 12 weeks by biomechanical tests and histologic analysis. Strikingly, at 6 weeks, an ACL failure load of 193 ± 24 N was recorded in the group repaired with PDGF-BB–coated sutures compared with a load of 136 ± 48 N for suture-only controls. Histologically, at 6 weeks, significant increases in both vascular density and collagen fibril content were found within the PDGF treatment group[35] (Fig 20-9).

Rotator cuff tendon

The rotator cuff is a composite of capsule, ligaments, and four tendons (Fig 20-10). The three most posterior tendons, which include the supraspinatus, infraspinatus, and teres minor, interdigitate to form a common insertion on the greater tuberosity of the proximal humerus. They are major contributors to shoulder abduction and external rotation strength. The subscapularis is located anteriorly and functions as an internal rotator.

The rotator cuff serves as a dynamic stabilizer of the glenohumeral joint. Injury to the rotator cuff is one of the most common reasons that patients seek the care of orthopedic surgeons.

Rotator cuff pathosis is actually a continuum ranging from edema and tendinitis to partial-thickness tears to full-thickness tears.[36] Controversy surrounds the pathogenesis of these developments. Intrinsic mechanisms, such as vascular and degenerative processes, combine with extrinsic factors, such as tensile overload, strain from abnormal mechanics, and impingement, to cause the symptoms of rotator cuff disease. Impingement syndrome, originally described by Neer,[36] identified the coracoacromial arch as the main cause of rotator cuff disease. He postulated that a decrease in subacromial space as a result of spurs or osteophytes causes impingement of the rotator cuff between the humeral head and the coracoacromial arch.

Animal studies using rat models have supported the role overuse plays in rotator cuff pathosis.[37] The authors compared rats placed on a running regimen versus rats limited to normal cage activity. Tendons in rats included in the exercise group demonstrated increased cellularity and loss of normal collagen fiber organization. Maximum stress and tissue modulus were significantly decreased at all time points studied.

Given the multitude of causes of rotator cuff pathosis, it is not surprising that these tears are very prevalent within the general population. Magnetic resonance imaging (MRI) studies have shown that, among asymptomatic patients, 30% of people older than 40 years will have a tear, and up to 80% of people older than 60 years will have one.[38]

Recently, Yamaguchi et al[39] performed bilateral ultrasounds on 588 patients with unilateral shoulder pain to diagnose the presence and size of possible rotator cuff tears. They found that, by the age of 66 years, patients presenting with unilateral shoulder pain have a 50% likelihood of having bilateral tears. They also concluded that tear size correlates with pain, because painful tears were, on average, 5.4 mm larger than nonpainful tears.

Patients with rotator cuff disease usually complain of pain and weakness, especially when their shoulders are in a position of abduction, flexion, or external rotation. Pain is often localized to the lateral aspect of the shoulder. Night pain is highly suggestive of rotator cuff pathology. Tears usually occur in patients older than 40 years. On examination, weakness in forward flexion, abduction, or external rotation is suggestive of a rotator cuff tear, although it is not always specific for a particular muscle. So-called impingement signs, such as Neer impingement sign, Hawkins sign, and Neer impingement test results, are usually positive as well.

MRI has become the gold standard for radiographic evaluation of the rotator cuff (Fig 20-11), although ultrasound is being used more frequently. Initial studies showed that both modalities have excellent specificity for full-thickness tears; however, MRI was much more sensitive.[40] A more recent study by Teefey et al[41] suggested that MRI and ultrasound have comparable accuracy for identifying rotator cuff tears.

Once diagnosed, pathologic conditions of the rotator cuff can be treated in a variety of ways. Tendinitis and partial-thickness rotator cuff tears often respond well to nonoperative measures, such as anti-inflammatory medications, physical therapy, and rest. Unfortunately, established full-thickness tears lack the ability to heal spontaneously and usually require surgical repair.

Less than 10 years ago, almost all repairs were done through large incisions that violated the deltoid musculature. Although outcomes were successful in terms of patient satisfaction, the split in the deltoid muscle caused increased postoperative pain and delayed postoperative rehabilitation. To avoid these consequences, surgeons transitioned first to mini-open repairs and eventually to all-arthroscopic repairs. At this point, the clinical results of

open, mini-open, and all arthroscopic repairs are comparable.[42] However, despite almost uniformly successful clinical outcomes in patients treated surgically, often the repair does not actually heal.

Multiple studies have documented the healing rate after rotator cuff repair to range from 20% to 90%.[43–45] This is important because function and strength are statistically significantly improved in those patients in whom the cuff actually heals.[1,46] Initial work on improving the healing rate of repairs focused on enhancing the instruments used for the surgeries. Sutures used in the repairs now have very high tensile strengths. Suture anchors have excellent pullout strengths. In addition, tendon-grasping techniques, using special graspers, have become very reliable.

More recently, as the understanding of the anatomic footprint of the rotator cuff has expanded, surgeons have attempted to improve healing by performing more anatomic repairs. When arthroscopic repairs were initially performed, the torn tendon edge was reapproximated back to its insertion on the greater tuberosity via the use of suture anchors placed in a single row. The medial-lateral dimensions of the rotator cuff footprint were not adequately restored with a simple single row of anchors.[47]

Kim et al[48] published the results of a biomechanical study that looked at the effects of adding a second row of suture anchors to better re-create the normal anatomy of the tendinous insertion. They found that a double row of suture anchors increased the initial strength of the repair and, more importantly, the surface area for healing. A recent clinical follow-up of double-row repairs showed that, after an isolated lateral row repair, 52% of the footprint remained uncovered. With the addition of a medial row of anchors, there were no residual deficits in coverage of the footprint.[49]

With the advances in surgical techniques described, the biomechanical environment for repairs has been nearly optimized. However, healing is still not at 100%. For this reason, surgeons and scientists are now looking for ways to augment the biologic process of healing of the tendon back to its bony insertion.

PDGF-BB, with its documented role in the tendon-healing process throughout the body, has been studied as a possible enhancer of rotator cuff tendon repairs. Kobayashi et al[12] determined the expression of various growth factors during the healing of acute rotator cuff tears in rabbits. PDGF was expressed between days 7 and 14 of healing, confirming its presence during the repair process.

Dines et al[50] performed some of the first studies using PDGF-BB to enhance the repair of rotator cuff tendon

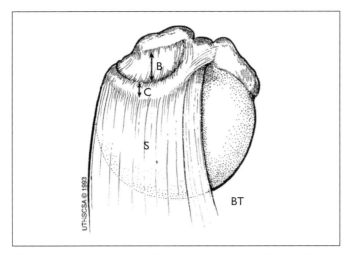

Fig 20-10a Superior view of the supraspinatus (S) covering the humeral head. (B) Intertubercular groove; (C) supraspinatus insertion; (BT) biceps tendon.

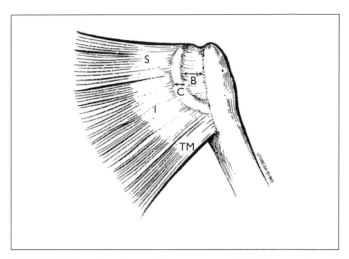

Fig 20-10b Posterior view of the rotator cuff. (S) Supraspinatus; (I) infraspinatus; (TM) teres minor; (B) intertubercular groove; (C) supraspinatus insertion.

Fig 20-11 T2-weighted MRI showing a tear in the supraspinatus tendon.

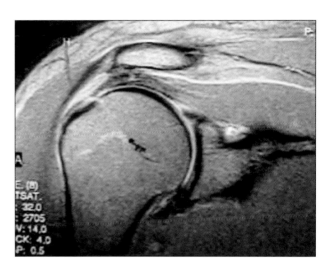

healing in a rat model. Rat tendon fibroblasts (RTF) were isolated and initiated in culture by explant outgrowth. Once RTFs were serially cultured and expanded, they were transduced with genes for PDGF-BB by a retroviral vector. Cells containing the active gene were selected by incorporation of a neomycin resistance gene added to the construct. Northern blot analysis and enzyme-linked immunosorbent assay confirmed gene expression.

To test whether PDGF-BB gene–transfected RTF cells would modulate the metabolism of surrounding tissue, the RTF cells were seeded on a bioabsorbable polymer scaffold and cultured. The two constructs were then assembled in apposition (two-layered construct) in culture. Tested configurations included single-construct

(RTF/0, control 1), nontransduced RTF (RTF/RTF, control 2), and RTF + PDGF-BB/RTF (experimental). Constructs were incubated and then pulse labeled with tritiated proline to assess collagen synthesis.

Enzyme-linked immunosorbent assay and Northern blot confirmed gene expression. RTF cells rapidly attached to polymer scaffolds and formed highly cellular tissue constructs within the polyglycolic acid scaffolds by 5 days after seeding. RTF constructs incubated alone exhibited a baseline level of collagen synthesis (control 1). This activity was increased 1.5 fold by placement of a similar construct in apposition (control 2). There was up to a 10-fold increase in collagen synthesis in native RTF when apposed to constructs containing PDGF-BB at both the 48- and

72-hour time points. In this study, Dines et al[50] demonstrated that tendon fibroblasts could be tissue engineered to deliver therapeutic peptides to the local environment to stimulate a repair response.

In a subsequent part of the study,[50] the same procedure was performed to transduce the RTFs with the genes for PDGF-BB by retroviral vectors. After selection and expansion, they were seeded on a polymer scaffold and further cultured.

The supraspinatus tendons of rats were surgically transected and allowed to undergo an inflammatory phase of healing for 2 weeks (mimicking the clinical setting of a chronic rotator cuff tear). A second surgery was then performed to repair the original tear. Repair involved standard suture realignment (control group) or suture repair with the addition of a gene-modified tendon tissue construct (experimental group). Experimental repair utilized a tendon cell construct on a polyglycolic acid scaffold incorporated with the gene for promoting repair (PDGF-BB).

Repaired tissue was harvested 12 weeks postrepair and analyzed histologically. Rotator cuffs treated with standard suture repair exhibited results ranging from poor or no restoration to incomplete restoration of tendon architecture, whereas the repairs in the experimental group resulted in nearly complete or full restoration of the torn tendon architecture. Histologic analysis demonstrated restoration of the normal crimp patterning and collagen bundle alignment in the experimental group.

This was one of the first studies documenting the efficacy of PDGF-BB to augment tendon repair in a rat model of rotator cuff injury.[51] Currently, studies are underway to examine the effects of PDGF-BB on the biomechanical characteristics of tendon repair in larger animal models.

As the aging population remains more active, and the understanding of the natural history of rotator cuff repairs improves, more rotator cuff repairs will likely be performed. Despite very good clinical results from these repairs, structurally these repairs are of questionable integrity. Over the past few years, by using improved surgical techniques, surgeons have given repaired tendons a better chance to heal. This has resulted in better structural repair, but the healing rate is still less than 90%. The next innovation to improve healing rates will be the use of growth factors with documented roles in the healing process. PDGF-BB will likely be at the forefront of these efforts, especially in light of preliminary studies showing its beneficial effects in the rotator cuff–healing process.

Flexor tendons of the hand

The flexor digitorum superficialis (FDS) and flexor digitorum profundus (FDP) are connected to the muscles in the forearm and run along the palm and into the fingers. The FDP inserts on the distal phalanx of the finger and the FDS inserts on the middle phalanx. When pulled simultaneously, the tendons bend the fingers and allow the hand to grasp.

The FDS and FDP tendons are fairly exposed and vulnerable to injury. Athletic and work injuries that cause avulsions from the tendon insertion are quite common. These injuries can result from twisting, overstretching, or blows to the hand. Fingers caught and pulled during sports have acquired the name *jersey finger*. Injuries to the tendon also occur as lacerations from sharp objects. Knife cuts, power equipment accidents, and broken glass cause transections of either or both tendons.

Repair of the tendon within a few weeks of the injury is critical to prevent muscle and tendon retraction. Furthermore, to preserve flexion, hand surgeons assiduously avoid causing excessive scarring around the tendon. Each tendon in the hand travels through a system of pulleys lined by a synovium and bathed by synovial fluid. This system guides forces along the tendon to its insertion, and any scarring that occurs along the tendon length may prevent smooth tendon gliding through the pulleys. Twenty or more suturing techniques have been developed to minimize scarring and provide the strongest repair possible to transected tendons. Ruptures of the tendon from its attachment site are reconnected to their attachment site with small anchors, screws, or plates.

There is a growing appreciation for the role played by PDGF-BB and other growth factors during healing of the flexor tendon. Expression of PDGF-BB has been observed 10 days following the laceration of canine flexor tendon; a pronounced upregulation of PDGF occurs in the endotenon, composed of both dense collagen bundles and supporting tenocytes. Also, the epitenon and sheath bordering the cut tendon appear thickened. The hyperplasia represents an early point of regeneration, and, in part, may reflect chemotactic and proliferative cues provided by PDGF to tendon fibroblasts.[13]

This hypothesis has been tested in vivo with cultures of both rat and rabbit primary tenocytes grown with PDGF-BB in concentrations ranging from 1 to 50 ng/mL. Cells from both species exhibited increases in DNA synthesis, collagen production, and integrin receptor expression beginning at concentrations of 10 ng/mL.[52–55] Similar

Fig 20-12 Stimulation of avian fibroblasts with both PDGF-BB and mechanical load results in a synergistic upregulation of DNA synthesis. Cultured avian fibroblasts subjected to stretching on flexible plastic culture dishes respond with an increase in proliferation. (DPM) Disintegrations per minute; (S) serum stimulation as a positive control. (From Banes et al.[61] Reprinted with permission.)

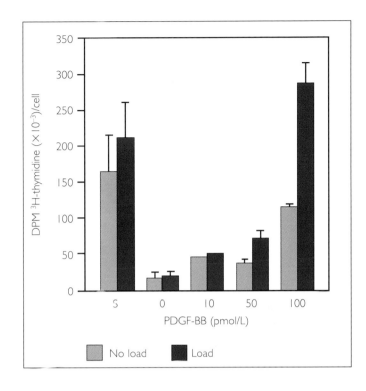

studies likewise found that the growth factors IGF-1 and bFGF potentiated cellular proliferation, matrix production, and angiogenesis.[22,56,57] Explant cultures treated with PRP elevate the expression of type I collagen, type III collagen, the proteoglycan decorin, and cartilage oligomeric matrix protein.[58] In vivo, IGF-1, bFGF, and PDGF likely work in concert to instruct the production of specific structural proteins and cell types in a time-appropriate sequence.

A few weeks after the flexor tendon has been physically reattached, the injured finger is treated with a regimen of passive movement exercises. The therapy reduces adhesion formation and assists with strengthening the tendon. An anabolic response to mechanical loading appears to lie behind the improvement in the tendon strength. Loading of the tendon upregulates collagen and IGF-1 transcripts and induces expression of VEGF and its receptor.[59,60]

Tendon motion also elevates the responsiveness of tenocytes to endogenous and applied growth factor sources. When avian flexor tendon fibroblasts were treated with both PDGF-BB and mechanical stretching, an enhanced and synergistic response in cell division was observed compared with mechanical loading alone[61] (Fig 20-12).

Discussion

Evolving technologies have substantially improved the outcomes of tendon surgical repair. For the rotator cuff, double-row versus single-row fixations produce higher initial pullout forces.[4,62] Another technique, transosseous bridging, provides more evenly distributed contact of the tendon with the tuberosity.[63] While these techniques optimize the physical reattachment and provide a favorable situation for healing, they contribute passively. Future advancements in tendon surgery are likely to come through the incorporation of active biologic agents, particularly growth factors such as PDGF-BB, in fixation devices.

At present, the most accessible source of growth factors is PRP. Yields of PDGF from concentrated PRP are usually in the range of 80 to 100 ng/mL, but a sufficient concentration for some tendons and local environments may be microgram-sized quantities.[58,64]

Indeed, several methods of growth factor delivery to the tendon have already been described. Rohrich and collaborators[65] described a method to attach growth factors with an amide linkage to a Mersilene suture (Ethicon).

When placed through rat Achilles tendon and cultured, surrounding fibroblasts proliferated in response to PDGF. Other investigators have explored the use of various injectable matrices, including polymerized fibrin, photo-polymerizable hydrogels, heparin hydrogels, and chitosan hydrogels to deliver growth factors.[19,66–68] In the selection of an appropriate carrier matrix, two criteria—rate of growth factor release and compatibility of the matrix with the tissue environment—are paramount.

Conclusion

Advances in tendon surgery and injury treatment are likely to come as a result of merging optimized surgical techniques and cytokines and growth factors. Among the growth factors known and available, PDGF occupies a prominent but not exclusive role.

Ongoing efforts to delineate the specific roles and effects of growth factors such as IGF-1, VEGF, TGF-β, and bFGF will in time provide a holistic picture of the interactions between growth factors and the biology of healing. With these new data, better devices will be designed to complement timing, degree, and specific growth factor expression that will allow surgeons to offer compromised patients therapies that mimic healthy tendon healing.

References

1. Kannus P. Structure of the tendon connective tissue. Scand J Med Sci Sports 2006;10:312–320.
2. Benjamin M, Toumi H, Ralphs JR, Bydder G, Best TM, Milz S. Where tendons and ligaments meet bone: Attachment sites ('entheses') in relation to exercise and/or mechanical load. J Anat 2006;208:471–490.
3. Kawamura S, Ying L, Kim HJ, Dynybil C, Rodeo SA. Macrophages accumulate in the early phase of tendon-bone healing. J Orthop Res 2005;23:1425–1432.
4. Boileau P, Brassart N, Watkinson DJ, Carles M, Hatzidakis AM, Krishnan SG. Arthroscopic repair of full-thickness tears of the supraspinatus: Does the tendon really heal? J Bone Joint Surg Am 2005;87:1229–1240.
5. Ahmed IM, Lagopoulos M, McConnell P, Soames RW, Sefton GK. Blood supply of the Achilles tendon. J Orthop Res 1998;16:591–596.
6. Gimbel JA, Van Kleunen JP, Lake SP, Williams GR, Soslowsky LJ. The role of repair tension on tendon to bone healing in an animal model of chronic rotator cuff tears. J Biomech 2007;40:561–568.
7. Meier SW, Meier JD. The effect of double-row fixation on initial repair strength in rotator cuff repair: A biomechanical study. Arthroscopy 2006;22:1168–1173.
8. Pasternak B, Fellenius M, Aspenberg P. Doxycycline impairs tendon repair in rats. Acta Orthop Belg 2006;72:756–760.
9. Fitzgerald BT, Hofmeister EP, Fan RA, Thompson MA. Delayed flexor digitorum superficialis and profundus ruptures in a trigger finger after a steroid injection: A case report. J Hand Surg [Am] 2005;30:479–482.
10. Scutt N, Rolf CG, Scutt A. Glucocorticoids inhibit tenocyte proliferation and tendon progenitor cell recruitment. J Orthop Res 2006;24:173–182.
11. Galatz LM, Silva MJ, Rothermich SY, Zaegel MA, Havliogu N, Thomopoulos S. Nicotine delays tendon-to-bone healing in a rat shoulder model. J Bone Joint Surg Am 2006;88:2027–2034.
12. Kobayashi M, Itoi E, Minagawa H, et al. Expression of growth factors in the early phase of supraspinatus tendon healing in rabbits. J Shoulder Elbow Surg 2006; 15:371–377.
13. Tsubone T, Moran SL, Amadio PC, Zhao C, An KN. Expression of growth factors in canine flexor tendon after laceration in vivo. Ann Plast Surg 2004;53: 393–397.
14. Affleck DG, Bull DA, Bailey SH, et al. PDGF(BB) increases myocardial production of VEGF: Shift in VEGF mRNA splice variants after direct injection of bFGF, PDGF(BB), and PDGF(AB). J Surg Res 2002;107:203–209.
15. Zymek P, Bujak M, Chatila K, et al. The role of platelet-derived growth factor signaling in healing myocardial infarcts. J Am Coll Cardiol 2006;48:2315–2323.
16. Chong AK, Ang AD, Goh JC, et al. Bone marrow-derived mesenchymal stem cells influence early tendon-healing in a rabbit achilles tendon model. J Bone Joint Surg Am 2007;89:74–81.
17. Caplan AI, Dennis JE. Mesenchymal stem cells as trophic mediators. J Cell Biochem 2006;98:1076–1084.
18. Lynch RM. Achilles tendon rupture: surgical versus non-surgical treatment. Accid Emerg Nurs 2004;12:149–158.
19. Sanchez M, Anitua E, Azofra J, Andia I, Padilla S, Mujika I. Comparison of surgically repaired achilles tendon tears using platelet-rich fibrin matrices. Am J Sports Med 2007;35:245–251.
20. Aspenberg P, Virchenko O. Platelet concentrate injection improves Achilles tendon repair in rats. Acta Orthop Scand 2004;75:93–99.
21. Virchenko O, Aspenberg P. How can one platelet injection after tendon injury lead to a stronger tendon after 4 weeks? Interplay between early regeneration and mechanical stimulation. Acta Orthop Scand 2006;77:806–812.
22. Bidder M, Towler DA, Gelberman RH, Boyer MI. Expression of mRNA for vascular endothelial growth factor at the repair site of healing canine flexor tendon. J Orthop Res 2000;18:247–252.
23. Zhang F, Liu H, Stile F, et al. Effect of vascular endothelial growth factor on rat Achilles tendon healing. Plast Reconstr Surg 2003;112:1613–1619.
24. Petersen W, Pufe T, Zantop T, Tillmann B, Mentlein R. Hypoxia and PDGF have a synergistic effect that increases the expression of the angiogenetic peptide vascular endothelial growth factor in Achilles tendon fibroblasts. Arch Orthop Trauma Surg 2003;123:485–488.
25. Gerich TG, Fu FH, Robbins PD, Evans CH. Prospects for gene therapy in sports medicine. Knee Surg Sports Traumatol Arthrosc 1996;4:180–187.
26. Millette E, Rauch BH, Kenagy RD, Daum G, Clowes AW. Platelet-derived growth factor-BB transactivates the fibroblast growth factor receptor to induce proliferation in human smooth muscle cells. Trends Cardiovasc Med 2006;16:25–28.
27. Mosier SM, Pomeroy G, Manoli A Jr. Pathoanatomy and etiology of posterior tibial tendon dysfunction. Clin Orthop Relat Res 1999;(365):12–22.
28. Rolf CG, Fu BS, Pau A, Wang W, Chan B. Increased cell proliferation and associated expression of PDGFRβ causing hypercellularity in patellar tendinosis. Rheumatology (Oxford) 2001;40:256–261.
29. Spindler KP, Imro AK, Mayes CE, Davidson JM. Patellar tendon and anterior cruciate ligament have different mitogenic responses to platelet-derived growth factor and transforming growth factor β. J Orthop Res 1996;14:542–546.
30. Vidali L, Chen F, Cicchetti G, Ohta Y, Kwiatkowski DJ. Rac1-null mouse embryonic fibroblasts are motile and respond to platelet-derived growth factor. Mol Biol Cell 2006;17:2377–2390.
31. Bornfeldt KE, Raines EW, Graves LM, Skinner MP, Krebs EG, Ross R. Platelet-derived growth factor. Distinct signal transduction pathways associated with migration versus proliferation. Ann N Y Acad Sci 1995;766:416–430.
32. Mishra A, Pavelko T. Treatment of chronic elbow tendinosis with buffered platelet-rich plasma. Am J Sports Med 2006;34:1774–1778.
33. Marumoto JM, Mitsunaga MM, Richardson AB, Medoff RJ, Mayfield GW. Late patellar tendon ruptures after removal of the central third for anterior cruciate ligament reconstruction. A report of two cases. Am J Sports Med 1996;24: 698–701.
34. Wolf RS, Lemak LJ. Revision anterior cruciate ligament reconstruction surgery. J South Orthop Assoc 2002;11:25–32.

35. Weiler A, Forster C, Hunt P, et al. The influence of locally applied platelet-derived growth factor-BB on free tendon graft remodeling after anterior cruciate ligament reconstruction. Am J Sports Med 2004;32:881–891.

36. Neer CS Jr. Anterior acromioplasty for the chronic impingement syndrome in the shoulder: A preliminary report. J Bone Joint Surg Am 1972;54:41–50.

37. Soslowsky LJ, Thomopoulos S, Tun S, et al. Neer Award 1999. Overuse activity injures the supraspinatus tendon in an animal model: A histologic and biomechanical study. J Shoulder Elbow Surg 2000;9:79–84.

38. Sher JS, Uribe JW, Posada A, Murphy BJ, Zlatkin MB. Abnormal findings on magnetic resonance images of asymptomatic shoulders. J Bone Joint Surg Am 1995;77:10–15.

39. Yamaguchi K, Ditsios K, Middleton WD, Hildebolt CF, Galatz LM, Teefey SA. The demographic and morphological features of rotator cuff disease. A comparison of asymptomatic and symptomatic shoulders. J Bone Joint Surg Am 2006;88:1699–1704.

40. Martin-Hervas C, Romero J, Navas-Acien A, Reboiras JJ, Munuera L. Ultrasonographic and magnetic resonance images of rotator cuff lesions compared with arthroscopy or open surgery findings. J Shoulder Elbow Surg 2001;10:410–415.

41. Teefey SA, Rubin DA, Hildebolt CF, Leibold RA, Yamaguchi K. Detection and quantification of rotator cuff tears. Comparison of ultrasonographic, magnetic resonance imaging, and arthroscopic findings in seventy-one consecutive cases. J Bone Joint Surg Am 2004;86A:708–716.

42. Bishop J, Klepps S, Lo IK, Bird J, Gladstone JN, Flatow EL. Cuff integrity after arthroscopic versus open rotator cuff repair: A prospective study. J Shoulder Elbow Surg 2006;15:290–299.

43. Galatz LM, Ball CM, Teefey SA, Middleton WD, Yamaguchi K. The outcome and repair integrity of completely arthroscopically repaired large and massive rotator cuff tears. J Bone Joint Surg Am 2004;86A:219–224.

44. Gartsman GM, Brinker MR, Khan M. Early effectiveness of arthroscopic repair for full-thickness tears of the rotator cuff: An outcome analysis. J Bone Joint Surg Am 1998;80:33–40.

45. Gerber C, Fuchs B, Hodler J. The results of repair of massive tears of the rotator cuff. J Bone Joint Surg Am 2000;82:505–515.

46. Harryman DT Jr, Mack LA, Wang Ky, Jackins SE, Richardson ML, Matsen FA III. Repairs of the rotator cuff. Correlation of functional results with integrity of the cuff. J Bone Joint Surg Am 1991;73:982–999.

47. Lo IK, Burkhart SS. Double-row arthroscopic rotator cuff repair: Re-establishing the footprint of the rotator cuff. Arthroscopy 2003;19:1035–1042.

48. Kim KC, Rhee KJ, Shin HD, Kim YM. Arthroscopic hybrid double-row rotator cuff repair. Knee Surg Sports Traumatol Arthrosc 2007;15:794–799.

49. Brady PC, Arrigoni P, Burkhart SS. Evaluation of residual rotator cuff defects after in vivo single- versus double-row rotator cuff repairs. Arthroscopy 2006;22:1070–1075.

50. Dines JS, Grande DA, Dines DM. Tissue engineering and rotator cuff tendon healing. J Shoulder Elbow Surg 2007;16(5 suppl):S204–S207.

51. Uggen JC, Dines J, Uggen CW, et al. Tendon gene therapy modulates the local repair environment in the shoulder. J Am Osteopath Assoc 2005;105:20–21.

52. Costa MA, Wu C, Pham BV, Chong AK, Pham HM, Chang J. Tissue engineering of flexor tendons: Optimization of tenocyte proliferation using growth factor supplementation. Tissue Eng 2006;12:1937–1943.

53. Thomopoulos S, Harwood FL, Silva MJ, Amiel D, Gelberman RH. Effect of several growth factors on canine flexor tendon fibroblast proliferation and collagen synthesis in vitro. J Hand Surg [Am] 2005;30:441–447.

54. Yoshikawa Y, Abrahamsson SO. Dose-related cellular effects of platelet-derived growth factor-BB differ in various types of rabbit tendons in vitro. Acta Orthop Scand 2001;72:287–292.

55. Harwood FL, Goomer RS, Gerlberman RH, Silva MJ, Amiel D. Regulation of $\alpha v\beta 3$ and $\alpha 5\beta 1$ integrin receptors by basic fibroblast growth factor and platelet-derived growth factor-BB in intrasynovial flexor tendon cells. Wound Repair Regen 1999;7:381–388.

56. Hsu C, Chang J. Clinical implications of growth factors in flexor tendon wound healing. J Hand Surg [Am] 2004;29:551–563.

57. Tsuzaki M, Brigman BE, Yamamoto J, et al. Insulin-like growth factor-I is expressed by avian flexor tendon cells. J Orthop Res 2000;18:546–556.

58. Schnabel LV, Mohammed HO, Miller BJ, et al. Platelet rich plasma (PRP) enhances anabolic gene expression patterns in flexor digitorum superficialis tendons. J Orthop Res 2007;25:230–240.

59. Olesen JL, Heinemeier KM, Haddad F, et al. Expression of insulin-like growth factor I, insulin-like growth factor binding proteins, and collagen mRNA in mechanically loaded plantaris tendon. J Appl Physiol 2006;101(1):183–188.

60. Nakama LH, King KB, Abrahamsson S, Rempel DM. VEGF, VEGFR-1, and CTGF cell densities in tendon are increased with cyclical loading: An in vivo tendinopathy model. J Orthop Res 2006;24:393–400.

61. Banes AJ, Tsuzaki M, Hu P, et al. PDGF-BB, IGF-I and mechanical load stimulate DNA synthesis in avian tendon fibroblasts in vitro. J Biomech 1995;28:1505–1513.

62. Smith CD, Alexander S, Hill AM, et al. A biomechanical comparison of single- and double-row fixation in arthroscopic rotator cuff repair. J Bone Joint Surg Am 2006;88:2425–2431.

63. Park MC, Cadet ER, Levine WN, Bigliani LU, Ahmad CS. Tendon-to-bone pressure distributions at a repaired rotator cuff footprint using transosseous suture and suture anchor fixation techniques. Am J Sports Med 2005;33:1154–1159.

64. Nishimoto S, Oyama T, Matsuda K. Simultaneous concentration of platelets and marrow cells: A simple and useful technique to obtain source cells and growth factors for regenerative medicine. Wound Repair Regen 2007;15:156–162.

65. Rohrich RJ, Trott SA, Love M, Beran SJ, Orenstein HH. Mersilene suture as a vehicle for delivery of growth factors in tendon repair. Plast Reconstr Surg 1999;104:1713–1717.

66. Sharma B, Williams CG, Khan M, Manson P, Elisseeff JH. In vivo chondrogenesis of mesenchymal stem cells in a photopolymerized hydrogel. Plast Reconstr Surg 2007;119:112–120.

67. Nakamura S, Ishihara M, Masuoka K, et al. Controlled release of fibroblast growth factor-2 from an injectable 6–O-desulfated heparin hydrogel and subsequent effect on in vivo vascularization. J Biomed Mater Res A 2006;78:364–371.

68. Zhang Y, Wang Y, Shi B, Cheng X. A platelet-derived growth factor releasing chitosan/coral composite scaffold for periodontal tissue engineering. Biomaterials 2007;28:1515–1522.

289

Index

Index